AF521695

Veterinary Biology and Medicine of Captive Amphibians and Reptiles

Veterinary Biology and Medicine of Captive Amphibians and Reptiles

LEONARD C. MARCUS, VMD, MD

Diplomate, American College of Veterinary Pathologists
Assistant Director of Health Services
State Laboratory Institute, Massachusetts Department of Public Health
Clinical Associate Professor of Preventive Medicine and Epidemiology
and Chief, Section of International Health
Tufts University School of Veterinary Medicine
Associate Clinical Professor of Pathology and of Pediatrics (joint appointment)
Tufts University School of Medicine
Lecturer, Department of Civil Engineering, Tufts University
Associate Staff, New England Medical Center
Affiliate, Angell Memorial Hospital

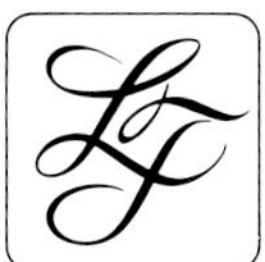

Lea & Febiger *Philadelphia 1981*

Library of Congress Cataloging in Publication Data

Marcus, Leonard C
Veterinary biology and medicine of captive amphibians and reptiles.

Includes index.
1. Amphibians—Diseases. 2. Reptiles—Diseases.
3. Veterinary medicine. I. Title.
SF997.5.A45M37 639.3'76 80–24859
ISBN 0–8121–0700–4

Published in Great Britain by Balliere Tindall, London

PRINTED IN THE UNITED STATES OF AMERICA

Print No: 3 2 1

To my father, Edward G. Marcus, who initiated and inspired my interest in biological science with walks in a city park before I was five years old.

Preface

From prehistoric time, people have held snakes and, to a lesser extent, other reptiles and amphibians in fear and awe. The serpent's role in the Garden of Eden, the deification of crocodiles by ancient Egyptians, and the legend, told by some American Indians, that the world rested on the back of a tortoise are some examples of the reptile's place in folklore and religion. The Asian snake charmer, the Hopi Indian dancing with rattlesnakes held in hands and mouth, and religious cults using or worshiping reptiles and amphibians have persisted to modern times.

An extension of this fascination with herpetofauna (reptiles and amphibians) is the practice of keeping these creatures as pets. This book is directed at the private veterinary practitioner who must advise people about the care of these pets and who must diagnose and treat these animals. Veterinary students should also find this text useful as a reference source.

Certain herpetofauna, especially newts, frogs, and turtles, are often used as laboratory animals. Problems in these laboratory colonies often occur epizootically. The housing, management, and facilities for laboratory animals are markedly different than for individual pets. There are even more variables in zoo medicine, where there is a greater variety and number of species and problems related to public display. Therefore, some of the advice offered in this book concerning individual pets may not be applicable to laboratory animal colonies or zoos.

In a similar vein, herpetologists, veterinary pathologists, and other biomedical scientists should find the text selectively useful as a reference source. However, I hope it will be judged primarily by how well it addresses the principal intended audience, the veterinary practitioner.

I want to express one other thought about what this book is not. It is not intended to encourage the indiscriminate keeping of reptiles and amphibians. I particularly disparage the keeping of endangered species, animals that do not thrive well in captivity, or dangerous animals, such as poisonous snakes. I am sure most veterinarians will agree with this sentiment. However, once faced with the problem of dealing with a sick pet, regardless of how appropriate or desirable that pet may be, most veterinarians would rather be able to offer some useful professional assistance, within reasonable limits of safety, than reject the case completely. I hope this book adequately provides the background and detailed information needed in the veterinary care of reptilian and amphibian pets.

Jamaica Plain (Boston), Massachusetts Leonard C. Marcus, VMD, MD

Acknowledgements

Professor Ernest Williams and Ms. Patricia Haneline in the Herpetology Department, Harvard University Museum of Comparative Zoology, provided specimens, access to literature, and taxonomic assistance. The Veterinary Pathology Division of the Armed Forces Institute of Pathology provided access to specimens and photographs. Angell Memorial Animal Hospital was a source of patients, and preparation and photography of specimens; Mr. Ernst Hoffman also helped in photography. Several individuals assisted in typing the manuscript during its fifteen years in preparation and the help of all is appreciated, but special thanks are due to Mrs. Christine Gunning and, in memoriam, to Ms. Mary Civaterese who put in many hours of work despite illness. Finally, many hours and weekends were taken from time I could have spent with my wife and children while I was working on this book. I hope to make up for some of that lost time now.

Contents

1 The Normal Amphibian and Reptile

INTRODUCTION

Although it is not possible to give exact figures, reptiles and amphibians are kept as pets in many American homes. It was estimated that 7 million turtles were raised for sale annually in the United States[6] prior to a ban on sale of baby turtles to prevent zoonotic salmonellosis (Chap. 3). Considering the number of iguanas, snakes, caimans, and American chameleons (or anole lizards) sold by pet stores, mail order supply houses, fairs, and circuses, the population of reptilian pets is considerable. According to figures released by the United States Department of Interior, 572,670 amphibians and 2,109,571 reptiles were imported into the United States in 1970. The great majority of these were intended for sale as pets, the rest for display in zoos or for laboratory use. The figures do not reveal how many of these animals survived long enough to be sold for their intended use. Mortality in shipment of these animals is very high owing to overcrowding, filthy conditions, deprivation of food and water, and exposure to the elements.

Psychiatrists may invoke such Freudian concepts as counterphobia and phallic symbolism to explain keeping reptilian pets, but there are more mundane reasons for this practice. Reptiles and amphibians can be interesting and practical pets, even if they lack the affection and intelligence of a dog or cat. They are clean, most of them are quiet, and they can be kept in a relatively small space, an important consideration for apartment dwellers. A boa constrictor can be an attractive conversation piece, and, even if it is not overly affectionate, it can give its owner a cozy hug. In addition, few other pets can be left untended in a cage while the owner leaves for a one- or two-week vacation. It is also advantageous that these animals are hypoallergenic.

As with any other pet, a reptile or amphibian should not be kept unless the owner is willing to take care of it. Most reptilian and amphibian pets are bought or captured by people who, though well-meaning, know little about their biology or care. As a result of improper husbandry, very few of these cold-blooded pets reach maturity. Another problem is that catching large numbers of any given species could decimate natural populations and result in a tilting of balances in nature. Indiscriminate release of unwanted pets in non-indigenous areas could also disrupt the environment.

Various species of sea turtles have been killed for food and their nesting habitats disrupted to the point where they are threatened with extinction. Baby sea turtles are occasionally kept as pets in saltwater aquariums. Since it is impossible to raise them to maturity in a house, keeping them should be discouraged unless the owner intends to release them within their natural range and habitat. Likewise, many crocodilian species are faced with extinction because of excess hunting and habitat destruction. These animals should not be kept as pets because they will not mature and reproduce in household captivity. The current fashion craze for reptilian skins may threaten other species with extinction. The International Union for Conservation of Nature lists 27 species of amphibians and 87 species of reptiles threatened with extinction (as of September, 1970). These should be held captive only by those licensed and qualified to do so.

Even the leopard frog *(Rana pipiens)*,* which we have taken for granted as a readily available laboratory animal, has declined in numbers at an alarming rate. There was an estimated 50% decrease in the United States frog population during the 1960s, mostly owing to destruction of habitat through drainage and construction and pollution of the environment with sewage and chemicals.[49] The annual harvesting of millions of frogs for laboratory use has also taken its toll.

A medium-sized leopard frog eats four grams of insects per day and the tadpoles consume a significant amount of detritus in fresh water.[49] The frogs and tadpoles are eaten by larger predators and thus form an important link in the food chain. Decimation of the frog population could well have ecological effects that may not be appreciated for many years, and then it may be too late to restore the balance.

The limited availability of frogs has caused one biological supply house to plea that fetal pigs be used for vertebrate anatomy courses. This laudable effort deserves acclaim because it reflects a concern and sense of responsibility too infrequently seen in the business world.*

Dangerous species, such as large crocodilians, snapping turtles, and poisonous snakes, should not be household items. Certainly, any veterinarian would be justified in refusing to handle a dangerous animal. Selection of appropriate reptilian pets is discussed by Evans,[41]

*The classification of leopard frogs has been revised. Animals that formerly were considered different geographic races of *R. pipiens* are now designated as different species *(R. pipiens, R. utricularia, R. berlandieri, R. blairi)*. Because this new designation is not widely recognized yet, the leopard frog is referred to as "*R. pipiens*" throughout this text. Reference to this revised classification and information on the commercial availability of leopard frogs and other amphibians can be found in Nace, G. W. and Rosen, J. K.: Sources of amphibians for research II. Herpetol. Rev., *10*:8–15, 1979.

*From Ann Arbor Biological Center, Catalog No. 101, 1976, p. 100.

and the precautions and husbandry techniques used in maintaining poisonous snakes in a serpentarium laboratory are discussed by Softly and Cockett.[83]

Serious amateur herpetologists study their interest with enthusiasm and intelligence and keep careful records on the health and activity of their specimens. Many large cities in the United States have herpetology clubs to which amateur and professional biologists belong. They are always pleased to find someone who is interested and competent to provide veterinary care.

Relatively little information about poikilothermic diseases is found in the curriculum of most veterinary schools or in the veterinary literature. Although some information can be found in books and journals devoted to laboratory animals, much of the pertinent information on diseases in reptilian and amphibian pets is found in the professional journals and amateur bulletins of herpetology, sources unfamiliar to most veterinarians.

Much of the published data on diseases of herpetofauna is based on clinical observation, rarely supported by adequate laboratory studies. Controlled scientific experiments of statistical validity are as rare as turtle's teeth. Thus, one is presented with a small mass of empirical data, much of it probably valid, but for the most part, unproven.

There is no less variation in the spectrum of diseases among cold-blooded hosts than there is among birds and mammals. Studies of species variation are so poor, however, that one must often be satisfied with enunciating principles of therapy for all lizards, all frogs, all snakes, or even all reptiles and amphibians, as if they were one homogeneous group.

Knowledge of reptilian and amphibian disease has suffered not only from lack of trained personnel, but also from lack of funds for research. These animals, with few exceptions (e.g., species used for leather or human food), do not have enough inherent fiscal value to warrant grant support. Even if their diseases could be used as models for higher species, it is usually more appropriate to study disease in homeothermic animals. This is particularly true if one's objectives are in applied, rather than basic, science.

Finances also hinder clinical studies. How thorough (and, therefore, how expensive) a work-up and therapy will the owner of a fifty-cent turtle support? People do keep some very rare and valuable specimens, however, that are economically worth as much study as would be invested in comparably priced livestock. These economic considerations limit what a practitioner can do in a practical way, and they are largely responsible for limitations of knowledge in the field. Nevertheless, I hope veterinarians will investigate reptilian and amphibian pathology further and perform and report controlled experiments whenever possible.

Reptilian and amphibian anatomy, physiology, and pathology differ enough from mammalian and avian forms that some review of these differences is in order. This may seem far removed from the bread-and-butter of practice, but some basic knowledge of structure and function in these animals is necessary if one is to handle their disease processes intelligently. It is also important to have some knowledge of the classification of reptiles and amphibians in order to understand their similarities and differences, and the diversity within the two classes.

Phylogenetics

Amphibians and reptiles, which collectively can be referred to as **herpetofauna,** are uniquely important links in the evolutionary chain. The Amphibia form a major intermediate step in the development of higher terrestrial life from the strictly aquatic fishes. Amphibians have not made a complete break from their ancestral home, however, for most of them must spend at least part of their life in water. Reptiles are the first major vertebrate group to have members that are completely terrestrial. (Some amphibians are also completely terrestrial.) Reptiles are the most highly developed cold-blooded vertebrates and are the ancestors of the homeotherms, the birds and mammals.

The unique biological apparatus vital for existence on terra firma shows its initial development in the herpetofauna. This accounts in large measure for the interest in this relatively small group of animals by zoologists and biomedical specialists, e.g., embryologists. Because the vital functions and structure of reptiles and amphibians are so homologous to higher forms, they have been widely used in anatomy and physiology laboratories. Therefore, a veterinarian in private practice may occasionally be called as a consultant to advise care and treatment of a laboratory colony of frogs and turtles. These creatures are also commonly used in the household laboratories of budding scientists of high-school age.

There are three major living groups (subclasses or orders, depending on the exact classification scheme used) of the Class Amphibia. Gymnophiona contains the caecilians, which are limbless, burrowing creatures of the tropics. Since they are rarely kept as pets and little is known about their diseases, nothing more will be said about the Gymnophiona. We are primarily concerned with the salamanders (Caudata or Urodela) and frogs and toads (Salientia or Anura). The terms **urodeles** and **anurans** will be used in the following chapters in referring to these two groups.

There are four orders with living representatives in the Class Reptilia. One of these orders, Rhynchocephalia, is represented by a single species, the tuatara, a lizard-like reptile from New Zealand, which is now facing extinction. Little more will be said of this animal, for it is most unlikely to appear in an American veterinary hospital. Reptilian orders which will be considered are Chelonia (turtles and tortoises), often referred to as **chelonians**, Crocodilia (alligators, caimans, crocodiles, and gavials), referred to collectively as **crocodilians**, and Squamata, subdivided into two suborders: Lacertilia or Sauria (lizards) and Ophidia or Serpentes (snakes). For a detailed classification of the herpetofauna, consult standard zoology and herpetology texts.[10,75]

Table 1–1. Some Differential Features Between Reptiles and Amphibians

AMPHIBIA	REPTILIA
1. Most species have metamorphosis from egg to larva to adult.	1. No distinct metamorphosis; the young generally resemble the adult in form.
2. Skin moist and glandular (except most adult toads, few salamanders).	2. Skin dry and cornified, glands few, never generalized.
3. No external scales.	3. Skin usually has scales or scutes.
4. Skull with 2 occipital condyles.	4. Skull with 1 occipital condyle.
5. Heart 3-chambered (1 ventricle, 2 atria).	5. Heart imperfectly 4-chambered (ventricles imperfectly divided; division almost complete in crocodilians).
6. Gills present at some stage of metamorphosis; some respiratory exchange through skin and buccal mucosa in many species; lungs in most adult amphibia.	6. Respiration by lungs; cloacal respiration in aquatic turtles.
7. Ten pairs of cranial nerves.	7. Twelve pairs of cranial nerves.
8. No embryonic membranes.	8. Amnion, chorion, yolk sac, allantois.
9. Mesonephric kidney (adult amphibian; pronephric kidney in larval stage).	9. Metanephric kidney.

It may be helpful to compare reptiles and amphibians, pointing out some major differences between the two groups (Table 1–1).

APPLIED ANATOMY AND PHYSIOLOGY

Detailed discussion of organ structure and function is not within the scope of this work; texts that deal specifically with these subjects should be consulted.[3,10,22,23,48,54,73,75,78] Coulson and Hernandez have published a number of metabolic studies of the alligator, summarized by them in 1971.[23]

It may be helpful in considering the following data on normal structure and function to think in terms of evolutionary adaptation, with development occurring in a stepwise manner from larval to adult amphibian to reptile to a creature that could live on dry land. The move from aquatic to terrestrial habitation was a major evolutionary step and required many changes in all organ systems. Within this evolutionary framework the following discussion will emphasize selected areas of clinical importance.

GROWTH, METAMORPHOSIS, AND LONGEVITY

Many reptiles and amphibians, particularly snakes, tend to increase in size throughout much of their life, although growth is slowed markedly at some point in maturation and usually stops before termination of the natural life span. It is possible that some species, e.g., crocodiles and pythons, may grow as long as they live, although at a much slower rate as they grow older. This is in contrast to mammals, in which growth ceases with closure of the epiphyses relatively early in the life of the individual, and the period of growth is more sharply defined than it is in herpetofauna. In reptiles, the epiphyses may never unite. Indeed, some reptiles lack epiphyses.[53]

*Table 1–2.** Longevity

NAME	YEARS	NAME	YEARS
AMPHIBIANS		Tiger salamander (*Ambystoma tigrinum*)	11
Congo eel (*Amphiuma means*)	27	Bullfrog (*Rana catesbeiana*)	16
Hellbender (*Cryptobranchus alleganiensis*)	29	Leopard frog (*R. pipiens*)	6
Mudpuppy (*Necturus maculosus*)	9	American toad (*Bufo americanus*)	10–15
American newt or eft (*Notophthalmus* [*Diemictylus, Triturus*] *viridescens*)	3	South African clawed toad (*Xenopus laevis*)	15
		Tree frog (*Hyla arborea*)	14
REPTILES		Fence lizard (*Sceloporis undulatus*)	4
American alligator (*Alligator mississippiensis*)	56	Anole (*Anolis* sp.)	3
Caiman (*Caiman niger*)	28	Galapagos tortoise (*Testudo elephantopus*)	100–150
Boa constrictor (*Constrictor constrictor*)	23	Box turtle (*Terrapene carolina*)	83–88
Cottonmouth moccasin (*Agkistrodon piscivorus*)	21	Snapping turtle (*Chelydra serpentina*)	20
Rattlesnakes (*Crotalus* sp.)	12–22	Painted turtle (*Chrysemys picta*)	11
Garter snake (*Thamnophis ordinata*)	11	Red-eared turtle (*Pseudemys scripta*)	7
Rat snakes (*Elaphe* sp.)	17–23		
Bull snake (*Pituophis catenifer*)	18		

*Derived from Tables 126 & 127 in Growth, Fed. Amer. Soc. Exper. Biol. 1963, 454–457.

The herpetofauna generally live longer than mammals of similar size. Longevity records, rounded in years, of various representative species are given in Table 1–2.

It is often claimed that the largest pythons, tortoises, and crocodilians live for two or three centuries. This might be true, but such reports are usually difficult to prove.[51]

Reptiles are born or hatched looking like miniature adults. They develop by growth and maturation of the various organ systems basically in the pattern seen in mammals. Many amphibians, on the other hand, go through **metamorphosis**. In frogs and toads there is, typically, a change from egg to free-living larva, or tadpole, to adult. In some tropical anuran species the tadpole is not free-living, but develops within the egg membrane, small adult forms eventually emerging from the egg. Most frog and toad eggs are deposited in water, but in some tropical species eggs are carried by the female, young adult forms eventually popping out of her skin (literally).

Development of a tadpole is divided into three phases. **Premetamorphosis** starts with emergence from the egg; towards the end of premetamorphosis the hind legs appear, but this period is mainly characterized by an increase in size with little morphologic change of the tadpole form. This is followed by **prometamorphosis** in which there is maturation of organ systems as well as continuation of growth. Prometamorphosis ends with the emergence of the forelegs and is followed by a **climactic phase** in which the tail and gills are resorbed, the mouth widens, and the adult form is assumed.

The metamorphic process is controlled by the hypothalamic-pituitary-thyroid axis and is dependent on increasing levels of thyroid hormone for normal development. According to the theory of metamorphosis-activation,[37] thyroid activity is relatively low in premetamorphosis. During prometamorphosis, thyroid hormones act by a positive feedback mechanism on the hypothalamus. Hypothalamic neurosecretory activity causes increased secretion of pituitary thyrotrophic hormone by decreasing the sensitivity of the pituitary to thyroid hormone. Thus, increasing levels of thyroid hormones increase neurosecretion of the hypothalamus, which causes increased output of thyrotrophic hormone by the pituitary gland which, in turn, further stimulates secretion by the thyroid. This positive feedback continues until a critical level of maturation when the hypothalamus loses its positive sensitivity to thyroid hormones. At this time (climax) the thyroid-pituitary axis behaves in a negative feedback manner, as in mammalian physiology.

Details of metamorphosis vary considerably among anuran species. Time of development from egg to adult varies from one month in the spadefoot toad *(Scaphiopus hammondii)* to two or three years in the bullfrog *(Rana catesbeiana)*.

Frieden has written an interesting and informative review on the biochemistry of amphibian metamorphosis.[44] A summary of some of the major developmental changes from tadpole to adult frog or toad is given in Table 1–3.

Table 1–3. Summary of Metamorphic Development of Frogs and Toads

BODY PART OR FUNCTION	TADPOLE	ADULT
Extremities	Tail; hind legs emerge in premetamorphosis, forelegs in prometamorphosis.	Tail resorbed; legs fully developed.
Diet	Algae, aquatic life. Food is predominantly vegetable matter.	Insects, worms.
Digestive tract	Mouth narrow, gut long.	Mouth widens; tongue elongates; stomach, liver and pancreas increase in size; intestine is shortened. Pancreatic and intestinal secretions increase.
Respiration	Gills. (Respiratory exchange may also occur across skin and mucous membranes.)	Lungs. (Respiratory exchange may also occur across skin and mucous membranes.)
Heart	One atrium, 1 ventricle.	Two atria, 1 ventricle.
Nitrogenous excretion	Chiefly ammonia. Pronephric kidney functional in young tadpoles; mesonephros becomes functional in older tadpoles.	Chiefly urea. Mesonephric kidney.
Hemoglobin	Stronger tendency to bind O_2; no Bohr effect.	Greater tendency to release O_2, which increases with decreased pH (Bohr effect).

Among the urodeles (salamander-like amphibians) metamorphosis is much simpler and roughly corresponds to climax in anuran metamorphosis. The larvae generally resemble adult forms including limb structure, which develops in embryogenesis. Salamander larvae possess gills that are lost in maturation in most species. The adults have lungs. There is a family (Plethodontidae) of **lungless salamanders** that lack both gills and lungs as adults.

A few urodeles retain gills throughout life. This situation, in which sexual maturity is reached in a larval form, is called **neoteny**. The mudpuppy *(Necturus maculosus)* is neotenic. *Ambystoma tigrinum*, which is found from Canada to Mexico, develops into the adult tiger salamander in most of its range, but is neotenic in Mexico and Colorado. The reproducing larva is known as the **axolotl**. Complete metamorphosis can be induced in the axolotl by administration of thyroid extract.[15] In other neotenic species, arrest in development may be due to diminished end-organ response to thyroxin rather than a deficiency of the hormone.[75]

Musculoskeletal System

Osteology is of considerable importance in taxonomy and paleontology, but deserves limited attention for our practical purposes. Detailed studies of the reptilian skeletal system are available.[10,48,76,79]

The amphibians were the first animals to develop a sternum. Their ribs are poorly developed and do not reach the sternum. In snakes, the sternum is lacking and ribs are found through the length of the body except for the tail and at the level of the first one or two cervical vertebrae. Differences in structure of the thoracic cage are significant in such procedures as necropsies and cardiac puncture.

Turtles, which also lack a sternum, have eight cervical vertebrae capable of a great range of motion; their ribs and 10 fused thoraco-lumbo-sacral vertebrae are incorporated in the **carapace** (dorsal shell). The carapace and **plastron** (ventral shell), which are joined laterally by the shell **bridge**, are composed largely of bony dermal plates which are covered with cornified epidermal scales. The shell accounts for approximately 30% of the turtle's weight, but it may be relatively less in the larger chelonians. There are 54 scales or epidermal shields on most turtle shells: 16 on the plastron and 38 on the carapace, including six which are unpaired, forming a mid-dorsal row. Some individual variation does occur. The anatomy and phylogeny of the turtle shell has been reviewed by Zangerl.[92]

Many lizards are able to break off part of their tails in a process called **autotomy**. The break occurs through a **fracture plane** in the body of a caudal vertebra. The amputated segment continues to twitch, attracting the attention of would-be predators while the lizard makes its escape. The tail grows back, minus the caudal vertebrae, but with a cartilaginous rod. Some amphibians can even regenerate limbs.

The skeleton of salamanders does not ossify completely. Even in old animals cartilage persists in the pelvic and pectoral girdles, in the carpus, and in the tarsus.[15,16]

Snakes have between 160 and 400 vertebrae, the number being relatively constant for any species, although some individual and sexual variation does occur. The number of vertebrae corresponds to the number of transverse scales on the ventral surface of the snake. The suppleness and mobility of the Ophidian body are possible because adjacent vertebrae can flex 25° laterally, 13° ventrally, and 12° to 18° dorsally. The complex attachments of muscles to each other and to vertebrae of varying distances from each other also allow suppleness and mobility. Muscular attachments also connect vertebrae to ribs, ribs to each other, ribs to ventral scales, and adjacent ventral scales to each other.

Salamanders may increase the number of caudal vertebrae during adult life. In contrast, caudal vertebrae in the tadpole fuse during metamorphosis to form a coccyx in the adult frog or toad.

Legs are lacking, of course, in snakes and limbless lizards. In some species of lizards vestigial limbs are present and either front or rear limbs may be lacking externally, although vestiges of pelvic and shoulder girdles are present. Pythons and boas have vestigial pelvic girdles represented externally by black, horny structures which should not be mistaken for abnormal growth (Fig. 1–1). They project like spurs on either side of the cloaca, are larger in males than in females, and are said to be used by the male to stimulate the female before coitus.[10]

Bellairs describes four different means of locomotion in snakes.[10] In **lateral undulatory locomotion** the snake moves by making a series of lateral flexions, pressing the convex side of the curves it forms against projections in its surroundings, such as plants or stones. **Concertina movement** is much slower, but permits the snake to traverse tunnels or troughs. In this form of locomotion the body is thrown into a series of S-shaped curves with the convex edge of the caudal curves pressing against the sides of the tunnel while the head advances by straightening of the cranial end of the body (Fig. 1–2). **Sidewinding** is a form of locomotion especially well developed in snakes living on sandy deserts. The sidewinder rattlesnake, *Crotalus cerastes*, is a prime example. In sidewinding, the long axis of the snake's body is kept at an oblique angle to the direction in which the snake is going. The head end is looped towards the desired direction, the neck takes purchase on the sand, and the rest of the body is shifted in the direction of travel in a stepwise series of parallel tracks (Fig. 1–3). Thick-bodied snakes such as boas, pythons, and large vipers and rattlesnakes can creep along in **rectilinear locomotion** in which the ventral scales from fore to aft are successively lifted, and the edge gains purchase on the ground and pushes the body forward in a straight line.

Lateral undulatory locomotion is the most rapid means of traveling over land by snakes; the racers and whipsnakes (*Coluber* and *Masticophis* spp.) can achieve 4 miles per hour and African mambas (*Dendraspis* spp.) are said to be capable of moving at 7 miles per hour. Rectilinear locomotion is the slowest means of movement. A useful point to remember is that snakes have great difficulty moving over smooth, polished surfaces, so it may simplify handling procedures if

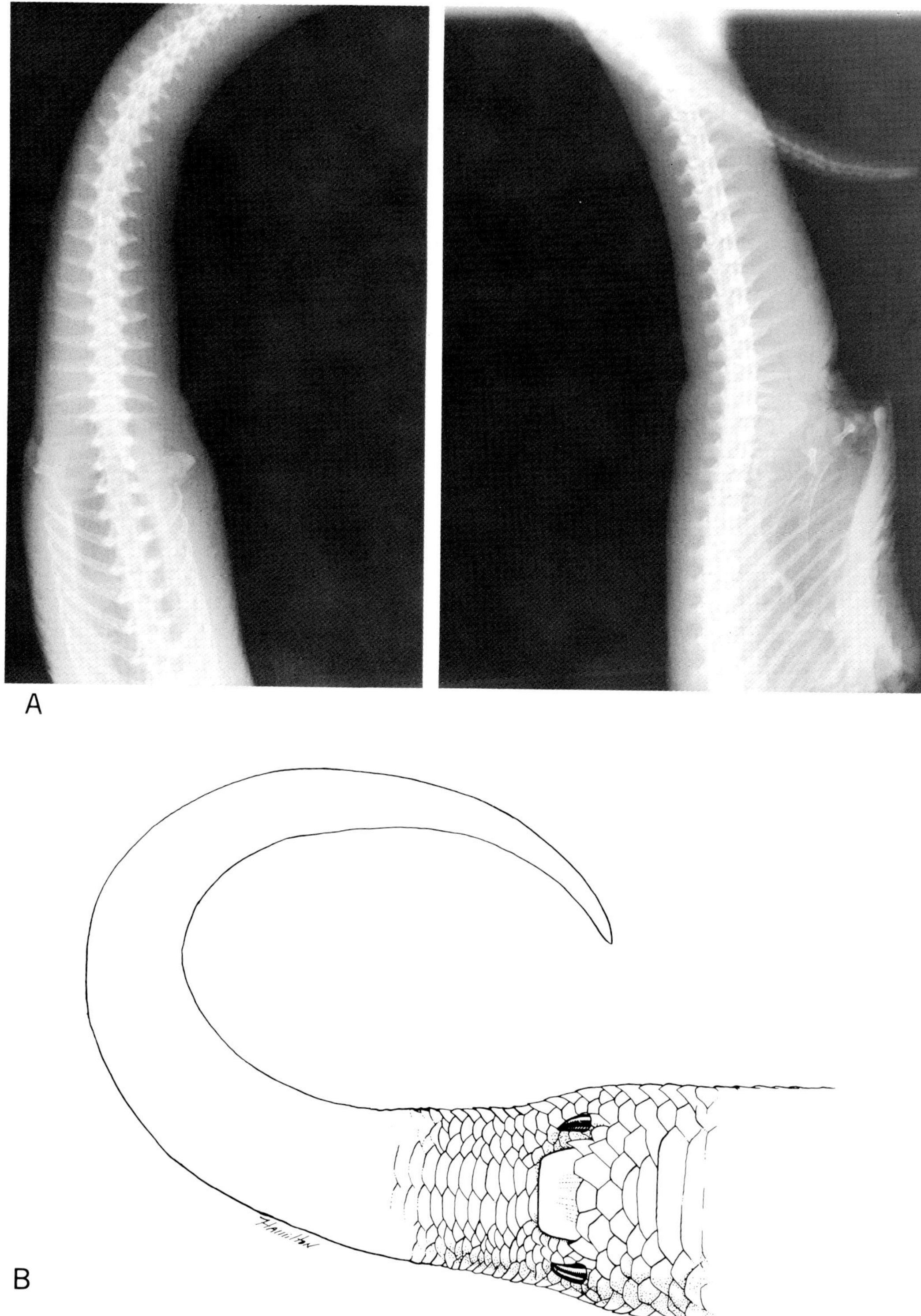

Fig. 1–1. **A.** Radiograph of a boa constrictor demonstrating the vestigial pelvic bones. Caudal direction to the top. Dorsoventral view (left), lateral view (right). **B.** Line drawing of the tail region of the boa constrictor in the radiograph above, showing the black "spurs" lateral to the cloaca. (Figures 1–1A and B courtesy of Dr. Howard E. Evans, Department of Anatomy, New York State College of Veterinary Medicine.)

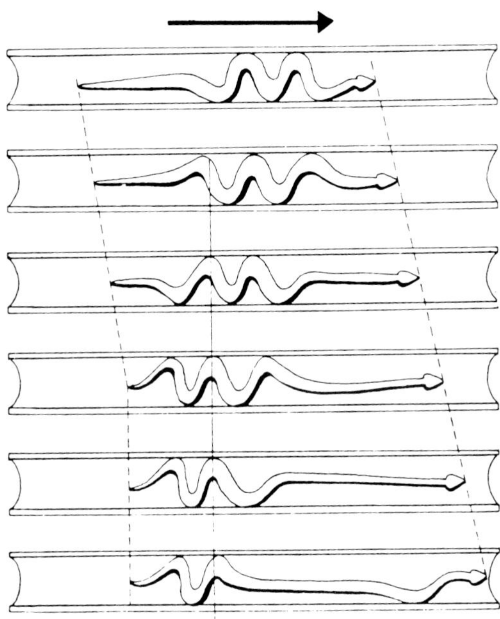

Fig. 1–2. Snake crawling through a narrow trough using concertina movement. (Modified from Gans. From the Life of Reptiles by Angus Bellairs. Published by Universe books, New York, 1970.)

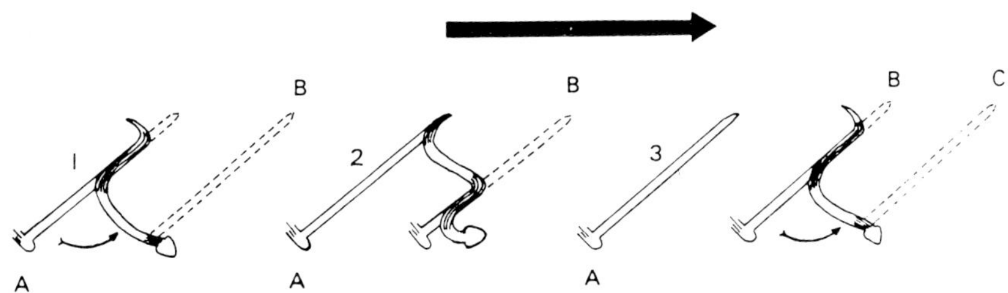

Fig. 1–3. Diagram showing principle of sidewinding. The shaded parts of the snake only are in contact with the ground. The solid parts of the track with impressions left by the head have already been made while the parts in interrupted lines will be made presently. **A** and **B** are the same tracks in the three successive phases of movement shown (numbered 1, 2 and 3); **C** (in 3) is the next track which will be made. The solid arrow shows the direction in which the snake as a whole is travelling. In real life the sidewinder uses a more complicated system of coils. (Modified from Gans. From The Life of Reptiles by Angus Bellairs. Published by Universe Books, New York, 1970.)

they are placed on such a surface while restraint is achieved with a snake hook or pinning stick.

Lizards have many peculiar adaptive mechanisms of locomotion. Geckos and anole lizards have setae with suction cups on their digital pads which give an almost adhesive quality to their feet, permitting some of these creatures to climb vertically up a sheet of glass and to run horizontally upside down across a ceiling. Most lizards move around on all four limbs, but some, e.g., the collared lizard *(Crotaphytus collaris)* and basilisks (*Basiliscus* sp.), are capable of running at considerable speed on their hind limbs. In contrast, African chameleons (*Chameleo* spp.) creep along branches at a snail's pace, holding on with pincer-like opposing claws and a coiled prehensile tail.

Several lizards and one snake, the golden tree snake *(Chrysopelea ornata)*, an Oriental rear-fanged snake, are capable of gliding. The best known aerobatic reptiles are the "flying dragons" (*Draco* spp.) of India and Malaya. These lizards, which average a little over a foot in length, have folded skin that can be expanded laterally, supported by rays of elongated ribs. Using these "wings," the lizards can launch themselves from branches and glide up to 20 yards from tree to tree. The golden tree snake can leap from a tree and glide to the ground, its belly being pulled in and its body held straight for maximum gliding efficiency. No modern reptile is capable of true flight.

A unique feature of amphibians is that they store calcium in **paravertebral lime sacs**, structures that envelop the spinal ganglia. A decrease in calcium content of these sacs occurs during metamorphosis, the element apparently being released for mineralization of the skeleton. Schlumberger and Burke have described the anatomy of the lime sacs in frogs and have commented on their probable function.[82]

Some lizards, e.g., *Phelsuma* spp., have organs on the sides of their neck called **chalk sacs**. These sacs may serve as a site of calcium storage, but their true function is uncertain.

Circulatory System

Tadpoles have a heart with one atrium and one ventricle, basically similar to the heart in fish. The interatrial septum develops during metamorphosis. Most adult amphibians have two atria and one ventricle. Muscular ridges project into the ventricular cavity and functionally separate oxygenated from deoxygenated blood. This functional separation of two bloodstreams is maintained in amphibians by a spiral valve dividing the truncus arteriosus, oxygenated blood being directed into the systemic arches while deoxygenated blood is sent to the pulmonary arteries. The lungless salamanders have an incomplete interatrial septum and lack pulmonary vessels.

Reptiles are the first animals to develop an interventricular (I–V) septum. The I–V septum is incomplete in turtles, lizards, and snakes (Fig. 1–4). Complete mixing of oxygenated and deoxygenated blood in the ventricle is avoided in these reptiles and in amphibians by current flows (Fig. 1–5). The I–V septum is complete in crocodilians except for a

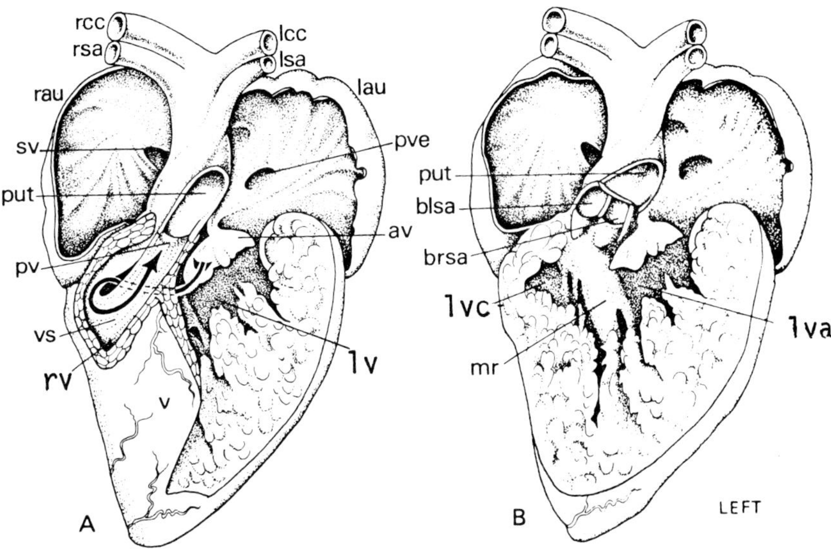

Fig. 1–4. Heart of green lizard *(Lacerta viridis)* dissected from ventral aspect. After Foxon et al. **A**, Ventral wall is removed from the two auricles and the greater part of the ventricle to show the ventral chamber and origin of the pulmonary trunk. Arrow shows flow of blood from left ventricle to right ventricle and pulmonary trunk. **B**, Ventral wall, interventricular septum, and base of pulmonary trunk are removed to show the whole of the left ventricle and the origin (or base) of the left and right systemic arches. **ao**, dorsal aorta; **av**, left auriculo-ventricular valve; **blsa**, base of left systemic arch (with valve); **brsa**, base of right systemic arch (with valve); **da**, ductus arteriosus (probably nonfunctional in *Lacerta*); **dc**, ductus caroticus; **eca**, external carotid artery; **fp**, foramen of Panizza; **ica**, internal carotid artery; **lau**, left auricle; **lcc**, left common carotid artery (carotid arch); **lpa**, left pulmonary artery; **lsa**, left systemic (aortic) arch; **lv**, left ventricle; **lva**, part of left ventricle (cavum arteriosum) on left of muscular ridge; **lvc**, part of left ventricle (cavum venosum) on right of muscular ridge; **mr**, muscular ridge or secondary septum; **ola**, opening of left auricle; **ora**, opening of right auricle; **put**, pulmonary trunk; **pv**, pulmonary valve; **pve**, pulmonary vein; **rau**, right auricle; **rcc**, right common carotid artery (arch); **rpa**, right pulmonary artery; **rsa**, right systemic (aortic) arch; **rv**, right ventricle; **sbc**, subclavian artery; **sv**, opening of sinus venosus; **v**, ventricle; **vs**, ventricular septum. (From The Life of Reptiles by Angus Bellairs. Published by Universe Books, New York, 1970.)

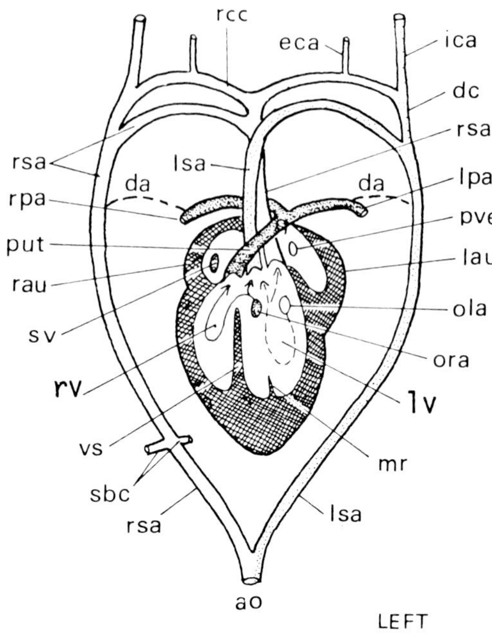

Fig. 1–5. Diagram showing circulation of blood in the heart and great vessels of the lizard *(Lacerta)* in ventral view. For the sake of clarity the main (incomplete) interventricular septum **(vs)** and secondary septum **(mr)** are shown as if in the vertical plane. Arrows indicate destinations of bloodstreams; deoxygenated blood is shown by continuous arrow lines and dark stipple, oxygenated blood by broken lines and unshaded areas, and mixed blood in left systemic arch **(lsa)** in light stipple. Modified from Bellairs. Other abbreviations are the same as those in Figure 1–4. (From The Life of Reptiles by Angus Bellairs. Published by Universe Books, New York, 1970.)

small opening, the **foramen of Panizza**, at the base of the septum near the origin of the two aortic arches (Fig. 1–6).

In many of the herpetofauna, systemic (oxygenated) blood enters the **sinus venosus** before entering the right atrium. In many reptiles, the sinus venosus is incorporated into the right atrium. The sinus venosus acts as a cardiac pacemaker in most, if not all, amphibians and reptiles.[90] The pulse, which is much slower in poikilotherms than in homeotherms, is in the range of 20 to 35 beats per minute in most active reptiles and becomes almost imperceptible in hibernating herpetofauna.

Reptiles have two persistent aortic arches. The right and left arches fuse caudal to the apex of the heart forming a single abdominal aorta (see Figs. 1–5 and 1–6). Because of current flows across the incomplete I–V septum, the right arch carries oxygenated blood and the left arch carries some deoxygenated blood. The introduction of deoxygenated blood into the systemic circulation via the left aortic arch presumably makes reptilian circulation less efficient than the avian and mammalian systems. The right and left arches are named for the location of their course outside the heart. Both systemic arches arise from the left

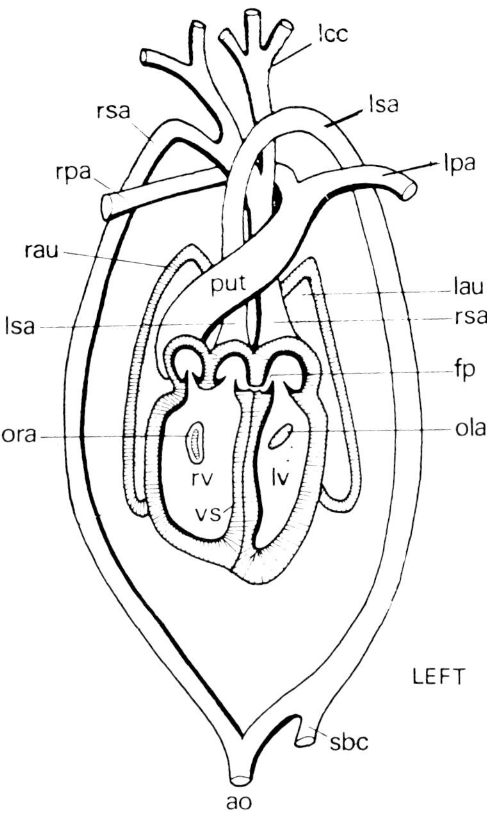

Fig. 1–6. Diagram showing crocodilian heart and great vessels in ventral view. **sbc**, coeliac artery. The subclavians arise from the carotid stems. Other abbreviations are the same as those in Figure 1–4. After Hughes. (From The Life of Reptiles by Angus Bellairs. Published by Universe Books, New York, 1970.)

ventricle in most reptiles other than crocodilians. The origin of the right arch is to the left of the left arch, with the two arterial trunks spiralling around each other to reverse this relationship as they emerge from the heart (see Figs. 1–4 and 1–5). The origin of the left arch may override the incomplete septum. Crocodilians, which have a complete I–V septum, have a right aortic arch arising from the left ventricle and a left arch arising from the right ventricle, the vessels twisting around each other as they emerge to reverse their relative positions. Much, if not all, of the blood entering the left aortic arch in crocodilians is shunted from the left ventricle through the foramen of Panizza, so both aortic arches carry oxygenated blood and separation of pulmonary and systemic circulation is well maintained in these animals. In all reptiles the right systemic arch predominates in size and functional capacity over the left. In most snakes the right common carotid artery is reduced in size or absent. Oxygenated blood is carried to the head via the left common carotid artery which branches off the right systemic arch. The pulmonary trunk arises from the right ventricle in all reptiles.

I had the opportunity to examine the hearts of two adult male Komodo dragons *(Varanus komodoensis)*. Blood in the pulmonary veins entered the left atrium and then flowed into the left ventricle from which no arteries emerged. During systole, blood was pumped through an interventricular septal (IVS) opening into the right ventricle (Figs. 1–7 and 1–8) where it hit a muscular ridge and was thus directed out the two aortas. The right aorta was about twice the diameter of the left (Fig. 1–9). Spiralling and fusion of the aortic trunks occurred as described previously for other reptiles. Systemic venous blood returned via the anterior and posterior venae cavae to the right atrium and thence to the right ventricle from which it was ejected through the pulmonary trunk which twisted from right to left in front of the two aortas (see Fig. 1–9).

Either side of the IVS opening was guarded by a flap valve studded by coarse verrucae on the side facing the opening (see Fig. 1–8). These flap valves had their base of attachment at the fibrous annulus. During ventricular diastole, the flap valves apparently closed the IVS opening. During systole, they swung craniad, closing the atrioventricular (A–V) openings. The septal flap valves had no chordae tendonae. A mural A–V valve leaflet with chordae tendonae was on the left, but no additional A–V valve leaflets were on the right. Two semilunar valves guarded the opening to each aorta and pulmonary trunk. A few verrucae were on the arterial side of the pulmonary semilunar valves, with more present on the left leaflet than on the right. A single coronary artery ostium was found behind the right semilunar valve leaflet of the right aorta.

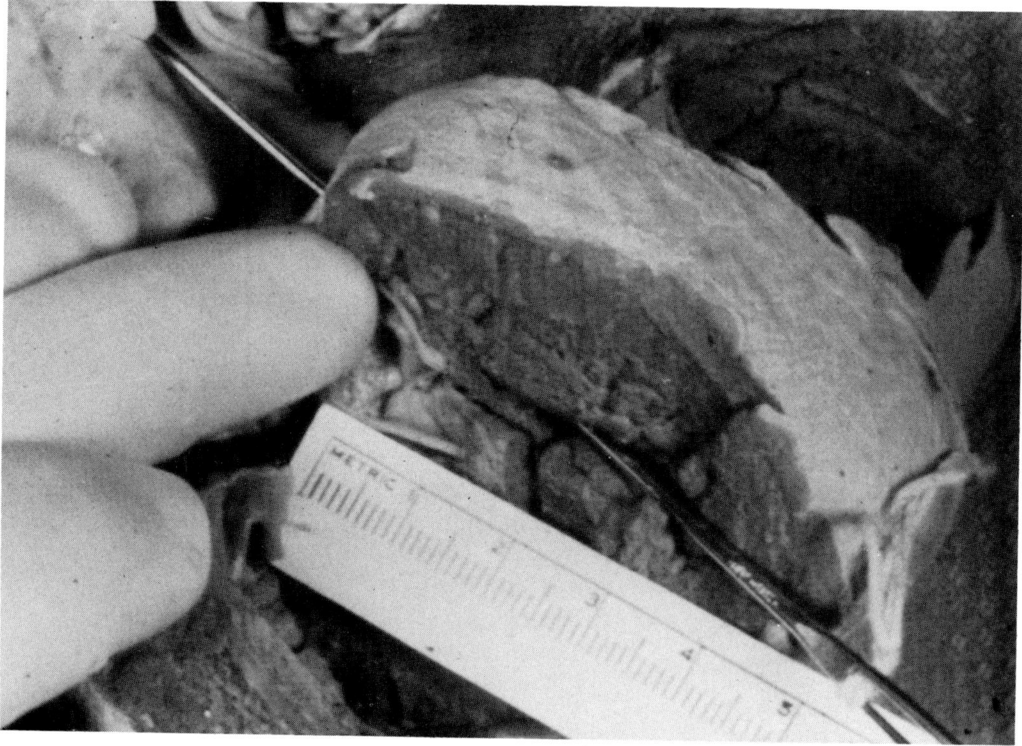

Fig. 1–7. Heart, Komodo dragon *(Varanus komodoensis)*. The probe passes from the left ventricle (ruler), through the interventricular septal opening to emerge in the right ventricle and out the aortic outflow tract (upper left). Both aortic arches and the pulmonary artery emerged from the right ventricle in two adult Komodo dragons examined by the author. Muscular ridges in the right ventricular chamber shunted oxygenated and deoxygenated blood into the appropriate outflow tracts. (Armed Forces Institute of Pathology Accession No. 1134021.)

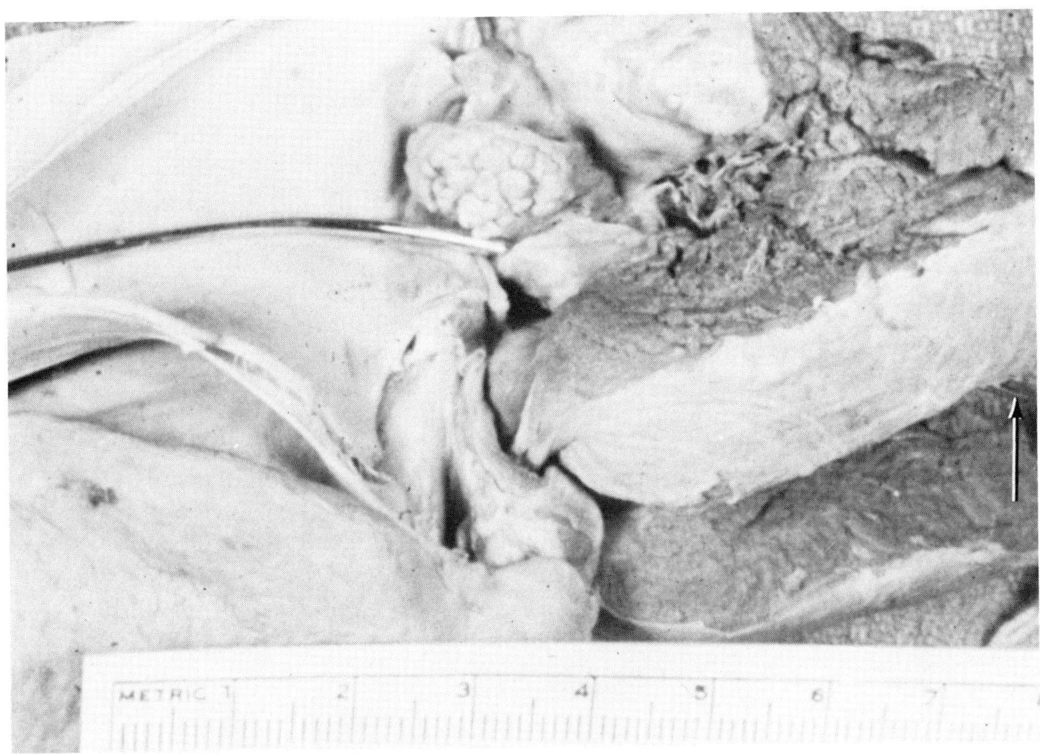

Fig. 1–8. Heart, Komodo dragon *(Varanus komodoensis)*. The end of the probe on the right (arrow) is in the left ventricular chamber. The probe passes through the opening in the interventricular septum into the right ventricle and up the aortic outflow tract (on the left). A verrucous valve (above probe, middle of picture) on either side of the septal opening closes that opening during diastole. These valves swing craniad during systole to act as atrioventricular valves. (Armed Forces Institute of Pathology Accession No. 1134021.)

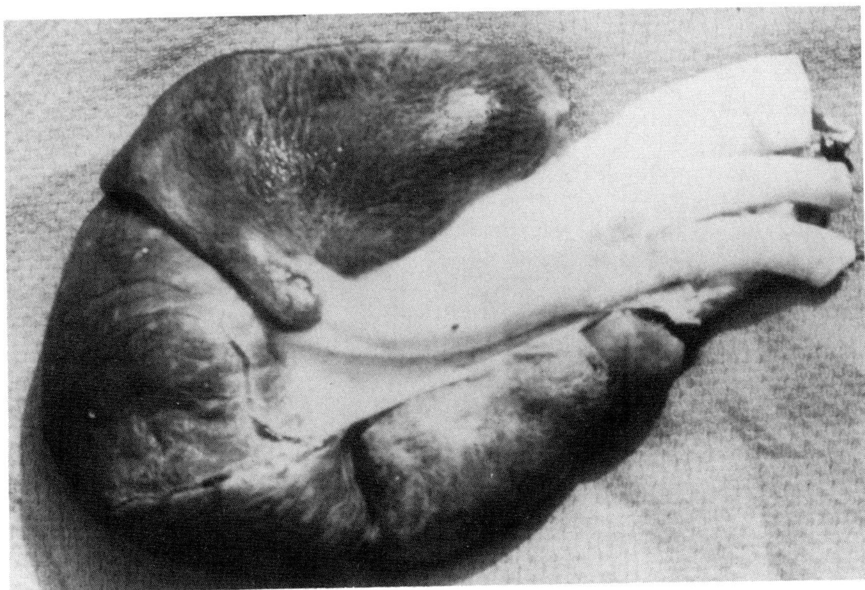

Fig. 1–9. Ventral view, heart of an adult Komodo dragon *(Varanus komodoensis)*. The largest vessel, towards the top of the picture, is the right aortic arch. The pulmonary artery crosses in front of the aortic trunks. Its cut end is towards the bottom of the picture. The vessel in the middle is the left aortic arch. (Courtesy of Dr. Richard Montali, National Zoological Park.)

More work needs to be done on the physiology of reptilian circulation. It is possible that different shunting mechanisms occur during hibernation, rest, exercise, diving, or other special activity. For example, when turtles or alligators submerge in water, apnea results in increased pulmonary vascular resistance and shunting of blood from right to left, bypassing the lungs.[26,88,89] This right to left shunt plus selective vasoconstriction help maintain adequate circulation in vital organs such as the brain. The physiology of diving in sea snakes and some other reptiles was reviewed by Heatwole.[55a]

Lymphoid and Hematopoietic Systems: Hematology and Immunology

The return of lymph to the venous system is aided in amphibians and reptiles by pulsating **lymph hearts**, which are muscular dilatations in the major lymphatic trunks.[35] Lymph nodes make their first phylogenetic appearance in some amphibians, e.g., *Bufo marinus*.[40] With the exception of the snapping turtle, *Chelydra serpentina*, most reptiles do not have lymph nodes, but they do have lymph follicles in the gastrointestinal tract and spleen. Tonsils have been demonstrated in some reptiles, e.g., the alligator.[50]

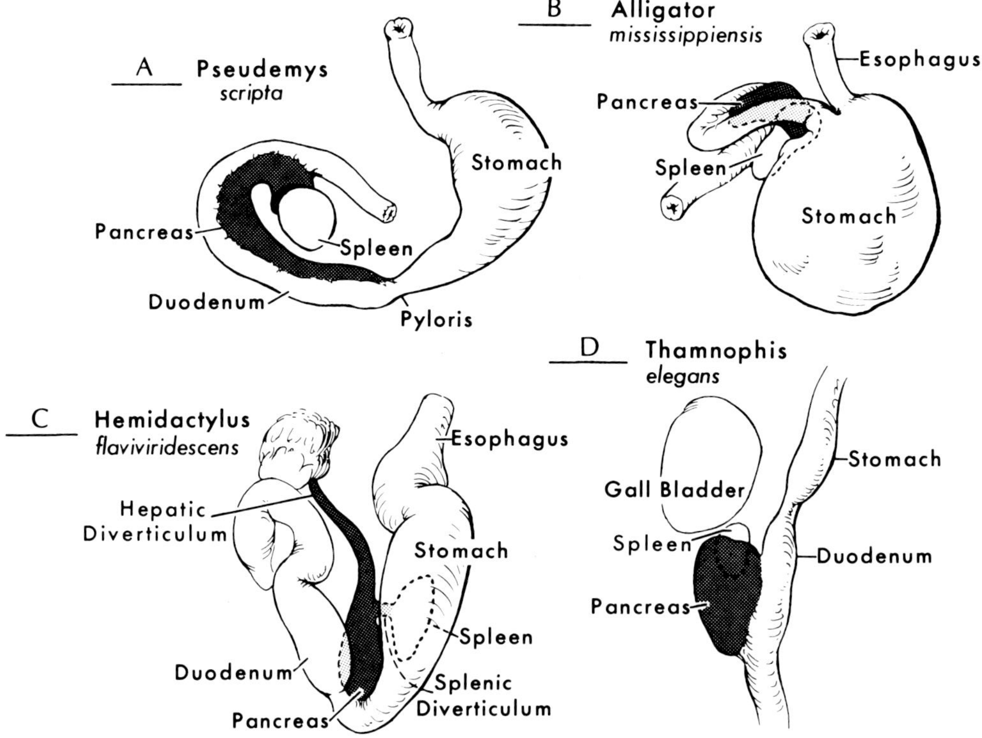

Fig. 1–10. Diagrammatic representations of the gross anatomy of the pancreas and spleen in various living reptiles. **A**, *Pseudemys scripta*, a turtle; **B**, *Alligator mississippiensis*, a crocodilian; **C**, *Hemidactylus flaviviridis*, a lizard; **D**, *Thamnophis elegans*, a snake. (From Miller, M.R. and Lagios, M.D.: Biology of Reptilia, Vol. III. New York, Academic Press, 1970.)

The bursa of Fabricius has not been demonstrated in most herpetofauna. However, lymphoid tissue resembling the avian bursa has been found in the cloacal region of the alligator and snapping turtle.[20]

The spleen of most snakes is intimately attached to the pancreas, and the combined structure appears as a red nodule (the spleen) on a white ovoid mass (the pancreas) (Fig. 1–10). In the Boidae the spleen and pancreas may be separate. A thymus is found in amphibians and reptiles, and its anatomy in reptiles has been reviewed by Bockman.[13]

Reptiles and amphibians mount an antibody response to antigenic stimulation, and they reject allografts. Antibody production in herpetofauna is temperature-dependent. In his informative review on immunity in reptiles, Cohen indicates that various steps in antibody synthesis can be separated by manipulation of temperature in these animals, making them, potentially, very useful laboratory models in which to study immune mechanisms.[20] Evans demonstrated greater antibody response in desert iguanas, *Dipsosaurus dorsalis*, and chuckwallas, *Sauromalus obesus*, at 35° C than at 25° C or at 40° C.[38,39] The temperature at which animals were held in the week following immunization was especially important. The toad *Bufo marinus* also has better antibody response at 25° and 35° C than at 15° C. Evans used *Salmonella typhosa* H antigen. The temperature of optimal antibody response in herpetofauna may vary with the particular animal species and antigen used.

Frogs *(Rana temporaria)* immunized with suspensions of killed *Pseudomonas fluorescens* produced no demonstrable antibodies as long as they were kept at 8° C. When they were transferred to 20° C, agglutinins were formed. Frogs that were kept at 20° C after immunization produced antibodies, but their titers dropped after they were moved to 8° C. This study indicates that the acquisition of the ability to produce specific antibody is separate from the actual production, and the latter function is more affected by temperature.[12]

Isoantigens and isoantibodies are demonstrable in poikilotherms.[57] Blood grouping can be done by hemagglutination as Frair has done in turtles.[43]

Precipitins can be transferred from maternal circulation to developing eggs.[69] The protective value of such passive antibody transfer in neonatal reptiles has not been investigated. The ontogeny of the immune response in cold-blooded vertebrates has been reviewed by DuPasquier.[33]

Equivalents of IgG and IgM are found in amphibian and reptilian sera. IgM is usually present in greater relative and absolute concentration than it is in mammals. Since herpetofauna are less capable of mounting an anamnestic response than are mammals, repetitive challenge with some antigens may elicit a macroglobulin response each time.[66] A complement system in amphibians has also been demonstrated.[66]

A fascinating aspect of herpetologic immunology is the question of seasonal variation in immune response: How does this vary with ambient temperature and hormonal fluctuations? This is not just an academic question, but could have public health and epidemiologic significance if herpetofauna prove to be significant reservoirs of such human diseases as eastern, western, and Japanese B encephalitides and leptospirosis (Chap. 3). The capacity of the agents causing these diseases to survive in hibernating reptiles has been demonstrated. I suspect that suppression of immune mechanisms during hibernation is significant in maintaining infections over winter.

Techniques of blood collection are discussed in Chapter 2.

The average reptilian hematocrit is approximately 29. Lower values (24 to 27) are typical of freshwater species, higher values (31 to 32) are found in marine turtles, and intermediate values (29 to 30) are typical of terrestrial reptiles (Table 1–4).[85] Erythrocytes of reptiles and amphibians are biconvex, oval, and nucleated, although a few anucleated erythroplastids can be found (numerous in some salamanders). Amphibians have the largest red blood cells among the vertebrates, with the maximum size found in a urodele, *Amphiuma tridactylum*, whose erythrocytes measure $65.3\mu \times 36.6\mu$.[55] The general rule is, the lower the animal is in the phylogenetic scale, the larger its erythrocyte, and, the bigger the red cell, the lower the red cell count. Among reptiles, lizards have the smallest erythrocytes and the highest red cell counts, whereas turtles have the lowest erythrocyte counts and the biggest red cells. (The largest red cell among reptiles is found in the most primitive member of the class, the tuatara.) Physiologic variation in red cell count occurs seasonally in reptiles, e.g., an increase just before winter and a decline in spring as hibernation ends and the mating season begins.[30] A relative anemia may be seen in tropical species during the mating season.[1] Seasonal anemia probably contributes to the increase in morbidity seen in captive frogs during the spring breeding season.[63]

Thrombocytes are smaller than erythrocytes, oval- to spindle-shaped, and nucleated. Leucocytes of the granulocytic, monocytic, and lymphocytic series are found, but accurate differential cell counts are best done by those familiar with white blood cell morphology in the given species. Total and differential cell counts, serum electrolytes, and other blood constituents vary not only with species, but also with seasonal activity (e.g., hibernation, mating).[22,64] For example, many reptiles in temperate climates have maximal lymphocyte and minimum eosinophil counts in the summer and the reverse situation in the winter.[30] Pienaar wrote a unique monograph on the hematology of some South African reptiles which includes physiologic data and some pathologic findings.[77] A brief review of reptilian hematology has been written by Frye.[45]

The chief center for hematopoiesis in the tadpole is the kidney. In the adult frog, blood cells are formed primarily in the spleen, and, to a lesser extent, in the bone marrow and liver. In reptiles, hematopoiesis occurs in the same organs as in the adult frog, but there is relatively more activity in the bone marrow. In adult salamanders the spleen is the chief hematopoietic organ. Blood cell formation in turtles has been

Table 1–4.* Body Fluid Partitioning in Reptiles

	FRESHWATER REPTILES (4 CROCODILIAN SPECIES, SNAPPING TURTLE)	MARINE TURTLES (5 SPECIES)	TERRESTRIAL REPTILES (GOPHER TORTOISE, IGUANA, BOA, GOPHER SNAKE)
Hematocrit X (range)†	26 (18–32)	31.5 (26–38)	30 (22–37)
Specific gravity, plasma X (range)†	1.023 (1.020–1.025)	1.030 (1.028–1.033)	1.028 (1.020–1.032)
Plasma volume (% of body weight) X (range)†	3.6 (2.8–4.8)	4.4 (3.5–5.4)	4.1 (3.1–5.3)
Blood volume (% of body weight) X (range)†	4.9 (3.8–6.1)	6.6 (5.2–7.9)	6.0 (4.7–7.3)
Extracellular fluid volume (% of body weight) X (range)†	15 (12.9–18.1)	19 (16.8–21.0)	16.8 (14.0–19.8)
Interstitial fluid volume (% of body weight)	11.5	14.6	12.7
Total body H_2O (% of body weight) X (range)†	73 (71.0–74.4)	65 (63.0–66.7)	70.4 (68.0–72.9)
Intracellular fluid volume (% of body weight)	58	45.8	53.7

*Adapted from Thorson, T.B.: Body fluid partitioning in Reptilia. Copeia, 592–601, 1968.
†X = mean or average value.

described and beautifully illustrated in an article by Jordan and Flippen.[61]

Blood Chemistry (see also pp. 31 to 32)

The metabolic rate of poikilothermic vertebrates is generally lower than in homeotherms. The resultant applications in biochemical experimentation have been documented by Coulson and Hernandez.[23]

The chemical composition of blood in reptiles is subject to physiologic fluctuations unmatched in birds and mammals. Rapid chemical changes occur with feeding, temperature variation, and diving. More gradual but prolonged changes occur with seasonal cyclic events, e.g., mating and hibernation.

The following discussion of blood chemistry of reptiles is abstracted from a chapter by Dessauer[27] to which the reader is referred for further details and references. The text by Coulson and Hernandez[22] should be consulted for studies on biochemistry of the alligator.

The plasma of most reptiles is colorless or straw-colored, but in iguanids and African chameleons it may be bright orange or yellow due to carotenoid pigments, and it may be greenish yellow in pythons and the fer-de-lance *(Bothrops jararaca)* due to carotenoids and riboflavin.

The osmolarity of blood in most crocodilians and freshwater turtles approximates the normal human value of 283 ±11 mol/liter, but is higher in most other reptiles. Compared to the normal human blood pH of 7.40, turtles tend to have higher (more alkaline) values, whereas snakes and lizards tend to have lower values. Marked changes in blood pH can occur in reptiles physiologically. A rise in temperature or a state of excitement can lower the pH significantly. Burrowing and diving reptiles can survive prolonged periods of hypoxia and acidosis. Turtles can remain submerged for an entire winter with their metabolic rate greatly reduced in the hypothermic state of hibernation.

A marked physiologic alkalosis occurs in alligators after eating owing to anion shifts, with bicarbonate replacing chloride in the blood as the latter ion is secreted in gastric juice as hydrochloric acid. Thus, there can be a postprandial reversal of the numerical values for fasting plasma chloride and bicarbonate (112 and 20 mmol/liter, respectively) (Fig. 1–11).

Amphibian blood glucose levels are relatively low, averaging 34 to 79 mg/dl in anurans.[72] Glucose levels in reptiles are higher (50 to 200 mg/dl) and subject to marked physiologic variation.[72] A temperature rise causes an increase in blood glucose in alligators, but a decrease in the pond turtle, *Emys orbicularis*. Hypoxia, as induced in diving, causes physiologic hyperglycemia and anaerobic glycolysis in aquatic turtles. Glucose given to reptiles per os is rapidly absorbed, but the rate at which blood glucose returns to the fasting level is temperature-dependent and "normal" glucose tolerance curves would differ for various reptilian species at each temperature range. Many reptiles, especially those from temperate climes, have marked seasonal variations in blood glucose, the general pattern being a decrease in late summer and autumn as fat and glycogen storage is accelerated.

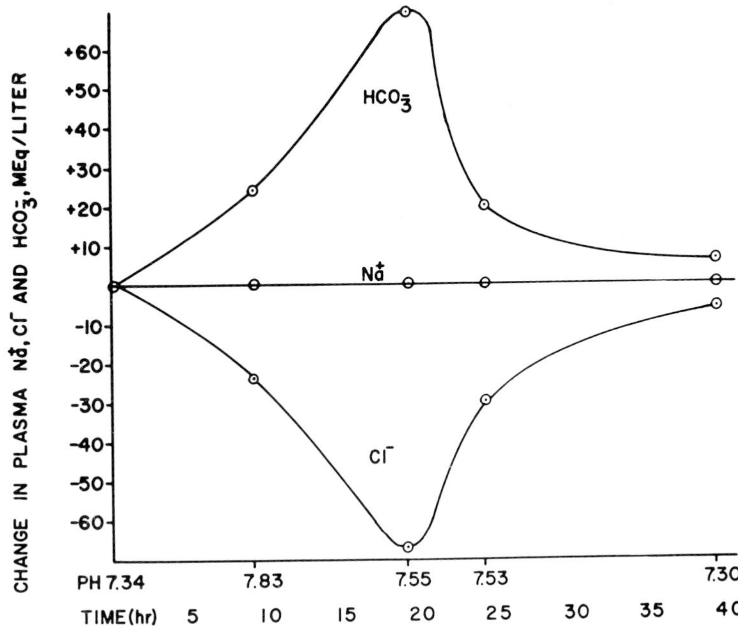

Fig. 1–11. A representative alkaline tide of a single alligator. The alligator was fed at time 0 and the blood was analyzed at 0 hour, 9 hours, 20 hours, 24 hours, and 40 hours. Blood pH was variable and, by itself, would be an unreliable index of the true alkalinity because handling the alligator caused it to hyperventilate. (From Coulson, R.A. and Hernandez, T.: Reptiles as research models for comparative biochemistry and endocrinology. J. Am. Vet. Med. Assoc., 159:1672–1677, 1971.)

Total plasma protein of reptiles ranges from 3 to 7 g/dl. Plasma proteins include albumin, globulins, lipoproteins, enzymes, and various components of the clotting system.

Reptilian blood clots slowly because its intrinsic thromboplastin activity is low and there is a strong effect from a natural circulating antithrombin factor. It is likely that slow clotting is needed to compensate for sluggish blood flow.[52]

Respiratory System

Larval and some adult amphibians respire with gills. Gills are especially prominent in salamander larvae, but they are often covered by an operculum in tadpoles. Most adult amphibians and all adult reptiles depend on lungs for breathing. In addition, there is respiratory exchange across the skin and buccal mucosa in many amphibians. Adult *Plethodontidae* (lungless salamanders) are entirely dependent on these latter routes for gas exchange. Cutaneous respiration can be the sole route of oxygen uptake for amphibians during hibernation. In some species cutaneous respiration is facilitated by the presence of capillaries within the epidermis. All amphibians depending on cutaneous respiration must be kept moist or they will die. Cutaneous respiration is found in many reptiles, especially some sea snakes.[55a]

Some freshwater turtles have a pair of accessory bladders off the dorsal wall of the cloaca which may have some respiratory exchange function, e. g., during hibernation. The respiration of soft-shelled turtles (Trionychidae) is exceptional among reptiles. About 70% of their oxygen uptake during submergence occurs through their leathery shell and 30% occurs across the pharyngeal mucosa from which many richly vascularized papillae project.[10] Some lizards also have pharyngeal respiration, though they depend mainly on pulmonary gas exchange.

The lungs of most reptiles and amphibians are simple sacs attached to bronchi with internal ridging similar in appearance to the mucosal surface of a ruminant's reticulum, the degree and complexity of the ridging varying by species. Crocodilians' lungs are somewhat more complex, being divided into chambers supplied by parabronchi. Extensions of the lung similar to avian air sacs are found in some lizards. The left lung is reduced or absent in most snakes; in the Boidae (boas and pythons) the left lung is present, but is smaller than the right lung. In some lizards one lung may be considerably larger than the other. The cranial part of the lung is involved in respiratory exchange in snakes, the caudal part being a thin-walled air sac. The lung volume of sea snakes is conspicuously larger than that of terrestrial snakes.[55a]

Reptiles lack a diaphragm; they have a single **pleuroperitoneal** body cavity. A membranous diaphragm-like structure in turtles at least partially separates thoracic and abdominal cavities.

The glottis in snakes is an elevated slit-like opening in the rostral part of the floor of the mouth just caudal to the root of the tongue (see Fig. 2–5). The glottis and opening of the esophagus are sufficiently distant from each other that it is a simple procedure to pass an endotracheal tube or to put a feeding tube into the esophagus of a snake by direct observation. There is no problem about "going down the wrong pipe." The glottis of turtles is also easily visualized, but it is more difficult to intubate or force-feed a turtle because of its ability to withdraw into its shell.

Digestive System and Feeding

The organs and compartments of the digestive tract are similar to the mammalian pattern.

The hinge joint for the jaws in reptiles is formed by a convexity in the **quadrate** bone in the upper jaw and a concavity in the **articular** bone (caudal part of the mandible) in the lower jaw, thus reversing the curvatures found in the temporomandibular joint of mammals (Fig. 1–12). The kinetics of jaw movement in lizards is complex: not only can the lower jaw be lowered, but the upper jaw can be moved forward and upward. This unique range of motion is owing to 1) the mobility of the pterygoids, paired bones in the caudal aspect of the roof of the mouth, which can move forward and back in a longitudinal (craniocaudal) plane and 2) to joints in the skull which permit some movement of the upper jaw around the fixed occipital segment. Presumably, such mobility helps in the shifting of prey to the throat, as can be appreciated if you watch a lizard grasp food and move it to the back of its mouth in a series of gulps with back and forth movements of its head.

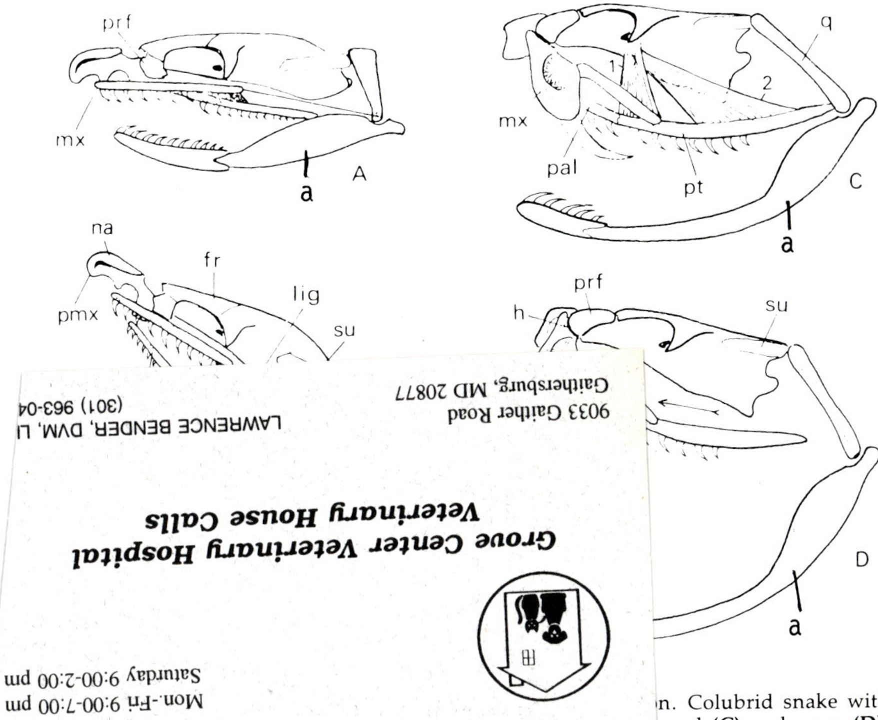

Fig. 1–12. ...n. Colubrid snake with ... closed **(C)** and open **(D)**, showing method of fang **(fa)** erection with independent movement of quadrate **(q)** and pterygoid **(pt)** bones. The muscles shown in **C** are the levator **(1)** and the protractor **(2)** pterygoidei. Arrows in **D** show direction of movement of bones as mouth opens. The small inset shows a viper about to strike, head drawn back, fangs erect, and jaws agape. **a**, articular part of mandible; **ec**, ectopterygoid (transpalatine); **fa**, fang; **fr**, frontal; **h**, hinge between prefrontal and maxilla; **ij**, intramandibular joint; **lig**, ligament (quadrato-maxillary); **mx**, maxilla; **na**, nasal; **pal**, palatine; **pmx**, premaxilla; **prf**, prefrontal; **pt**, pterygoid; **q**, quadrate; **su**, supratemporal. (From The Life of Reptiles by Angus Bellairs. Published by Universe Books, New York, 1970.)

The jaws of snakes are capable of a greater range of motion than that found in lizards. The quadrate bones of snakes are long and slant down and back, so the hinge joint of the jaw (quadrato-articular joint) is caudal to the occiput with the mouth closed (Fig. 1–13, Fig. 1–12, A, C). The dorsal aspect of the quadrate articulates with the **supratemporal** bone which also has some pivotal mobility. When the mouth is opened, the supratemporal and quadrate bones swing down and forward (ventro-rostrally) as the lower jaw is depressed (see Fig. 1–12, B, D). There is no mandibular symphysis in snakes; the right and left lower jaws move independently. Thus, the snake's mouth can gape open so wide that it can swallow prey larger in diameter than itself. The teeth are arranged in a double row (on the maxilla and palatine bones) in the upper jaw and curve backwards in both the upper and lower jaw, which prohibits escape of prey. The food item is grasped, usually at the head end, and the snake virtually crawls over it by advancing its oral grip on first one side, then the other.

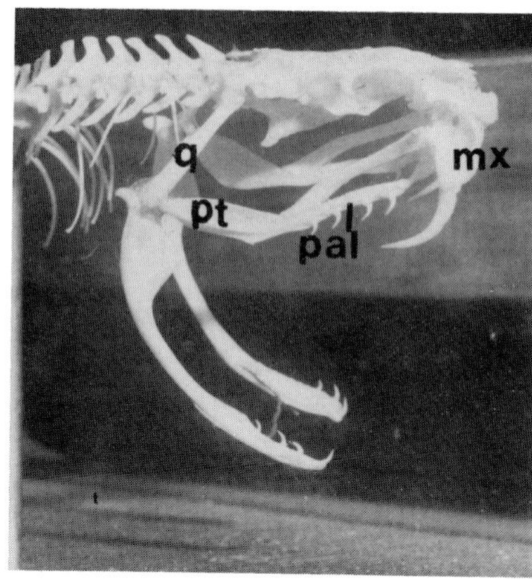

Fig. 1–13. Skull of rattlesnake (*Crotalus* sp) with mouth open. Note the lack of a mandibular symphysis. **mx**, maxilla; **pal**, palatine; **pt**, pterygoid; **q**, quadrate.

The muscles that close the jaws are innervated by the mandibular division of the trigeminal nerve and are much more powerful than the depressor mandibulae muscles that open the mouth and are innervated by the facial nerve.

Further details on skull structure and the kinetics of jaw movement are very well described by Bellairs.[10]

Turtles lack teeth but can bite effectively with horny beaks. Frogs and toads may have teeth or teeth-like structures in their upper jaws. In most herpetofauna the teeth are uniform in shape and structure **(homodont)**, but some lizards have teeth that differ in shape from front to back **(heterodont)**, and some snakes and two lizards (gila monster, *Heloderma suspectum*, and Mexican beaded lizard, *H. horridum*) have specialized teeth for injecting venom. These teeth are in the lower jaw of the two poisonous lizards and in the upper jaw of all poisonous snakes. Two families, the Hydrophidae (sea snakes)* and Elapidae (cobras, kraits, mambas, coral snakes), have a pair of short, erect, rigid fangs in the front of the upper jaw (Fig. 1–14). In the family Viperidae, the two subfamilies, Viperinae (true vipers) and Crotalinae (pit vipers), have long, curved, hinged fangs enclosed in a sheath (see Fig. 1–14). The fangs fold back when the mouth is closed and become erect in striking. Movement of these fangs can be individually controlled by the viperine snakes. The remaining group of poisonous snakes, the Opisthoglypha, have grooved fangs on the posterior parts of the upper jaw. Most of the snakes in the latter group are mildly poisonous and only a few, such as the boomslang *(Disphylidus typus)*, are dangerous to man.

*The family Laticaudidae (sea kraits) has recently been separated from the Hydrophidae.[55a] The venom apparatus of these two families is similar.

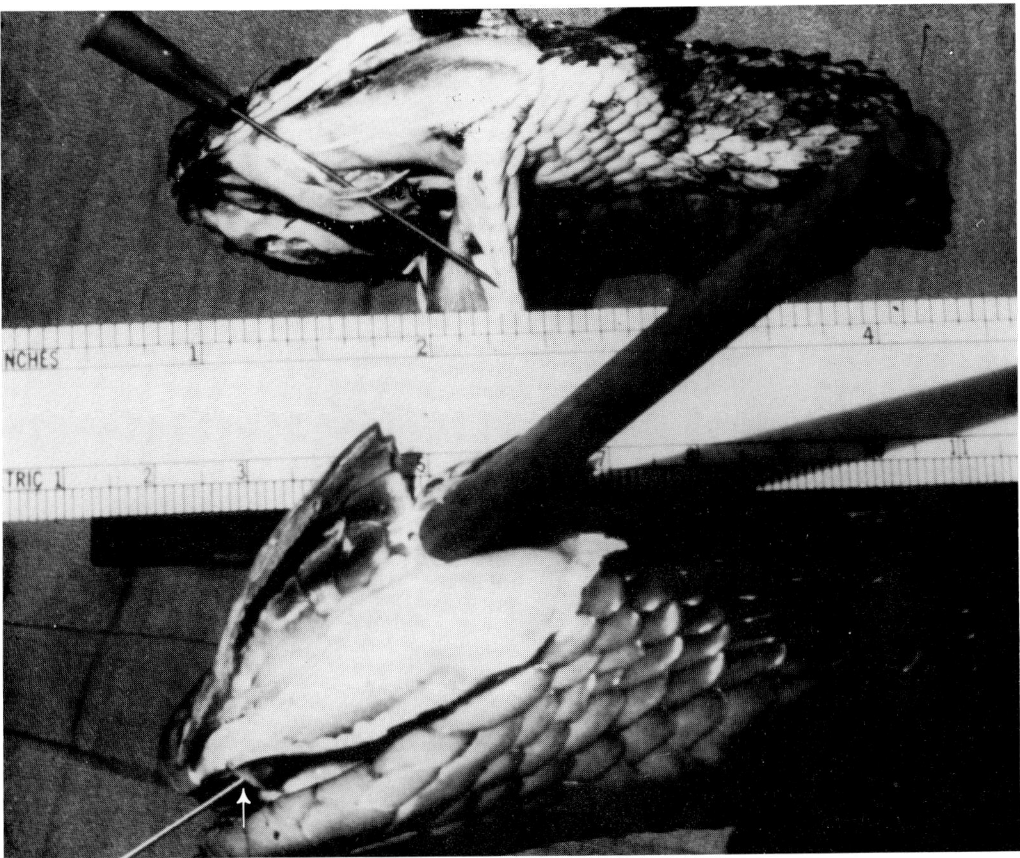

Fig. 1–14. Head of a viper (puff adder, *Bitis arietans*) (top) and a cobra (*Naja* sp.) (bottom) dissected to show the venom apparatus. The sheath over the viper's fang has been cut to demonstrate the length of the fang and its resting position, curved against the roof of the mouth when the mouth is closed. The poison fang of the cobra is short and erect (arrow).

The teeth of snakes, crocodilians, and most lizards are continuously and regularly replaced, a condition termed **polyphyodonty**, and a reptile may go through many sets of teeth in its lifetime. Two practical points should be derived from this fact. 1) The age of the animal cannot be judged by the wearing of the teeth. 2) Poisonous snakes cannot be rendered permanently harmless by pulling their fangs. The microscopic, gross, and developmental anatomy of reptilian dentition has been reviewed by Edmund.[34]

Poison glands are modified salivary glands. As a broad generalization, it may be said that the poisons of the Elapidae are paralytic agents (neurotoxins), whereas poisons of the Viperidae are hemolytic and necrotizing agents. This is an oversimplification, however, and anyone who works with poisonous snakes should be thoroughly familiar with the toxicology and therapy of snake bites appropriate for the given species. Practicing veterinarians would be well advised to leave poisonous animals alone. They should not be kept as pets.

Occasionally, the veterinarian is called upon to render a poisonous snake harmless or **venomoid** (the venom apparatus retained but rendered nonfunctional). The safest, simplest, and most rapid technique is to divide the poison ducts and ligate or cauterize the cut ends.[59] After the snake is under surgical anesthesia (Chap. 2) a 1 to 1.5 cm incision is made parallel to the gum line through the skin of the upper jaw, between two rows of scales, about half-way between the ventral edge of the upper lip and ventral aspect of the eye. The duct is subcutaneous and readily isolated (Figs. 1–15 and 1–16). The snake will not be able to kill its prey after this operation and should be offered food items that are dead, though preferably still warm, especially for pit vipers, which depend in part on thermal sensation to detect their prey. The operation does nothing to alter the snake's disposition; a venomoid viper or pit viper is still able to inflict nasty puncture wounds with its fangs. Extirpation of the poison glands is possible, but the surgery is longer, more complicated, and more disfiguring, and most snakes do not survive long afterwards.[17] The gross and microscopic anatomy of crotaline venom glands has been described by Kochva and Gans.[65]

In poisonous snakes the poison duct leads to hollow or grooved fangs in the upper jaw. The Gila monster *(Heloderma suspectum)* and the Mexican beaded lizard *(H. horridum)* have multilobulated venom glands beneath the skin in the lateral aspect of the rostral half of the lower jaw. Each lobe is drained separately by its own duct. In the poisonous lizards the venom runs into the space between gums and lips. The venom probably rises in grooves in the lizard's teeth by capillary action and is inoculated by chewing on the victim rather than by rapid injection, as in viper or pit viper envenomation. (Elapids poison their prey by a chewing action, necessitated by the shortness of their fangs.)

Several elapid species, including the African ringhals *(Hemachatus haemachatus)*, the African black-necked cobra *(Naja nigricollis)*, and the

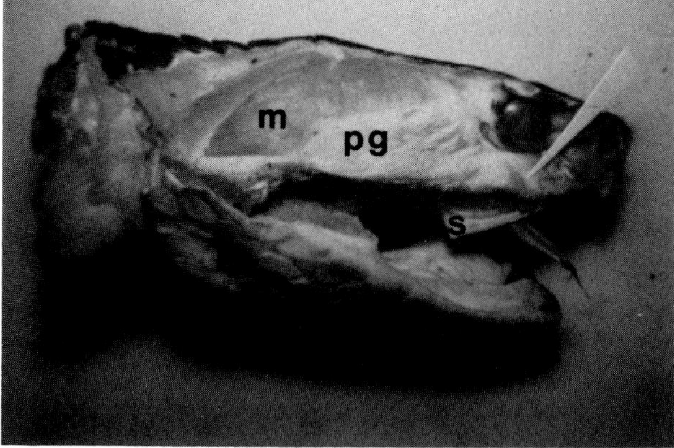

Fig. 1–15. Head of cottonmouth moccasin *(Agkistrodon piscivorus)*, with skin removed. Venom duct is indicated by the pointer. White tissue caudal to the duct is the connective tissue capsule of the poison gland (p.g.). **m**, muscle; **s**, incised fang sheath. (Armed Forces Institute of Pathology photograph. Accession No. 1058160.)

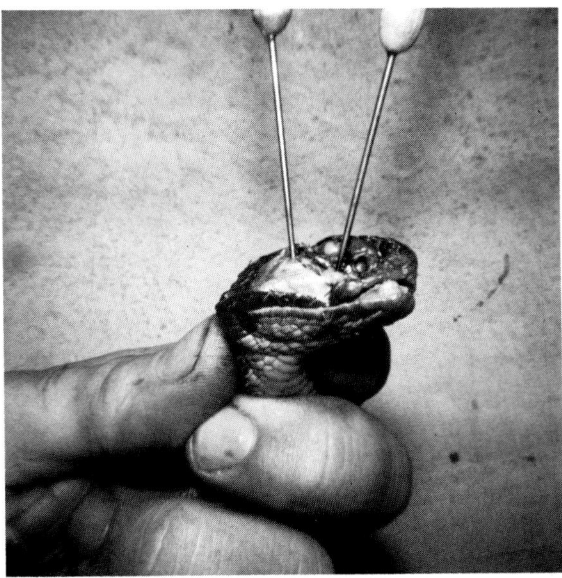

Fig. 1–16. Timber rattlesnake *(Crotalus horridus)*. Dissection of poison gland (ventral to probe on the left) and venom duct (indicated by probe on right, between the eye and pit).

Indian cobra *(N. naja)* can forcefully eject venom through their fangs and direct the spray with great accuracy for more than two meters. I was hit in the face by the venom of a spitting cobra at a distance of more than three meters, at which distance the liquid was dissipated into a spray of fine droplets. Fortunately, I was protected by eyeglasses. Severe burning, temporary blindness, and possible systemic poisoning can result when the poison gets into the eyes, which is where the snake aims. Anyone who must handle these dangerous creatures would be well advised to wear glasses, goggles, or some form of face mask to protect his eyes. The safest procedure is to anesthetize a poisonous snake before handling it, for example, by giving it an inhalant anesthetic in an enclosed box (Chap. 2).

The tongues of some anuran amphibians are lacking (e.g., *Xenopus laevis*, the South African clawed toad) or immobile, but most toads and frogs have a protrusible sticky tongue that is attached rostrally in the lower jaw and is used to catch insects. The tongue of all snakes and some lizards (e.g., the monitors) is forked (see Fig. 3–48) and retractable into a sheath at its base. Its constant flickering action is probably used to bring odorous particles to **Jacobson's organ** in the roof of the mouth for olfactory evaluation, the forked tip presumably bringing the scent to both openings of this organ (see p. 45). True chameleons have protrusible tongues that can be stretched as long as the rest of the body and tail to catch insects. The caudal part of the chameleon's tongue is folded in accordian pleats when at rest; it contains a hollow central tendon that rapidly slides over a well-lubricated cartilaginous core. The caudal pleats are unfolded as the tongue shoots forward in about 1/25 of a second to catch its prey. The tongue of turtles and crocodilians is not protrusible. Taste buds are found in the tongues of at least some reptiles and amphibians. In no reptile is the tongue used as an offensive weapon, contrary to common folklore.

Crocodilian stomachs are divided into two compartments. The first is the gizzard which is muscular and may contain swallowed stones; the second compartment is the glandular stomach.

In conformity with the shape of the body, all the viscera in snakes are elongated. The alimentary tract is a tube with some "kinking," but nowhere near the complexity of coiling found in more squat forms, such as the turtle. In herpetofauna, as in mammals, herbivores tend to have a longer intestinal tract than carnivores. Most tadpoles have a diet rich in plant material and their intestinal tract is relatively long and coiled. During metamorphosis the tube becomes relatively short and straight, an adaptational change appropriate for the insectivorous habits of adult frogs and toads. The stomach of tadpoles is primarily a storage organ; it develops a digestive function similar to that in mammals as the adult stage is reached. Except for snakes, most reptiles have a cecum. This is the first phylogenetic group in which this organ is seen.

The digestive juices of herpetofauna are very effective. Chitinous remnants of insects, hair, horn, and feathers may be found in their feces, the rest of the prey, including bones, being dissolved, digested, and absorbed.

Many herpetofauna can vomit, this reflex being especially active in snakes. Many frogs and toads can evert their stomachs so the gastric mucosal lining may actually protrude from the mouth, a rather emphatic and decisive way to reject a meal.

The liver of reptiles and amphibians normally contains melanin which may give the organ a black-spotted or streaked appearance. The liver of many herpetofauna in temperate climes enlarges in the fall, before hibernation, due to increased glycogen storage. All reptiles and most, if not all, amphibians have gallbladders.

Amphibians are the first class of vertebrates in which the pancreas appears as a discrete, separate organ. The pancreas of snakes is a white, ovoid structure intimately attached to the spleen in most species. The anatomy of the reptilian pancreas has been reviewed by Miller and Lagios[71] (see Fig. 1–10).

Fat is stored in the abdominal cavity as discrete masses of adipose tissue, the **fat bodies**. Reptiles and amphibians have relatively little subcutaneous fat. It is likely that the fat bodies are a nutrient reservoir that can be mobilized to meet energy demands during periods of starvation or hibernation. The fat bodies reach maximum development in the fall and are maximally depleted during the spring breeding season.

The digestive and urogenital tracts of reptiles and amphibians exit by a common canal, the cloaca.

Urinary System and Fluid Balance

The adult amphibian kidney is derived from the mesonephros, whereas reptiles, like higher vertebrates, have metanephric kidneys.

The kidneys of reptiles and amphibians are flattened, lobulated (never bean-shaped), elongated organs lying parallel and adjacent to the lumbar and sacral vertebrae. In lizards the caudal ends of the kidneys are found caudal to the cloaca, extending between the origin of the tail muscles. Crocodilian kidneys have two lobules; each lobule is supplied by a branch of the ureter.

Venous blood from the pelvis, hind legs, and caudal part of the abdomen perfuses the reptilian and amphibian kidney via a **renal portal system**. Kidneys of the herpetofauna are also perfused by one or more renal arteries. The nephron in the reptile consists of a glomerulus and a renal tubule divisible into six segments. In many snakes and lizards the sixth segment in the male is modified as a sex gland known as the **renal sex segment**. The renal sex segment is prominent throughout the year in snakes in temperate climates; in lizards it undergoes seasonal hypertrophy at the time of spermiogenesis.[11,42,70] Zwart presents an informative review of the anatomy, physiology, and pathology of the reptilian kidney.[93] Deyrup has reviewed water balance and renal function in amphibians.[29]

The herpetofauna include species which are primarily marine, aquatic, or terrestrial, and many which are amphibious. Many amphibia are aquatic as larvae, but terrestrial or amphibious as adults. Each kind of habitat presents a different problem in salt and water balance (Table 1–4).

The total body water and intracellular fluid volume of marine turtles and various terrestrial reptiles are lower than in freshwater reptiles; extracellular fluid volume (plasma and interstitial fluid) is higher in the marine and terrestrial reptiles than in freshwater forms. [85] As shown in Table 1–4, values for terrestrial reptiles are intermediate between those for freshwater and marine species.

Isotonic saline solution for most amphibians is 0.7% NaCl and approximately 0.8% NaCl for many of the (nonmarine) reptiles commonly kept in captivity. A Ringer's solution suitable for many (nonmarine) reptiles is 8.1 g NaCl, 0.22 g KCl, 0.20 g $NaHCO_3$ and 0.20 g $CaCl_2$ dissolved in 1000 ml sterile distilled water.[84]

Many marine reptiles, e.g., marine iguanas *(Amblyrhynchus cristatus)* and sea turtles, and some terrestrial lizards excrete excess salt through **salt glands**. These are orbital glands in sea turtles and nasal glands in lizards. A sublingual salt gland has been described in sea snakes by Dunson, et al.[32] Terrestrial reptiles have no sweat glands and lose very little moisture through the skin. They produce a highly concentrated urine. Most of their water loss occurs through the respiratory tract. Adult toads (*Bufo* sp.) are dry-skinned and largely terrestrial. Toads and turtles, such as *Chrysemys (Pseudemys)* and *Terrapene* sp., conserve water by reabsorbing it from the urinary bladder.

Aquatic amphibians have a skin that is freely permeable to water. Electrolyte balance is maintained by active "pump" mechanisms. Indeed, the frog skin is a standard model for studying transport across biological membranes. Frogs (*Rana* spp.) have very large glomeruli to facilitate the filtration and excretion of water.

*Table 1–5.** Blood Urea and Uric Acid in Reptiles

	UREA (MG/DL)	URIC ACID (MG/DL)
CHELONIA		
Snapping turtle *(Chelydra serpentina)*	96	2
Painted turtle *(Chrysemys picta)*	37	2
Red-eared turtle *(Pseudemys scripta)*	22	1
Box tortoise *(Terrapena carolina)*	30	2
Green (sea) turtle *(Chelonia mydas)*	52	8
SAURIA		
Anole *(Anolis carolinensis)*	7	8
Iguana *(Iguana iguana)*	1	5
SERPENTES		
Black snake *(Coluber constrictor)*	4	6
Kingsnake *(Lampropeltis getulus)*	2	6
Water snake *(Natrix sipedon)*	3	6
Cottonmouth moccasin *(Agkistrodon piscivorus)*	5	6
Asp viper *(Vipera aspis)*	10	4
Western diamond-back rattlesnake *(Crotalus atrox)*	1	2
Timber rattlesnake *(C. horridus)*	11	3
Prairie rattlesnake *(C. viridis)*	0	2
CROCODILIA		
American alligator *(Alligator mississippiensis)*	0	3

*Adapted from Dessauer, H.C.: Blood chemistry of reptiles: physiological and evolutionary aspects. *In* Biology of the Reptilia. Edited by C. Gans and T.S. Parsons. Academic Press, New York, 1970.

The principal nitrogenous waste products of herpetofauna vary with the animal's natural environment. Although ammonia is toxic to most vertebrates, it is efficiently and safely excreted by primitive aquatic vertebrates because it is very soluble and freely diffusible in water. The principal nitrogenous waste product of young tadpoles is ammonia, whereas in adult frogs it is urea, with transition occurring during metamorphosis. Sea turtles excrete uric acid, urea, and ammonia. The ratio of these products varies by species. Freshwater turtles that spend most of their time in water excrete approximately equal quantities of ammonia and urea; turtles that are more amphibious in their habits excrete relatively more urea. Uric acid is the principal nitrogenous waste product of terrestrial tortoises.[74]

Alligators mainly excrete ammonia, but also some uric acid. Terrestrial reptiles, which must conserve water, primarily excrete highly concentrated uric acid which is eliminated by tubular secretion and, to a lesser extent, by glomerular filtration. Normal blood levels of urea and uric acid in some reptiles are shown in Table 1–5.

Most amphibians and many reptiles have a urinary bladder, but this organ is missing in crocodilians, snakes, and some lizards.

Reproductive System

Ovaries and testes are paired internal organs in reptiles and amphibians. Differentiating their sex by superficial examination is often difficult. In many chelonians, e.g., the box tortoise *(Terrapene carolina)*,

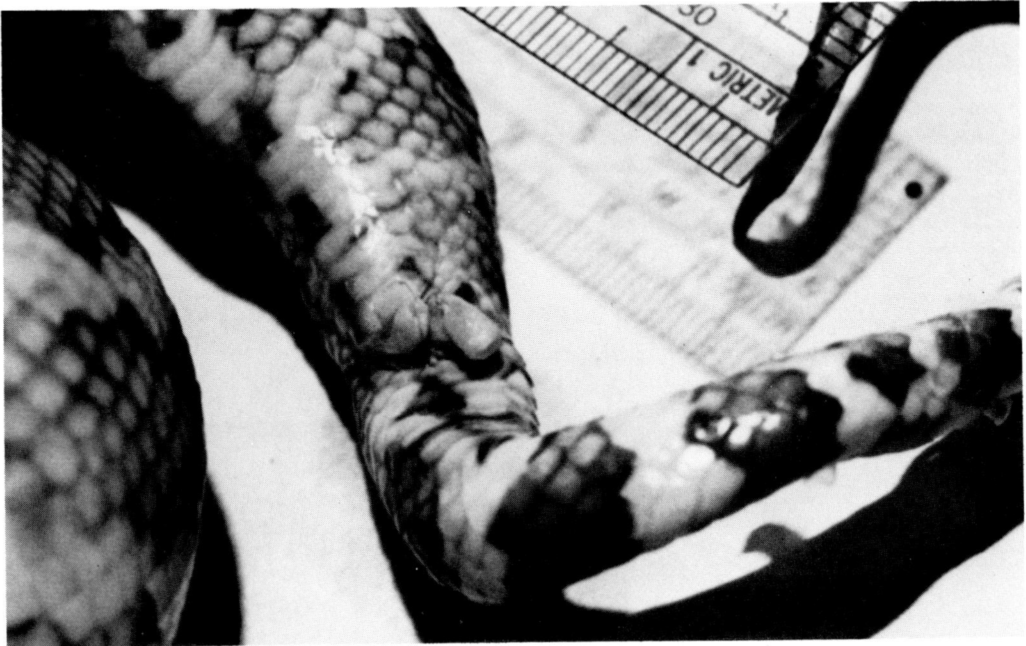

Fig. 1–17. Everted hemipenes of male carpet python *(Morelia argus)*. (Courtesy of Harvard University Museum of Comparative Zoology.)

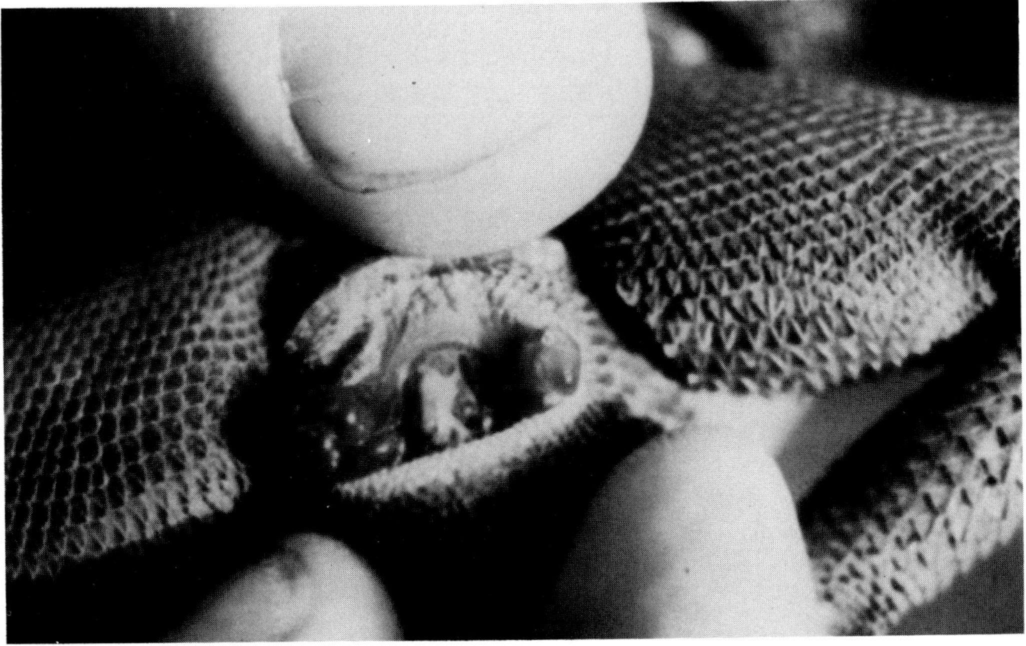

Fig. 1–18. Eversion of hemipenes in a male rainbow lizard *(Agama agama)*.

the male has a slightly concave plastron. Another secondary sex characteristic of the box tortoise is that the iris is red in the male and brown in the female. In many chelonians the males have longer tails and claws than the females and their cloacal aperture may be more caudally situated.

In lizards and snakes the male has paired **hemipenes**, copulatory organs, which can be extruded from the cloaca (Figs. 1–17, 1–18, and 1–19). Only one hemipenis is inserted into the female cloaca at the time of mating. The appearance of the hemipenes varies by species; they may be forked, elaborately folded, or covered with spines or papillae. In snakes, the hemipenes are everted as they are extruded.

Crocodilians and turtles have a single extrusible penis. The sex of mature crocodilians can be determined by digital palpation of the penis through the cloaca.[14] (Good luck!)

In most crocodilians and lizards the male is larger than the female, but the reverse is true in many species of snakes. In many snakes, the male has a body that tapers evenly all the way to the tip of the tail, whereas the female's body is constricted just distal to the cloaca. Sex can be more definitively determined in snakes by measuring the depth of the paracloacal sacs. A lightly lubricated flexible probe, such as a standard dissecting probe, is inserted into the opening of the sac, located at the lateral mucocutaneous margin of the cloaca. The depth of insertion is marked and measured against the ventral tail scales. The depth of sacs in female snakes is usually three to five scales; in males, seven to twelve.

Among amphibians there may be considerable sexual dimorphism, with males differing from females in voice, color, size, or skeletal structure. In bullfrogs *(Rana catesbeiana)*, the tympanum in the male is much larger than in the female (Fig. 1–20). The male frog of many species has **nuptial pads**, protuberances on the prepollex region of the foreleg, which help him grasp the female in amplexus.

In most salamanders the male can be identified by the presence of villous papillae in the cloaca (Fig. 1–21).

There is less sexual dimorphism among reptiles than among amphibians but varying secondary sex characteristics are found. In many lizards the male has a different (usually brighter) color than his mate, and some male lizards are adorned with dorsal or caudal crests, throat fans, or horns. Femoral pores may be more prominent in male lizards (see p. 48). Texts dealing with the natural history and identification of herpetofauna go into the details of sexual dimorphism among species.

Eight species of whiptailed lizards *(Cnemidophorus* sp.) are all female and reproduce parthenogenetically.[24,67] The Caucasian rock lizard *(Lacerta saxicola)* also reproduces by parthenogenesis.[25]

With very few exceptions, fertilization is external in frogs and toads, with the male emitting sperm as the female releases her eggs. Frog eggs typically form a jelly-like mass; toads usually lay their eggs in gelatinous strings. In most species embryogenesis and the emergence of a tadpole occur in fresh water. The females of some South American

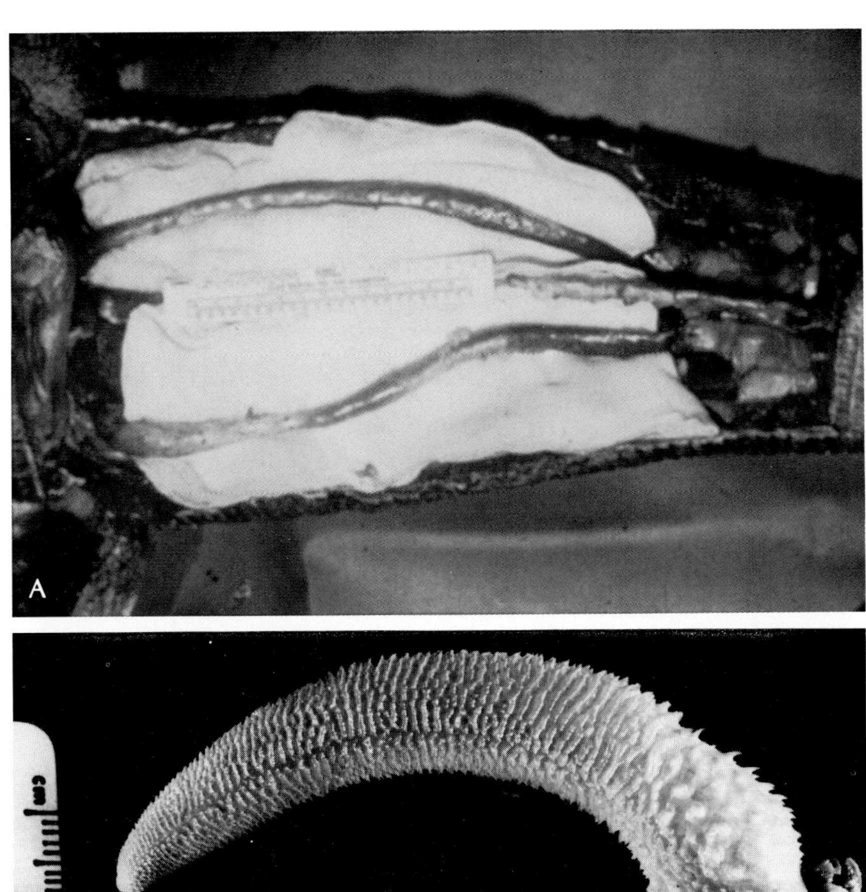

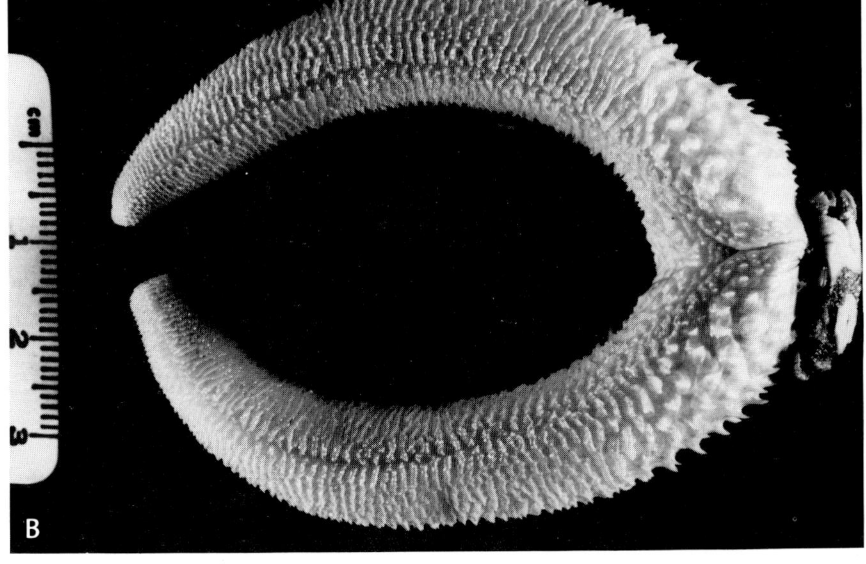

Fig. 1–19. **A.** Dissection of hemipenes (overlying white cloth) of adult male Komodo dragon (*Varanus komodoensis*). Base of tail is to the left. (Armed Forces Institute of Pathology Accession No. 1134021.) **B.** Dissected hemipenes of a western diamondback rattlesnake (*Crotalus atrox*). (Photograph courtesy of Dr. Howard E. Evans, Department of Anatomy, New York State College of Veterinary Medicine.)

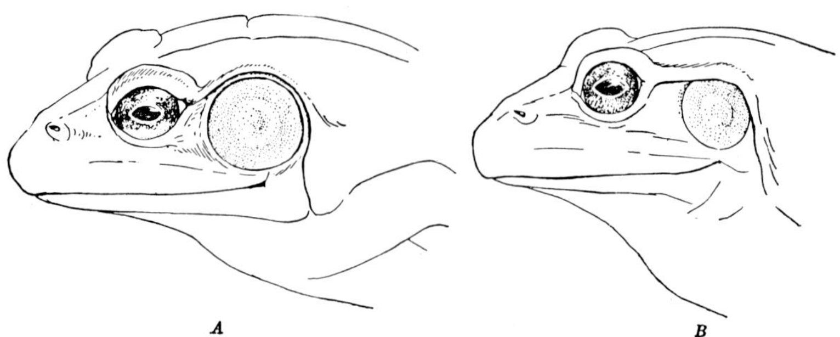

Fig. 1–20. Sexual dimorphism in the Bullfrog *(Rana catesbeiana)*. The tympanum is markedly larger in the male **(A)** than in the female **(B)** of the Bullfrog and allied species. (From Noble, G.K.: The Biology of the Amphibia. New York, McGraw-Hill, 1931. Reprinted by Dover Publications, 1954.)

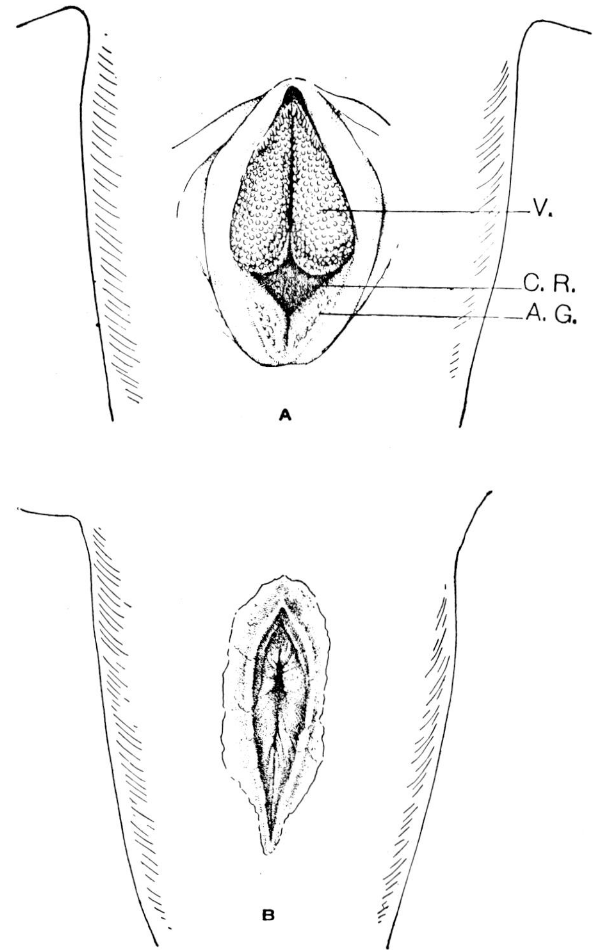

Fig. 1–21. The cloacal orifice of a male **(A)** and a female **(B)** salamander, *Desmognathus fuscus*, showing the villosities which serve to distinguish the males of most species of salamanders from the opposite sex. **A.G.**, abdominal gland; **C.R.**, cloacal roof, region of pelvic gland; **V.**, villosities of the cloacal glands. (From Noble, G.K.: The Biology of the Amphibia. New York, McGraw-Hill, 1931. Reprinted by Dover Publications, 1954.)

species, e.g., the Surinam toad *(Pipa pipa)*, carry the developing eggs on their backs.

In most salamanders fertilization is internal: The female places a sperm packet or **spermatophore** into her cloaca after it is deposited by the male during courtship. The sperm are stored in the **spermatotheca**, a series of tubules in the roof of the female cloaca. Sperm storage also is found in some female reptiles, up to several years in some species. This could account for reproduction in captivity in animals which could not have mated for some time.

In temperate climates snakes and lizards generally mate in the spring and the young are born or hatch in late summer. Some lizards may lay several clutches of eggs in a breeding season. Spring is also the season for most amphibians from temperate zones to mate and oviposit.

It has been suggested that the male renal sex segment (see p. 31) in some snakes, e.g., garter snakes (*Thamnophis* spp.) and water snakes (*Natrix* spp.), produces a secretion at the end of ejaculation which congeals in the female cloaca, forming a temporary plug. This plug might function to retain sperm in the oviduct and to obstruct copulation of the same female by other males.[28]

Many reptiles have specific mating behavioral patterns analogous to courtship in higher forms. Such patterns may include combat between rival males, which in snakes consists of interwining of their bodies, the two males wrestling for the favor of their lady fair. To those unfamiliar with the love life of serpents such fighting may be mistaken for coitus. Some turtles and crocodilians normally mate in water and a suitable aquatic environment must be provided for these species if they are to reproduce in captivity. The likelihood of some herpetofauna breeding in captivity is improved by keeping the sexes separated for a few weeks prior to the mating season.

Reproductive adaptations in amphibians associated with environmental conditions have been reviewed by Gallien,[47] and the reproductive physiology of reptiles has been reviewed by Miller.[70]

Sperm production and release are seasonal in frogs in temperate zones and are regulated by the ambient (seasonal) temperature, which in turn controls gonadotropin secretion by the pituitary. There is also seasonal variation in the sensitivity of the seminiferous tubules to gonadotropin. The end result of this internal and external regulation of the male reproductive system is that sperm is normally released only during the spawning season.[87]

The great majority of amphibians are **oviparous** (egg layers), but African toads in the genus *Nectophrynoides*[47] and a few salamanders are **ovoviviparous**, which means that fertilized eggs with shells are retained and larvae develop internally. Most reptiles, including all crocodilians and chelonians, lay eggs, but some snakes, including all vipers (Viperidae), boas (Boidae), water snakes (*Natrix* sp.), and garter snakes (*Thamnophis* sp.), and some lizards, e.g., horned toads *(Phrynosoma* spp.), give birth to living young, i.e., they are **viviparous**. Actually, there are gradations between egg laying and live bearing in lizards and snakes, for eggs may be retained until embryogenesis is advanced, with ovoviviparous species hatching the eggs internally. In other species a true placenta is formed. The amount of respiratory, nutritional, and excretory exchange across the placenta varies with species. The blood urea of garter snakes (*T. sirtalis*) increases from five to 10 mg/dl during pregnancy owing to transplacental clearance.[27]

The herpetofauna have the greatest reproductive capacity among the vertebrates higher than fish in the phylogenetic scale. The egg mass of a toad may contain thousands of eggs, and the Indian and reticulated pythons may lay a clutch of up to 100 eggs. The anaconda (*Eunectes murinus*), which is viviparous, may have as many as 42 babies in a litter and water snakes (*Natrix* spp.) may have as many as 100. In nature, young reptiles and amphibians are subject to heavy predation and relatively few in a clutch or litter reach maturity.

A veterinarian may be asked how to hatch a clutch of reptilian eggs. The two most important factors are control of temperature and control of humidity. Embryogenesis will not occur at too high or too low temperatures and sublethal excess heat may result in anomalies such as stunted tails.[18] Evans recommends keeping lizard eggs between 24° and 29°C (75° and 85°F) between layers of loose moist peat moss or rotted wood.[41] One could also use sterile sand containing 8% water, by weight,[18] layers of soaked newspaper from which excess water has been wrung out, or moist vermiculite. The same incubating conditions used for lizards can be used for snake or turtle eggs. The container should provide for adequate circulation of air because too much dampness may cause the eggs to be destroyed by mold. If moisture is inadequate, the eggs become dehydrated. The eggs of geckos and land tortoises should be incubated at drier conditions than for other reptiles.[7] Reptilian eggs do not have to be turned during incubation.

The hatching reptile escapes from the egg with the aid of a midrostral egg tooth in the case of snakes and lizards (paired in geckos) or an egg caruncle on the tip of the snout of chelonians and crocodilians. The egg tooth or caruncle is shed soon after hatching.

The total gestational/hatching period averages six to 12 weeks in most reptiles. Some oviparous species may retain eggs until embryogenesis is advanced, so the external incubation period for these eggs is short.

In contrast to mammals and lizards in which the female is homogametic (XX) and the male heterogametic (XY), amphibian and snake males are homogametic (designated WW) and the females heterogametic (designated WZ). Sex chromosomes have not been identified in turtles, crocodilians, and boid snakes.[10]

Endocrine System

The basic structure and function of the endocrine glands in herpetofauna are similar to those in higher vertebrates. Hormone function in reptiles and amphibians has some unique features in terms of target organs involved, e.g., in the processes of metamorphosis (see p. 7), and ecdysis, and changes in skin color (see pp. 39, 48 to 50).

The hypothalamic-pituitary-thyroid axis controls amphibian metamorphosis. Anterior pituitary hormones other than thyrotropin have not been well studied in reptiles and amphibians.

The pars intermedia of the pituitary produces melatonin, a polypeptide hormone that causes dispersion of melanin granules in melanophores, resulting in darkening of the skin, e.g., when the animal is placed on a dark background. In reptiles skin color is also under nervous control, which accounts for pigmentary changes in certain lizards with altered states of arousal.

Phylogenetically, the amphibians are the first animals to develop significant antidiuretic hormone function from the neurohypophysis. This fact is appropriate in an evolutionary sense because, as the first terrestrial vertebrates, they faced important problems in water conservation.

The thyroid is a single organ in snakes, turtles, and some lizards. It is bilateral in crocodilians and most lizards and the two lobes, located in the middle of and ventral to the trachea, are usually joined by an isthmus.[68] In turtles and snakes the thyroid is anterior to the pericardium, near the base of the heart (Fig. 1–22). In most amphibians the thyroid is paired, and accessory thyroid tissue may be found. In anurans the thyroids are close to the hyoid cartilages.

Thyroid activity is lowest during hibernation and maximal during the mating season. At the preferred body temperature (Chap. 2), thyroid hormones regulate metabolic rate in reptiles, but this effect may not be demonstrable at lower temperatures.[68] The thyroid helps control ecdysis in reptiles (see p. 49). This relationship is direct in lizards, but inverse in snakes.[68]

Amphibians are the most primitive vertebrates with distinct, organized parathyroids. These glands are usually found near the thymus or ultimobranchial bodies in herpetofauna and do not migrate into the thyroid as they do in mammals. Two pairs of parathyroids are found in turtles and snakes; lizards and crocodilians have one or two pairs.[19]

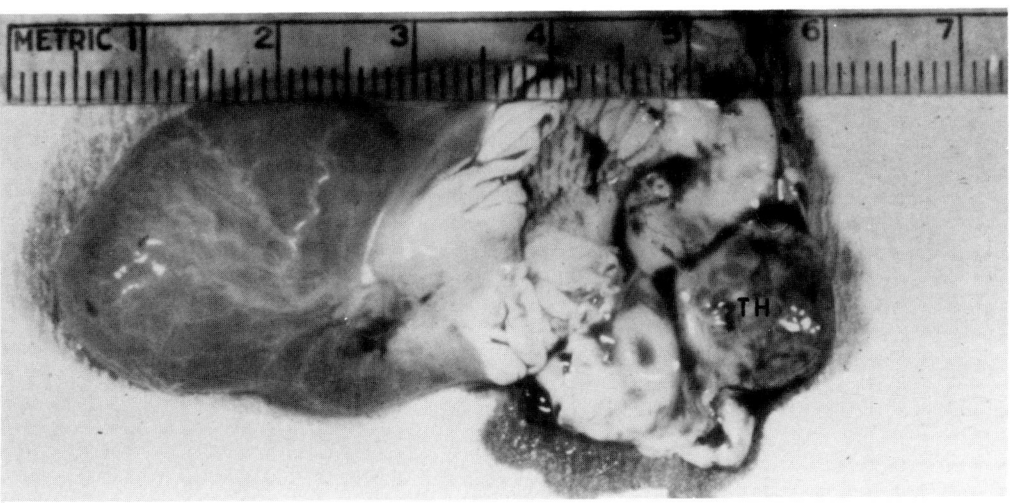

Fig. 1–22. Thyroid gland **(TH)** at base of the heart of cottonmouth moccasin *(Agkistrodon piscivorus)*. (Armed Forces Institute of Pathology Accession No. 1058160.)

Islets of Langerhans are found in the pancreas of herpetofauna, particularly in the splenic pole of the pancreas of snakes. Reptilian islets contain alpha and beta cells and secrete insulin and glucagon. Amphibians, such as the California newt *(Taricha torosa)* only have beta cells and only secrete insulin.[71,72] Normal fasting blood sugar of urodeles is about 24 mg/dl, whereas in lizards the average is 90 to 110 mg/dl (see p. 22).[72] Pancreatectomy causes diabetes (hyperglycemia) in some herpetofauna, but in lizards it causes hypoglycemia, apparently because removing the source for glucagon has a greater influence than removing the source of insulin.[10,58,72]

The equivalents of mammalian cortical and medullary tissue are intermingled in the adrenal glands of herpetofauna, or their relative positions may be the reverse of the mammalian situation, i.e., "cortical" cells may be surrounded by chromaffin cells. Chromaffin tissue can also be found alongside autonomic nerves and the great vessels. The reptilian adrenal has an arterial and a portal venous blood supply. In turtles the gland is closely adherent to the kidney, but in other reptiles it may be closer to the gonads or genital ducts.[46]

Nervous System

Phylogenetically, development of the basal ganglia is first seen in the amphibians, and development of the cerebral cortex begins in the reptiles. In both groups, the midbrain is the principal center of nervous integration, but the corpus striatum takes over some of this function in reptiles. Amphibians have cranial nerves I to X, whereas reptiles have I to XII. The spinal cord of reptiles ends near the tip of the tail, in contrast to the cauda equina arrangement in mammals. Herrick has written a detailed monograph on the anatomy of the brain of the tiger salamander, *Ambystoma tigrinum*.[56]

The telencephalon of lower vertebrates is smooth, with gyri and sulci becoming more apparent as one ascends the phylogenetic scale. The primary gross indication of cerebral edema in mammals is flattening of the brain surface, but the lack of convolutions in the amphibian or reptilian brain makes this difficult to discern.

A part of the diencephalon, the parapineal organ, has developed into a median **parietal eye** in the tuatara and certain lizards (Fig. 1–23). A rudimentary cornea, lens, and retina are in this third eye. The organ may be capable of photoreception, but its exact function is unknown. Lizards also have an intracranial pineal organ which contains photoreceptor-like cells. The pineal is absent in crocodilians. It is glandular in appearance in turtles and snakes, but its function is unknown. In amphibians the pineal complex contains a **frontal organ** which is thought to be a photoreceptor used in directional orientation and in setting circadian rhythms.[62] The structure and function of the pineal, parapineal, and other derivatives of the diencephalic roof in vertebrates have been of interest to comparative zoologists for many years. An excellent review of the subject is contained in the volume edited by Ariëns-Kappers, and Schadé.[4]

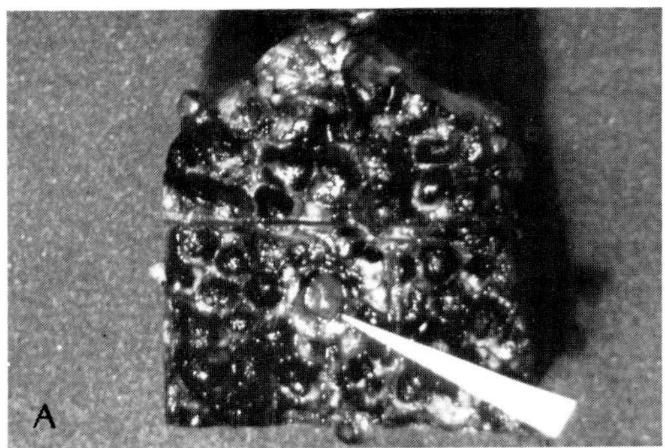

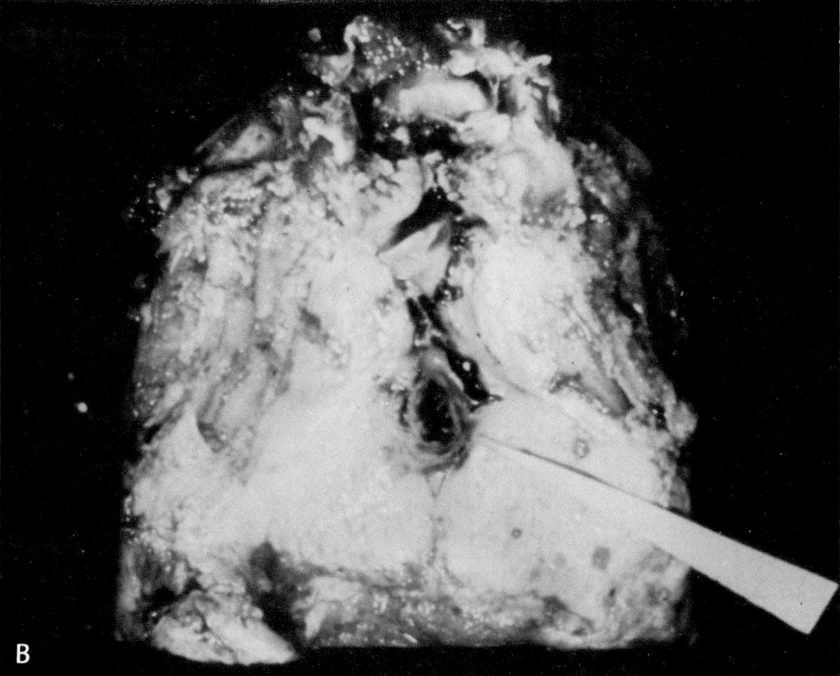

Fig. 1–23. Part of the calvarium of adult male Komodo dragon *(Varanus komodoensis)*. **A.** External surface. **B.** Internal surface. Pointer indicates the third or parietal eye. (Armed Forces Institute of Pathology Accession No. 1134021.)

The neurologically intact, healthy reptile or amphibian appears alert and has good muscle tone. A brisk withdrawal reflex should be evident after local noxious stimulation such as pinching. When the animal is placed on its back, it should also have a good righting response. This response may be delayed, i.e., some reptiles and amphibians may "play possum" when threatened. Some lizards, crocodilians, and frogs are seemingly "hypnotized" into remaining passively in dorsal recumbency when the abdomen is rubbed.

A common method of killing frogs in laboratories is to destroy the central nervous system by pithing. The frog is held with the neck flexed, with the prosector's index finger on the back of the animal's head, and his thumb on the back of the spinal column. A needle is inserted through the foramen magnum into the cranial cavity and then is directed caudad down the spinal column.

Special Senses

Much variation and modification of ocular structure are found in reptiles and amphibians. The eyes of cave-dwelling salamanders and some burrowing herpetofauna may be reduced to vestigial remnants.

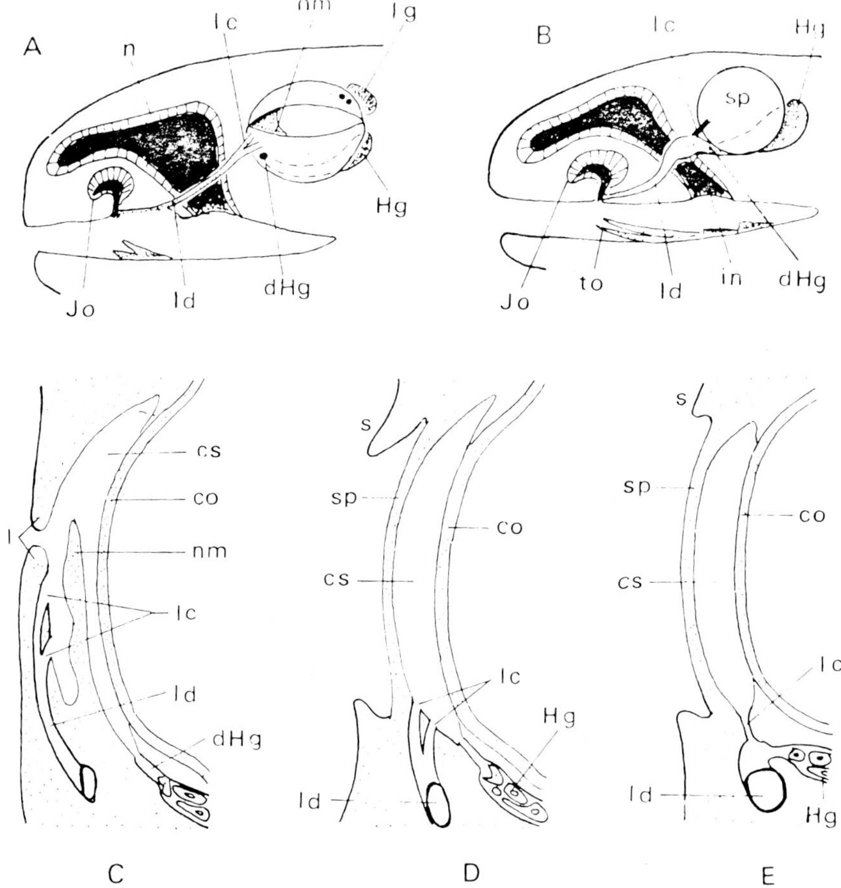

Fig. 1–24. **A, B,** Diagrams show Jacobson's organ, nose and lachrymal duct, from left side, partly in section, in typical lizard **(A)** and snake **(B)**. In the lizard there are two lachrymal canaliculi and the lachrymal duct opens in front into the duct of the organ of Jacobson, and often into a groove in the palate close by. In the snake the lachrymal duct opens into the duct of Jacobson's organ, the harderian gland leads directly into the lachrymal duct, and there is generally a single canaliculus. **C** to **E,** Diagrammatic transverse sections through front of eye of typical lizard **(C)** (eyelids, nictitating membrane, two lachrymal canaliculi); typical gecko **(D)** (spectacle instead of movable lids, no nictitating membrane, two canaliculi); snake **(E)** (spectacle, no nictitans, one canaliculus). **co**, cornea; **cs**, conjunctival space; **dHg**, duct of harderian gland; **Hg**, harderian gland; **in**, internal nostril; **Jo**, Jacobson's organ; **l**, eyelids; **lc**, lachrymal canaliculus; **ld**, lachrymal duct; **lg**, lachrymal gland; **n**, nasal sac; **nm**, nictitating membrane; **s**, projecting scale; **sp**, spectacle; **to**, tongue. (From The Life of Reptiles by Angus Bellairs. Published by Universe Books, New York, 1970.)

Aquatic animals may have a functional third eyelid, a transparent nictitating membrane. In contrast, all snakes and some lizards, e.g., most geckos and skinks, lack movable eyelids; their eyes are covered with a transparent **spectacle** (Fig. 1–24), formed by fusion of the lids in embryogenesis and shed at the time of ecdysis. In some lizards, a transparent window is found in the lower lid, permitting vision when the eye is closed. In the true chameleons the eyelids are fused except for a small central aperture. The eye is closed by movement of the upper lid in crocodilians and by the lower lid in other reptiles. Eye movements in chameleons and some other lizards are independent of each other.

In turtles and lizards, the sclera contains plates of cartilage or bone and **scleral ossicles** at the limbus may be demonstrable radiographically. The sclera of crocodilians contains cartilage but no ossicles.

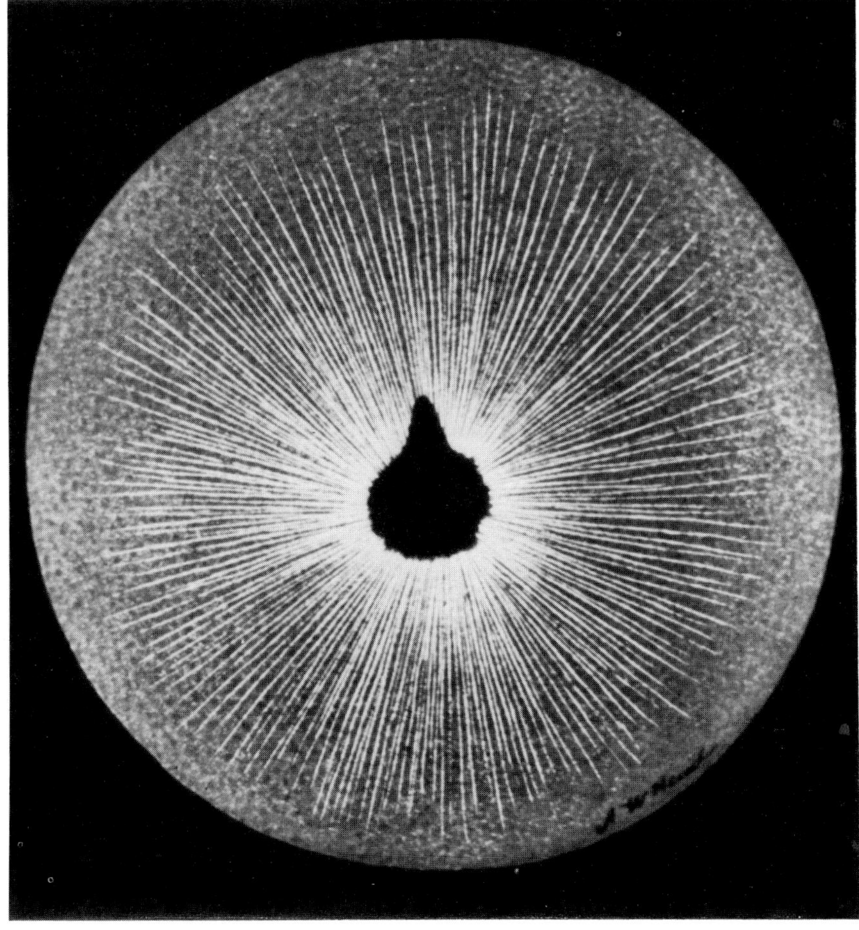

Fig. 1–25. Ocular fundus of Turkish gecko *(Hemidactylus turcicus)*. The orange-red fundus is uniformly stippled with small black spots. The pecten, which projects into the vitreous, obscures the optic disc. White medullated nerve fibers radiate from the margin of the disc. (From Wood, C.A.: The Fundus Oculi of Birds. Chicago, Lakewood Press, 1917.)

Bone and cartilage are lacking in snake eyes and no scleral ossicles are found in the eyes of modern amphibians.

A **conus papillaris**, homologous to the **pecten** in birds, is found in many reptiles and is readily seen with the ophthalmoscope as a black mass overlying the optic disc (Fig. 1–25). It is well developed in lizards (Fig. 1–26), rudimentary in some turtles, and absent in amphibians and in most snakes.

Reptiles may have one or two ophthalmic glands in their orbit. Most lizards and turtles have a harderian gland in the nasal aspect of the orbit and a temporally located lacrimal gland (see Figs. 1–24 and 3–81A). Crocodiles, snakes, and the tuatara only have the harderian gland.[36] (Underwood describes a lacrimal gland in crocodilians.[86]) Both glands are serous tubuloacinar organs whose secretions enter the conjunctival sacs. The ophthalmic glands undergo squamous metaplasia with hypovitaminosis A in turtles, and the swollen appearance of the eyes caused by these enlarging glands is usually the presenting sign of this common nutritional disorder (Chap. 3). Lacrimal ducts are absent in turtles, but in other reptiles they drain into the palate in the area of Jacobson's organ (see p. 45), usually by joining the duct of that organ. The openings of the lacrimal ducts may be blocked by exudate in cases

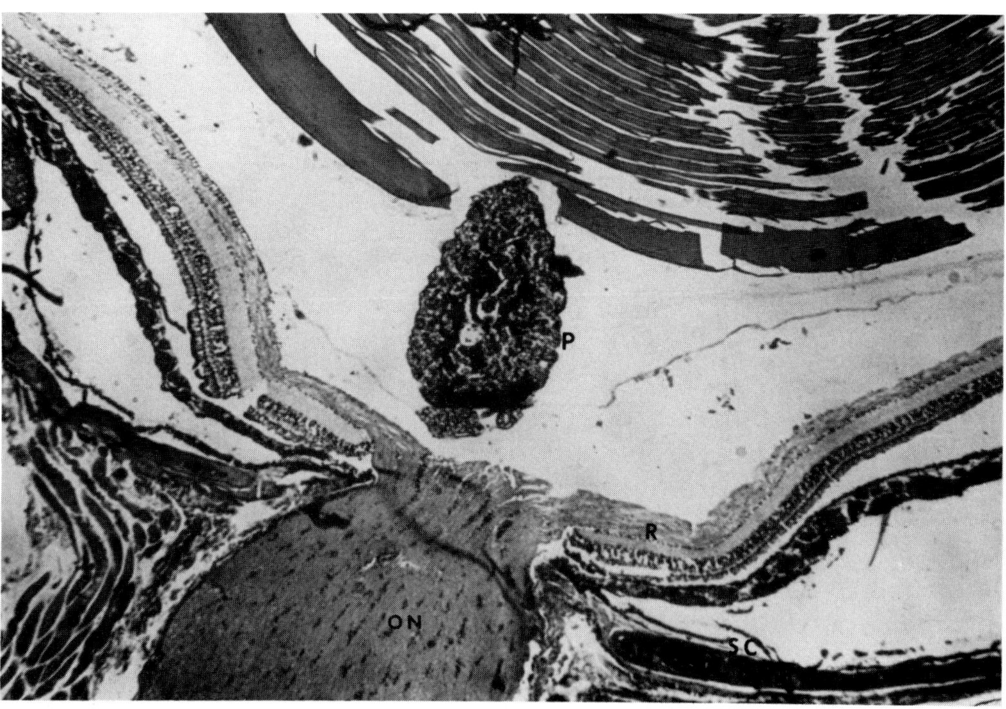

Fig. 1–26. Section through posterior segment of eye showing cone-shaped, heavily pigmented pecten **(P)** overlying the head of the optic nerve **(ON)**. Scleral cartilage **(SC)**, which ossifies in older animals, is seen to the right of the optic nerve. The lens, artifactually fragmented and displaced posteriorly, is at the top **(R, retina)**. Sudan plated lizard *(Gerrhosaurus major)*. (Armed Forces Institute of Pathology photograph.)

of ulcerative stomatitis, resulting in distention of the corneo-spectacular space (Chap. 3).

In the New World all nonvenomous snakes except boa constrictors have round pupils. Coral snakes also have round pupils, but all pit vipers have vertically slit pupils. The mildly poisonous rear-fanged snakes, a minor group in the New World, may have round or vertically slit pupils.

An interesting feature of the crocodilian eye is the presence of a tapetum. This layer is rich in guanine crystals which reflect light at night. Whatever functional value the tapetum may have for crocodilians is offset by the fact that hunters can readily spot their eyes in the glare of a flashlight, which makes hunting them easy and has contributed to their decimation.

Horned toads (more properly, horned lizards, *Phrynosoma* spp.) have the unique and unusual capacity to squirt droplets of blood from their eyes for several feet when they are alarmed. Presumably this is a defensive mechanism designed to confuse or startle an enemy.

Behavioral studies of conditioned responses indicate that lizards and turtles can perceive color, but chromatic perception seems to be lacking in crocodilians and snakes. Definite proof of this is problematical.

A fascinating essay on the anatomy and function of amphibian and reptilian eyes was written by Johnson.[60] This monograph includes color plates of the ocular fundus of many species. Many of these plates are reproduced and ocular physiology of these animals is further discussed from an evolutionary standpoint in the *Eye in Evolution*, edited by Duke-Elder.[31] Another excellent review of reptilian ocular anatomy was written by Underwood.[86] Extraocular photoreception by diencephalic organs was discussed previously (see p. 40).

Eyelids and external ear openings are lacking in all snakes and some lizards. If either of these structures is found in a limbless reptile, it must be a legless lizard rather than a snake. Snakes were once thought to be deaf, but they are very sensitive to vibration and it is likely that they can hear low-pitched airborne sounds.[9] Snakes have a middle ear, although its structure is greatly reduced compared to that of lizards. Turtles also lack an external ear; their tympanic membrane is covered by skin. The anatomy of the reptilian ear has been reviewed by Baird.[5]

Jacobson's organ is a peculiar part of the olfactory system in herpetofauna. In amphibians Jacobson's organ is thought to function in detecting waterborne odors; other olfactory tissue in the nasal passages functions on land. This organ is absent in crocodilians and modified or absent in turtles. In other reptiles Jacobson's organ is a specialized paired olfactory organ within the roof of the mouth lying on either side of the midline, enclosed in the vomer and septomaxillary bones (see Fig. 1–24). A duct on each side leads from the organ to the roof of the oral cavity. The flickering tongue of snakes and lizards brings odorous particles to Jacobson's organ, and branches of the olfactory nerve carry sensation from its receptor cells back to the brain. The anatomy of the nose and Jacobson's organ in reptiles have been reviewed in detail by Parsons.[76]

Sensory pits that act as thermoreceptors are found in some snakes.[8,9] They are most highly developed in the Crotalidae or pit vipers, which have an obvious pit or depression located bilaterally between the nostril and eye (Fig. 1–27). There is a larger opening to the pit rostrally (towards the nostril) and a smaller one caudally (towards the eye) (Fig. 1–28). The pit forms a hollow in the maxillary bone, a feature that distinguishes the skull of a pit viper from that of a true viper. A membrane about 10μ thick separates an inner and outer chamber. This **pit membrane** is innervated by branches of the ophthalmic and maxillary divisions of the trigeminal nerve.

Smaller, simpler pits with a single chamber are found along the upper and lower labial scales bordering the mouth in pythons and some boas (Fig. 1–29). They are innervated by the ophthalmic, maxillary, and mandibular branches of the trigeminal nerve.

These pits are very sensitive to focal changes in environmental temperature, and detect radiant heat from any source warmer than the general background. In pit vipers the sensory fields of the pits overlap, giving the animal three-dimensional heat perception. The pits apparently are an important means of locating prey, especially in nocturnal hunting.

Aquatic larval amphibians, adult salamanders, and some adult frogs have **lateral line organs,** which are receptors (also found in fish) sensitive to pressure waves. These organs also help maintain balance in water.

Integument

During the evolutionary development of terrestrial vertebrate life the structure of the skin had to undergo many modifications for survival in a new environment. Except for toads and a few adult salamanders,

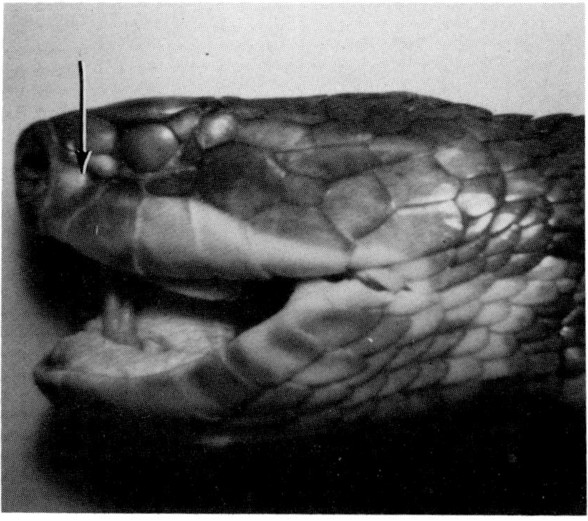

Fig. 1–27. Cottonmouth moccasin *(Agkistrodon piscivorus)* showing pit (arrow) located between nostril and eye. (Armed Forces Institute of Pathology photograph. Accession No. 1058160.)

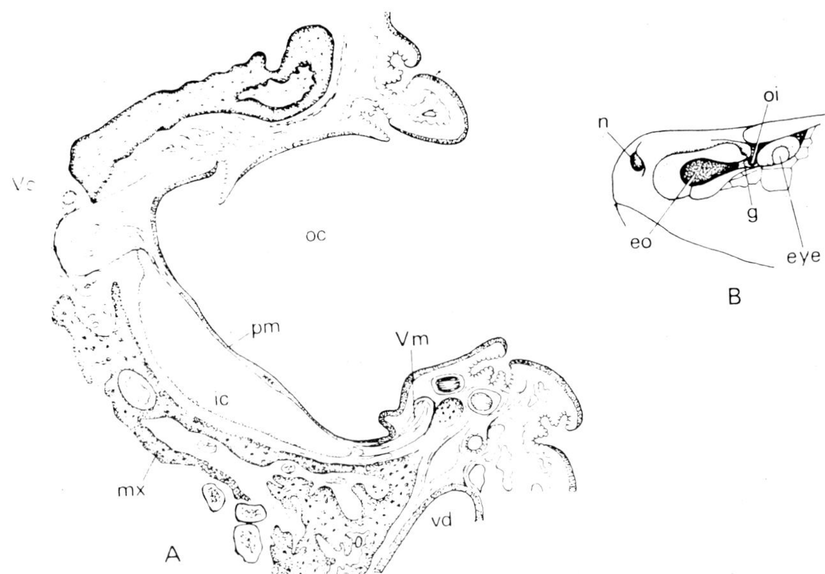

Fig. 1–28. **A**, Microscopic section through sensory pit of rattlesnake *(Crotalus terrificus)*. **B**, Left side of snout of bushmaster *(Lachesis muta)*. The flap of tissue partly covering the external opening of the pit is lifted up, showing the groove between the pit and eye, and the external opening of the inner pit chamber. (A and B after West, G.S. (1900) Quart. J. Microsc. Sci.) **ic**, inner chamber of pit; **eo**, external opening of pit; **g**, groove between pit and eye; **mx**, maxilla; **n**, nostril; **oc**, outer chamber of pit; **oi**, opening of inner pit chamber to exterior; **pm**, pit membrane; **vd**, venom gland duct; **Vm**, branch of maxillary division of trigeminal (Vth) nerve. **Vo**, branch of ophthalmic division of Vth nerve. (From The Life of Reptiles by Angus Bellairs. Published by Universe Books, New York, 1970.)

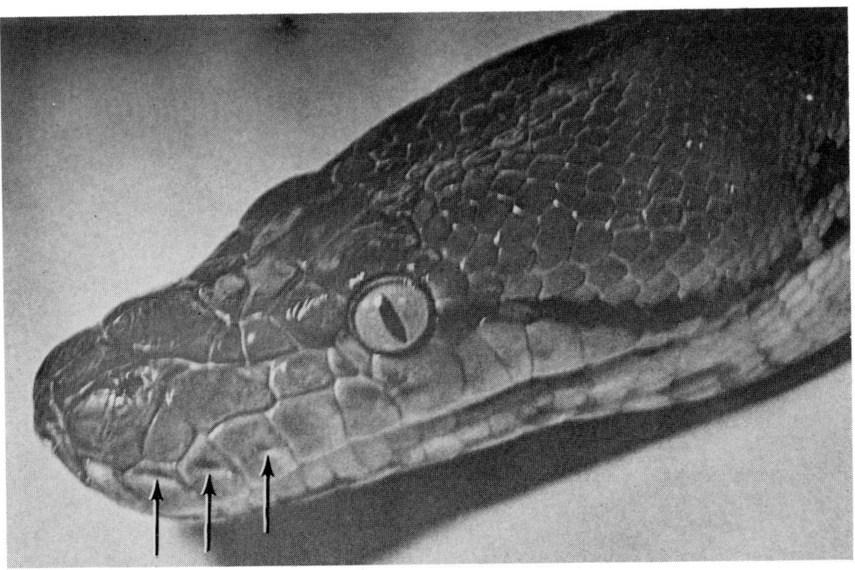

Fig. 1–29. Labial pits (arrows) of reticulated python *(Python reticularis)*.

amphibians have a moist, slimy skin. If kept in too dry an atmosphere amphibians soon die of dehydration. Most adult frogs and salamanders must have access to fresh water or, at least, to damp earth and vegetation. Amphibian skin is an important respiratory organ (see p. 23) and is important in maintaining water and electrolyte balance (see p. 31).

The amphibian skin is rich in glands of two types: granular and mucous. The former are often concentrated in cutaneous "warts." The contents of both types of glands may be highly irritating to mucous membranes, but the granular gland secretion is usually more toxic. South American Indians use certain toads as a source of poisons for their arrows. Some toads in the Southwestern United States are toxic enough to kill dogs that mouth them, though most dogs recover spontaneously. The toxin is thought to have an action similar to that of digitalis.[80] Secretions from the skin of some amphibians may be toxic for other amphibians. For example, secretions of the pickerel frog, *Rana palustris*, can kill other frogs and, therefore, this species should be caged by itself.

Reptilian skin is dry and, with certain exceptions (e.g., specific musk glands), is aglandular. A pair of scent glands is located in the inner aspect of the lower jaw and another pair is located in the cloaca of crocodilians of both sexes. Many lizards have a row of **femoral glands** on the ventrocaudal aspect of their thighs.[21] The holocrine secretion of these glands drains by way of **femoral pores**, which are tiny openings visible on the skin. They may be found in both sexes, but in some species femoral glands are better developed in males. Their function is unknown.

Reptiles are covered with **scales** or **scutes**, although, as an exception, soft-shell turtles have scales that are few and small. Scale pattern is specific, and therefore is used in classification and identification of reptiles.

Crocodilians and some lizards may have plates of bone in the dermis underlying their scales, providing a kind of armor plating. These bony plates, called **osteoderms** or **osteoscutes**, are readily visualized in radiographs (Fig. 1–30) and are a considerable barrier to incision during surgery. In some species these bony plates are not found on the ventral midline. Among the Amphibia, some frogs and toads have bone in the skin on their head or back. The turtle's shell is discussed on page 8.

The color of a reptile's or amphibian's skin is determined by distribution of three kinds of cells in the skin: **iridocytes** or **guanophores**, which contain guanine, a white material; **lipophores**, which contain red and yellow pigments; and **melanophores**, which contain melanin. A particularly fascinating aspect of herpetologic dermatology is the ability of certain species to change color. While this phenomenon is best known in Old World or true chameleons (family Chamaeleontidae) and so-called "New World chameleons" or anole lizards (*Anolis* spp.), it is also characteristic of many tree frogs (*Hyla* spp.) and some other lizards and amphibians. The ability to change color is dependent on the contraction and expansion of ameboid

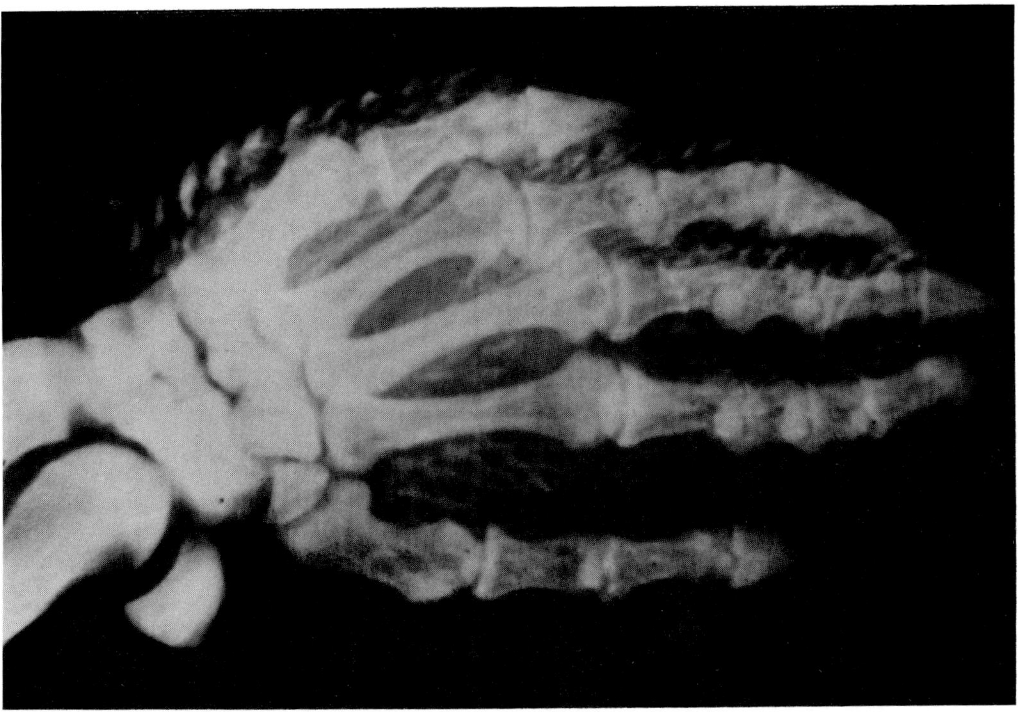

Fig. 1–30. Radiograph of front foot of mature male Komodo dragon *(Varanus komodoensis)* showing osteoderms. (Armed Forces Institute of Pathology Accession No. 1134021.)

processes of melanophores, with contraction producing a lighter shade and expansion a darker shade. Specific colors are dependent on the arrangement of the guanophores and lipophores in relation to the melanophores and to each other.[2] Stimuli to change color include temperature, intensity of ambient light, color of surroundings, and mood (anger, fright, or varying degrees of calm or excitement). Control of melanophore size is mediated partly through humoral control (intermedin or melanin dispersion hormone from the pars intermedia and epinephrine from the adrenal), and partly through nervous control. The relative importance of the various stimuli and mechanisms of mediation vary with different species, e.g., it is thought that color change in Old World chameleons is more dependent on nervous control, whereas in anole lizards it is more under endocrine control.

Members of the order Squamata shed the outer keratinized layer of skin periodically as they grow. In lizards the skin is usually shed in several large pieces. In snakes the skin is normally shed intact, including the spectacles over the eyes. The snake crawls out of his shed skin, turning it inside out. Before the beginning of **shedding** or **ecdysis** the snake's eyes appear dull. Snakes often refuse food at this time and become irritable. Shedding is facilitated by keeping the relative humidity at 50 to 60% and by providing the snake with a pan of water in which to soak and rough rocks on which to rub. Rattlesnakes add a new rattle each time they shed. If all rattles, including the terminal button, are present (they commonly are broken off), the number of rattles equals the number of ecdyses, which in turn depends on the growth rate of the snake. Frequency of ecdysis is proportional to the rate of growth. Therefore, young snakes shed more frequently than older ones.[58a] Many snakes in the temperate zone shed their skins an average of two to five times a year.

In chelonians and crocodilians desquamation of epidermis occurs gradually and piecemeal. Amphibians also molt, and the process is apparently under the control of the pituitary-thyroid axis.[81] Many frogs and salamanders eat their shed skin, and certain flukes that encyst in amphibians' skin depend on this peculiar habit for completion of their life cycle (see Table 3–3).

Although molting usually occurs piecemeal, it is not unusual to find the intact cast of an amphibian's limb in the cage. (This is especially common with the newts and toads.) If a client is concerned over such a finding, he should be reassured that it is a normal process.

REFERENCES

1. Acuña, M.L.: The hematology of the tropical lizard *Iguana iguana* Linnaeus: II. Seasonal variations. Herpetologica, *30*:299–303, 1974.
2. Alexander, N.J., and Fahrenbach, W.H.: The dermal chromatophores of *Anolis carolinensis* (Reptilia, Iguanidae). Am. J. Anat., *126*:41–56, 1969.
3. Andrew, W.: Textbook of Comparative Histology. Oxford University Press, New York, 1959.
4. Ariëns-Kappers, J., and Schadé, J.P.: Structure and Function of the Epiphysis Cerebri. Elsevier Publishing Co., New York, 1965.
5. Baird, I.L.: The anatomy of the reptilian ear. *In* Biology of the Reptilia. Edited by C. Gans and T.S. Parsons. Academic Press, New York, 1970, Vol. II, pp. 193–275.
6. Baker, E. F., Anderson, H. W., and Allard, J.: Epidemiological aspects of turtle-associated salmonellosis. Arch. Environ. Health, *24*:1–9, 1972.
7. Ball, D.J., and Bellairs, A.d'A.: Reptiles. *In* Handbook on the Care and Management of Laboratory Animals. Edited by UFAW. Williams & Wilkins, Baltimore, 1972, pp. 490–510.
8. Barrett, R., Maderson, P.F.A., and Meszler, R.M.: The pit organs of snakes. *In* Biology of the Reptilia. Edited by C. Gans and T.S. Parsons. Academic Press, New York, 1970, Vol. II, pp. 277–300.
9. Bellairs, A.: The sensory pits. *In* The Life of Reptiles. Edited by A. Bellairs. Universe Books, New York, 1970, Vol. II, pp. 386–389.
10. Bellairs, A.: The Life of Reptiles. Universe Books, New York, 1970, Vols. I and II.
11. Bishop, J.E.: A histological and histochemical study of the kidney tubule of the common garter snake *Thamnophis sirtalis* with special reference to the sexual segment in the male. J. Morphol., *104*:307–350, 1959.
12. Bisset, K.A.: The effect of temperature upon antibody production in cold-blooded vertebrates. J. Path. Bact., *60*:87–92, 1948.
13. Bockman, D.E.: The thymus. *In* Biology of the Reptilia. Edited by C. Gans and T.S. Parsons. Academic Press, New York, 1970, Vol. III, pp. 111–133.
14. Brazaitis, P.J.: The determination of sex in living crocodilians. Br. J. Herp., *4*:54–58, 1968.
15. Brunnst, V.V.: The axolotl *(Siredon mexicanum)*. I. As material for scientific research. Lab. Invest., *4*:45–64, 1955.
16. Brunnst, V.V.: The axolotl. II. Morphology and pathology. Lab. Invest., *4*:429–449, 1955.
17. Burke, T.J.: Extirpation of the viperid glandular venom apparatus. J. Zoo Anim. Med., *2*:13–17, 1971.
18. Bustard, H.R.: Tail abnormalities in reptiles resulting from high temperature egg incubation. Br. J. Herp., *4*:121–123, 1969.

19. Clark, N.B.: The parathyroid. *In* Biology of the Reptilia. Edited by C. Gans and T.S. Parsons. Academic Press, New York, 1970, Vol. III, pp. 235–262.
20. Cohen, N.: Reptiles as models for the study of immunity and its phylogenesis. J. Am. Vet. Med. Assoc., *159*:1662–1671, 1971.
21. Cole, C.J.: Femoral glands in lizards: a review. Herpetologica, *22*:199–206, 1966.
22. Coulson, R.A., and Hernandez, T.: Biochemistry of the Alligator. Louisiana State University Press, Baton Rouge, 1964.
23. Coulson, R.A., and Hernandez, T.: Reptiles as research models for comparative biochemistry and endocrinology. J. Am. Vet. Med. Assoc., *159*:1672–1677, 1971.
24. Cuellar, O.: Additional evidence for true parthenogenesis in lizards of the genus *Cnemidophorus*. Herpetologica, *24*:146–150, 1968.
25. Darevski, I.S.: Natural parthenogenesis in a polymorphic group of Caucasian rock lizards related to *Lacerta saxicola* Eversmann. J. Ohio Herpet. Soc., *5*:115–152, 1966.
26. Dawson, W.R.: Reptiles as research models in comparative physiology. J. Am. Vet. Med. Assoc. *159*:1653–1661, 1971.
27. Dessauer, H.C.: Blood chemistry of reptiles: physiological and evolutionary aspects. *In* Biology of the Reptilia. Edited by C. Gans and T.S. Parsons. Academic Press, New York, 1970. Vol. III, pp. 1–72.
28. Devine, M.C.: Copulatory plugs in snakes: enforced chastity. Science, *187*:844–845, 1975.
29. Deyrup, I.J.: Water balance and kidney. *In* Physiology of the Amphibia. Edited by J.A. Moore. Academic Press, New York, 1964, pp. 251–328.
30. Duguy, R.: Numbers of blood cells and their variation. *In* Biology of the Reptilia. Edited by C. Gans and T.S. Parsons. Academic Press, New York, 1970. Vol. III, pp. 93–109.
31. Duke-Elder, S. (Ed.): System of Ophthalmology Series. Eye in Evolution. C.V. Mosby Co., St. Louis, 1958, Vol. I.
32. Dunson, W.A., Packer, R.K., and Dunson, M.K.: Sea snakes: an unusual salt gland under the tongue. Science, *173*:437–441, 1971.
33. DuPasquier, L.: Ontogeny of the immune response in cold-blooded vertebrates. Curr. Top. Microbiol. Immunol., *61*:38–88, 1973.
34. Edmund, A.G.: Dentition. *In* Biology of the Reptilia. Edited by C. Gans, A. d'A. Bellairs, and T.S. Parsons. Academic Press, New York, 1969, Vol. I, pp. 117–200.
35. Elkan, E.: Observations on the lymphatic system of the South African claw footed toad (*Xenopus laevus* Daudin). Br. J. Herp., *2*:37–53, 1957.
36. Elkan, E., and Zwart, P.: The ocular disease of young terrapins caused by vitamin A deficiency. Path. Vet., *4*:201–222, 1967.
37. Etkin, W.: Metamorphosis. *In* Physiology of the Amphibia. Edited by J.A. Moore. Academic Press, New York, 1964, pp. 427–468.
38. Evans, E.E.: Antibody response in amphibia and reptiles. Fed. Proc., *22*:1132–1137, 1963.
39. Evans, E.E.: Comparative immunology. Antibody response in *Dipsosaurus dorsalis* at different temperatures. Proc. Soc. Exp. Biol. Med., *112*:531–533, 1963.
40. Evans, E.E., et. al.: Antibody formation and immunologic memory in the marine toad. *In* Phylogeny of Immunity. Edited by R.T. Smith, P.A. Mieschen, and R.A. Good. University of Florida Press, Gainesville, 1966, pp. 218–226.
41. Evans, H.E.: Keeping reptiles as pets. *In* Current Veterinary Therapy IV. Edited by R. W. Kirk. W.B. Saunders Co., Philadelphia, 1971, pp. 419–433.
42. Fox, W.: Seasonal variation in the male reproductive system of Pacific coast garter snakes. J. Morphol., *90*:481–554, 1952.
43. Frair, W.: Blood group studies with turtles. Science, *140*:1412–1414, 1963. (Reprinted, Int. Turtle and Tortoise Soc. J., *1*:30–32, 1967.)
44. Frieden, E.: The chemistry of amphibian metamorphosis. Sci. Am., *209*:110–118, 1963.
45. Frye, F.L.: Hematology of captive reptiles (with emphasis on normal morphology). *In* Current Veterinary Therapy, VI. Edited by R.W. Kirk. W.B. Saunders Co., Philadelphia, 1977, pp. 792–798.
46. Gabe, M.: The adrenal. *In* Biology of the Reptilia. Edited by C. Gans and T.S. Parsons. Academic Press, New York, Vol. III, 1970, pp. 263–318.
47. Gallien, L.: Endocrine basis for reproductive adaptations in Amphibia. *In* Comparative Endocrinology. Edited by A. Gorbman. John Wiley & Sons, Inc., New York, 1959, pp. 479–487.
48. Gans, C., Bellairs, A.d'A., and Parsons, T.S.: Biology of the Reptilia. Academic Press, New York, 1969, Vol. I.
49. Gibbs, E.L., Nace, G.W., and Emmons, M.B.: The live frog is almost dead. Bioscience, *21*:1027–1037, 1971.

50. Good, R.A., et al.: Morphologic studies on the evolution of the lymphoid tissues among the lower vertebrates. *In* Phylogeny of Immunity. Edited by R.T. Smith, P.A. Mieschen, and R.A. Good. University of Florida Press, Gainesville, 1966, pp. 149–168.
51. Graham, T.E., and Hutchison, V.H.: Centenarian box turtles. Int. Turtle and Tortoise Soc. J., *3*:25–29, 1969.
52. Hackett, E. and Hann, C.: Slow clotting of reptile bloods. J. Comp. Pathol., *77*:175–180, 1967.
53. Haines, R.W.: Epiphyses and sesamoids. *In* Biology of the Reptilia. Edited by C. Gans, A. Bellairs, and T.S. Parsons. Academic Press, New York, 1969, Vol. I, pp. 81–115.
54. Harris, V.A.: The Anatomy of the Rainbow Lizard. Hutchinson Tropical Monographs, London, 1963.
55. Hartman, F.A., and Lessler, M.A.: Erythrocyte measurements in fishes, amphibia and reptiles. Biol. Bull., *126*:83–88, 1964.
55a. Heatwole, H.: Adaptations of marine snakes. Am. Sci., *66*:594–604, 1978.
56. Herrick, C.J.: The Brain of the Tiger Salamander. University of Chicago Press, Chicago, 1948.
57. Hildemann, W.H.: Immunogenetic studies of poikilothermic animals. Am. Naturalist, *96*:195–204, 1962.
58. Houssay, B.A.: Comparative physiology of the endocrine pancreas. *In* Comparative Endocrinology. Edited by A. Gorbman. John Wiley & Sons, Inc., New York, 1959, pp. 639–667.
58a. Jacobson, E.R.: Histology, endocrinology and husbandry of ecdysis in snakes (a review). Vet. Med. Small Anim. Clin., *72*:275–280, 1977.
59. Jaros, D.B.: Occlusion of the venom duct of Crotalidae by electrocoagulation: An innovation in operative technique. Zoologica., *25*:49–51, 1940.
60. Johnson, G.L.: Contributions to the comparative anatomy of the reptilian and the amphibian eye, chiefly based on ophthalmological examination. Philos. Trans. R. Soc. Lond., B *216*:315–353, 1927.
61. Jordan, H.E., and Flippen, J.C.: Hematopoiesis in Chelonia. Folia Haematol., *15*:1–24, 1913.
62. Justis, C.S., and Taylor, D.H.: Extraocular photoreception and compass orientation in larval bullfrogs, *Rana catesbeiana*. Copeia, No. 1, 98–105, 1976.
63. Kaplan, H.M., and Crouse, G.T.: Blood changes underlying the seasonal resistance of frogs to disease. Copeia, No. 1, 52–54, 1956.
64. Kaplan, H.M., and Rueff, W.: Seasonal blood changes in turtles. Proc. Anim. Care Panel, *10*:63–68, 1960.
65. Kochva, E., and Gans, C.: Histology and histochemistry of venom glands of some crotaline snakes. Copeia, No. 3, 506–515, 1966.
66. Legler, D.W., et al.: Immunoglobulin and complement systems of amphibian serum. *In* Biology of Amphibian Tumors. Edited by M. Mizell. Springer-Verlag, Berlin-Heidelberg-New York, 1968, pp. 169–176.
67. Lowe, C.H., and Wright, J.W.: Evolution of parthenogenetic species of *Cnemidophorus* (whiptail lizards) in western North America. J. Ariz. Acad. Sci., *4*:81–87, 1966.
68. Lynn, W.G.: The thyroid. *In* Biology of the Reptilia. Edited by C. Gans and T.S. Parsons. Academic Press, New York, 1970, Vol. III, pp. 201–234.
69. Maung, R.T.: Immunity in the tortoise, *Testudo ibera*. J. Path. Bact. *85*:51–66, 1963.
70. Miller, M.R.: The endocrine basis for reproductive adaptations in reptiles. *In* Comparative Endocrinology. Edited by A. Gorbman. John Wiley & Sons, Inc., New York, 1959, pp. 499–516.
71. Miller, M.R., and Lagios, M.D.: The pancreas. *In* Biology of the Reptilia. Edited by C. Gans and T.S. Parsons. Academic Press, New York, 1970, Vol. III, pp. 319–346.
72. Miller, M.R., and Wurster, D.H.: The morphology and physiology of the pancreatic islets in urodele amphibians and lizards. Comparative Endocrinology. Edited by A. Gorbman. John Wiley & Sons, Inc., New York, 1959, pp. 668–680.
73. Moore, J.A. (Ed.):Physiology of the Amphibia. Academic Press, New York, 1964.
74. Moyle, V.: Nitrogenous excretion in chelonian reptiles. Biochem. J., *44*:581–589, 1949.
75. Noble, G.K.: The Biology of the Amphibia. McGraw-Hill Co., Inc., New York, 1931. Reprinted 1954, Dover Publications, Inc.
76. Parsons, T.S.: The nose and Jacobson's organ. *In* Biology of the Reptilia. Edited by C. Gans and T.S. Parsons. Academic Press, New York, 1970, Vol. II, pp. 99–191.
77. Pienaar, U.DeV.: Haematology of some South African reptiles. Witwatersrand Univ. Press, Johannesburg, 1962.

78. Prosser, C.L., and Brown, F.A., Jr.: Comparative Animal Physiology. 2nd Edition. W.B. Saunders Co., Philadelphia, 1961.
79. Romer, A.S.: Osteology of the Reptiles. University of Chicago Press, Chicago, 1956.
80. Russell, R.L.: Toad poisoning. *In* Current Veterinary Therapy. Edited by R.W. Kirk. W.B. Saunders Co., Philadelphia, 1966, pp. 621–622.
81. Scharrer, E.: General and phylogenetic interpretations of neuroendocrine interrelations. *In* Comparative Endocrinology. Edited by A. Gorbman. J. Wiley & Sons, Inc., New York, 1959, pp. 233–249.
82. Schlumberger, H.G., and Burke, D.H.: Comparative study of the reaction to injury. II. Hypervitaminosis D in the frog with special reference to the lime sacs. A.M.A. Arch. Pathol., *56*:103–124, 1953.
83. Softly, A., and Cockett, E.G.: Aspects of maintaining snakes as laboratory animals. J. Inst. Anim. Technicians, *17*:49–60, 1966.
84. Telford, S.R., Jr.: What do we know about the parasites in reptiles? Int. Turtle and Tortoise Soc. J., *1*:10–13, 37–38, 1967.
85. Thorson, T.B.: Body fluid partitioning in Reptilia. Copeia, No. 3, 592–601, 1968.
86. Underwood, G.: The eye. Biology of the Reptilia. Edited by C. Gans and T.S. Parsons. Academic Press, New York, 1970, Vol. II, pp. 1–97.
87. van Oordt, G.J., van Oordt, P.G., and van Dongen, W.J.: Recent experiments on the regulation of spermatogenesis and the mechanism of spermiation in the common frog, *Rana temporaria*. *In* Comparative Endocrinology. Edited by A. Gorbman. John Wiley & Sons, Inc., New York, 1959, pp. 488–498.
88. White, F.N.: Functional anatomy of the heart in reptiles. Am. Zool., *8*:211–219, 1968.
89. White, F.N.: Redistribution of cardiac output in the diving alligator. Copeia, No. 3, 567–570, 1969.
90. Wilber, C.G.: Some circulatory problems in reptiles and amphibians. Ohio J. Sci., *62*:132–138, 1962.
91. Wood, C.A.: The Fundus Oculi of Birds. Lakeside Press, Chicago, 1917.
92. Zangerl, R.: The turtle shell. *In* Biology of the Reptilia. Edited By C. Gans, A.d'A. Bellairs, and T.S. Parsons. Academic Press, New York, 1969, Vol. I, pp. 311–339.
93. Zwart, P.: Studies on Renal Pathology in Reptiles. Path. Vet., *1*:542–566, 1964.

2 Principles of Husbandry and Veterinary Care of Herpetofauna

General Principles of Diagnosis

Reptiles and amphibians are stereotyped in symptomatology; relatively few specific diseases can be diagnosed without laboratory assistance. Postmortem examination of captive specimens may fail to reveal the cause of death or may reveal such extensive disease that one wonders how these animals survived as long as they did.

In general, disease in reptiles and amphibians is manifested by listlessness (e.g., arboreal species may spend little time climbing), anorexia, weight loss, and dehydration. The latter two signs are evidenced in snakes and lizards by longitudinal tenting of the skin. Dehydration in frogs and salamanders is indicated by dryness of the skin and in any reptilian or amphibian species by dryness of the mouth and other mucous membranes. Because the oral mucosa is normally pale in many species its color cannot be relied upon as a measure of anemia.

Illness may alter the frequency and duration of shedding, most noticeable in snakes. Changes in the appearance of the droppings and the frequency of excretion may be observed in sick specimens. Histories obtained from the owner should detail changes in activity, appetite, excretion, and periodicity of ecdysis.

A reptile's or amphibian's body temperature varies with the ambient temperature. Fever, mediated endogenously, as occurs in homeotherms, is unknown in herpetofauna. However, reptiles can behaviorally evoke a febrile response to bacterial pyrogens, as demonstrated in the desert iguana *(Dipsosaurus dorsalis)*.[56]

In Chapter 3, specific diseases of herpetofauna are discussed and, for ease of presentation, are presented etiologically. Unfortunately, the practitioner rarely sees cases in which the cause of the problem is

Table 2–1. A Guide to Differential Diagnosis in Herpetofauna by Organ System and Chief Complaint or Physical Sign

ORGAN SYSTEM*	PROBLEM*	DIFFERENTIAL DIAGNOSIS*
I. INTEGUMENT		
Turtle shell	Fractures	Trauma
	Softening	Malnutrition
	Deformity	Malnutrition Congenital anomaly
	Necrosis	Algae
	Ulceration	Ulcerative shell disease
Skin	Cutaneous and subcutaneous swellings or nodules	Abscesses Mycobacterial infections Dermatophilosis Geotrichosis Mycoses *Dermocystidium* and *Dermosporidium* infections (Amphibia) Sparganosis Filariasis Myiasis Blister disease (snakes) Tumors
	Petechiae and erythema	Septicemia (including salmonellosis) Miscellaneous bacteria Molchpest (salamanders) Chlorine poisoning (frogs)
	Ulceration	Redleg (frogs) SCUD (turtles and frogs) Mycobacterial dermatitis "Scale rot" (cutaneous necrolysis, snakes) Chlorine poisoning (frogs)
	Sloughing	Ecdysis (normal) Molchpest (salamanders) Lead poisoning (frogs)
	Mold and other superficial growth	*Saprolegnia* infection Cutaneous protozoa
II. ALIMENTARY TRACT		
Mouth	Petechiae	Septicemia
	Ulceration	Ulcerative stomatitis
	Caseous exudate	Ulcerative stomatitis
	Gaping	Pneumonia Oral trematodiasis
Stomach	Vomiting and hematemesis	Helminthiasis (especially ascariasis and *Kalicephalus* spp.) Amebiasis Poisoning Behavioral anorexia Tumor Septicemia

Table 2–1. A Guide to Differential Diagnosis in Herpetofauna by Organ System and Chief Complaint or Physical Sign (continued)

ORGAN SYSTEM*	PROBLEM*	DIFFERENTIAL DIAGNOSIS*
Intestine	Diarrhea, melena	Helminthiasis Coccidiosis Amebiasis Bacterial gastroenteritis (including salmonellosis) Poisoning
	Constipation Intestinal obstruction	Amebiasis Helminthiasis Mycobacterial granuloma
III. RESPIRATORY TRACT	Nasal discharge, dyspnea, wheezing, abnormal breath sounds	Pneumonia (bacterial, mycotic, verminous, pentastomid)
IV. SKELETAL	Fractures	Trauma Osteomyelitis
	Deformities	Congenital defects Malnutrition
	Lameness	See Differential Diagnosis of Fractures and Deformities Gout
	Gangrene of extremities	Clostridial infection
V. NERVOUS	Convulsions, twitching, coma	Septicemia Flaccid paralysis Poisoning Dehydration, electrolyte imbalances Hypoglycemia
	Incoordination	Streptomycin toxicity Strigeid metacercariae
VI. EYE	Swelling	Corneospectacular swelling (snakes)
	Closed lids	Avitaminosis A (turtles)
VII. HEMATOPOIETIC	Anemia, anisocytosis, poikilocytosis	Septicemia Hemogregarines Malaria (*Plasmodium* spp.) Miscellaneous bloodborne organisms Seasonal anemia
VIII. ENDOCRINE	Enlarged thyroid	Nutritional goiter
IX. SYSTEMIC	Inanition, weight loss	Ulcerative stomatitis Pneumonia Mycobacterioses Amebiasis *Plistophora myotrophica* myositis (*Xenopus laevis*) *Kalicephalus infection* Maladaptation syndrome Hypovitaminosis A Neoplasia

*Page numbers for additional discussion of these conditions may be found in the index.

immediately evident. Therefore, Table 2–1 is offered as a guide to differential clinical diagnosis, based on chief complaints and findings on physical examination. The diagnoses listed are limited to entities mentioned in the book because they are the most common and/or best documented.

The same diagnostic principles can be applied to all vertebrates. It should be obvious, for example, that foreign bodies should be considered as a cause of obstruction of the alimentary tract and neoplasia should be in the differential diagnosis of fractures, vomiting, constipation, dyspnea, convulsion, and anemia in herpetofauna, just as they are in the dog or cat. Neoplasia (to name but one omission) has not been consistently included in the list of differential diagnoses. Table 2–1 is, by no means, definitive or complete.

Temperature and Humidity

Most herpetologic specimens thrive best in an ambient temperature between 24°C (75°F) and 26.6°C (80°F), though some tropical specimens may do well at temperatures up to approximately 37°C (99°F). Tropical species do not necessarily have higher thermal preferences, but they may have less tolerance for low temperatures than species from temperate climates. Some reptilian species tolerate a relatively narrow ambient temperature range, others a much wider range.[6]

Even tropical specimens will not survive prolonged elevated temperatures. Herpetofauna exposed to direct sunlight will die of dehydration or heat stroke. They must have access to shade.

Reptiles and amphibians survive temperatures near 5°C (near 40°F) for extended periods, living in a state of hibernation. Frogs are often kept in this torpid condition for weeks or months in the laboratory and require little or no food during this time. Such a state of suspended animation is rarely desirable in a private collection, though it may be useful for keeping animals temporarily, as when food supply runs short or the owner must leave the animals untended for some time.

Reptiles do not have the built-in thermostatic regulatory mechanisms of homeotherms, but they are able to remain remarkably thermostable in the wild by behavioral adaptation, e.g., seeking out sun or shade, orienting their bodies to get optimal radiation from the sun, clinging to cool or warm surfaces, or burrowing in sand or mud.[4] By sunbathing, the false swift *(Liolaemus multiformia)* of the high Andes can maintain a body temperature as much as 56°F above air temperature.[49] Animals that depend on environmental factors to control their body temperature are best described as **ectothermic**, a term more appropriate than **"poikilothermic"** or **"cold-blooded,"** although, out of habit, the latter terms are used throughout this section.

Within a given geographic area different species are found to maintain quite different body temperatures, e.g., the temperature of snakes is generally lower than that of lizards in the same geographic area. If a temperature gradient is available to captive herpetofauna, certain species tend to stay in warmer parts of the cage while others seem to prefer cooler zones.[39] Thermoregulatory behavior and temperature ranges of various American reptiles are discussed in detail by Brattstrom.[6]

Water is a good conductor of heat and is more thermostable than air, so the aquatic environment offers less variation in microclimate than is found on land. Therefore, a poikilotherm's body temperature will closely approximate the temperature of the water in the stratum in which it is immersed, but on land its body temperature may vary markedly from the apparent air temperature.

Pythons incubate their eggs by coiling around them. Investigators in the Bronx Zoo have demonstrated that certain species, such as the Indian python *(Python molurus)*, can maintain a body temperature as much as 7.3°C (13.1°F) above air temperature. This is done by rapid muscular contractions, up to 38 per minute.[31]

For many reptilian species there seems to be an ideal temperature range for activity, a lower range for rest, and a still lower range for hibernation. At a given temperature a reptile may be active enough to crawl or swim and feed, but the reptile may require a higher temperature for its digestive processes to function properly. Snakes will seek out warm areas while digesting a meal and cooler areas while shedding.[6,51] Grass snakes *(Natrix natrix)* do not digest frogs when kept at 5°C postprandially. At 15°C digestive processes are greatly retarded, but frogs are completely digested within 60 hours when grass snakes are kept at 25° or 35°C.[55]

The **preferred body temperature** is that temperature a reptile will voluntarily establish when a range of temperature is available. The preferred body temperature of most snakes, turtles, and nocturnal lizards is 25° to 32°C (77° to 89°F); for crocodilians and many diurnal lizards it is 32° to 37°C (89° to 99°F). It seems likely that some variation in temperature is necessary, and specimens should not be kept constantly at the preferred body temperature. Crocodilians and diurnal lizards are usually kept at 25° to 32°C and generally do well, although it might be better to give them voluntary access to the higher temperature range indicated above. At temperatures about 37°C, crocodilians may go into tetany as a result of hyperventilation. When spiny lizards *(Sceloperus occidentalis)* were kept at their preferred temperature for 13 weeks there was some mortality and all the lizards suffered from hyperthyroidism.[61] Prolonged exposure to one or two degrees above the preferred body temperature decreases spermatogenesis in lizards.[42]

In the wild, reptiles are obviously subject to diurnal and nocturnal variations in temperature, and this has a great influence on activity patterns. How often this daily variation in temperature is required for optimal survival in captivity is a moot, but important, point. In captivity, diurnal lizards that are exposed to alternating photoperiods generally select cooler temperatures during darkness and warmer temperatures when it is light.[52]

Behavioral selection of temperature by captive reptiles may be modified by the presence of humans, e.g., "shy" animals may refuse to emerge from hiding. Dominant lizards may select and defend a territory with a higher temperature gradient, and thus remain warmer, if caged with a subordinate animal than if alone. Hormonal states, e.g., pregnancy, may alter temperature selection. The influence and significance of these and other factors are incompletely understood.[52]

Teleologically, it would seem best to imitate conditions found in nature since the animals' physiologic processes and behavior patterns have evolved accordingly. In general, zoos keep species from temperate climes in air temperatures of 22° to 30°C (71° to 86°F) and tropical specimens at 25° to 35°C (77° to 95°F). Those species that have done well at these temperatures are the ones usually kept on display. Those that do not do well are referred to as "delicate," which may be more an admission of our ignorance than an indication of any inherent weakness in the species.

If a cage contains various media, e.g., a water pan, rocks and sand, a focal heat source such as a light bulb or heating coil (screened to prevent direct contact), and scattered areas of shade, the reptile can select the environment that suits it best at a given time. Peaker presents a useful discussion of thermal requirements of captive reptiles and reviews the pertinent literature on this topic.[48]

As a general rule, amphibians prefer a lower temperature range than reptiles. Most amphibians are active and feed well at 20° to 25°C (68° to 77°F). Few tolerate temperatures above 28°C (82.5°F) for very long.

Relative humidity has a marked effect on body temperature of amphibians. At low humidity, evaporation from the skin lowers the amphibian's temperature below that of the surrounding air, whereas at high humidity the amphibian's heat production cannot be dissipated by evaporation, so its body temperature rises above the ambient air temperature. The relatively dry-skinned toads and salamanders also rely on pulmonary function for evaporative heat loss. Reptiles are more dependent on heat loss through breathing than amphibians are because the dry reptilian skin inhibits (but does not totally prohibit) cutaneous evaporation. Lizards pant at an increasing rate as their temperature is raised. The efficiency and usefulness of evaporative heat loss are limited by the threat of dehydration when the process is carried too far.

A relative humidity between 35% and 70% is suitable for most specimens. Desert animals generally tolerate lower levels, and jungle animals generally prefer more humid conditions. Many herpetologists think that high humidity is necessary for normal ecdysis in snakes (Chap. 1), but Kauffeld contends that excess moisture is harmful and that it contributes to skin diseases.[38] He recommends maintaining a low humidity, even for water snakes.

It may be difficult for the herpetologist to obtain insects or other food items for his collection in the winter. Should he keep his specimens in a state of hibernation? Weight loss and significant mortality occur during natural hibernation,[28] and similar losses may occur during hibernation in captivity. In general, tropical species that normally do not hibernate should be kept warm and active all year long. Not enough is known about the effect of the presence or absence of annual hibernation periods on longevity, health, growth, and breeding of specimens from temperate climates. Inducing hibernation in them is optional.

Hibernation temperatures should be kept above freezing, but low enough to keep the animal torpid so that its metabolism is maintained at a very low level. A constant temperature range of 2° to 5°C (35° to 41°F) should be satisfactory for most species, and 4.4° to 6.7°C (39.9° to 44.1°F) should be satisfactory for toads.[15] A hibernaculum for frogs, probably adaptable for other aquatic species, can be constructed out of a garbage can and laundry basket (Fig. 2–1). Herpetofauna should not be fed for several days prior to induction of hibernation so there will be no undigested food in their gut to decompose.

Problems associated with too much or too little heat and humidity

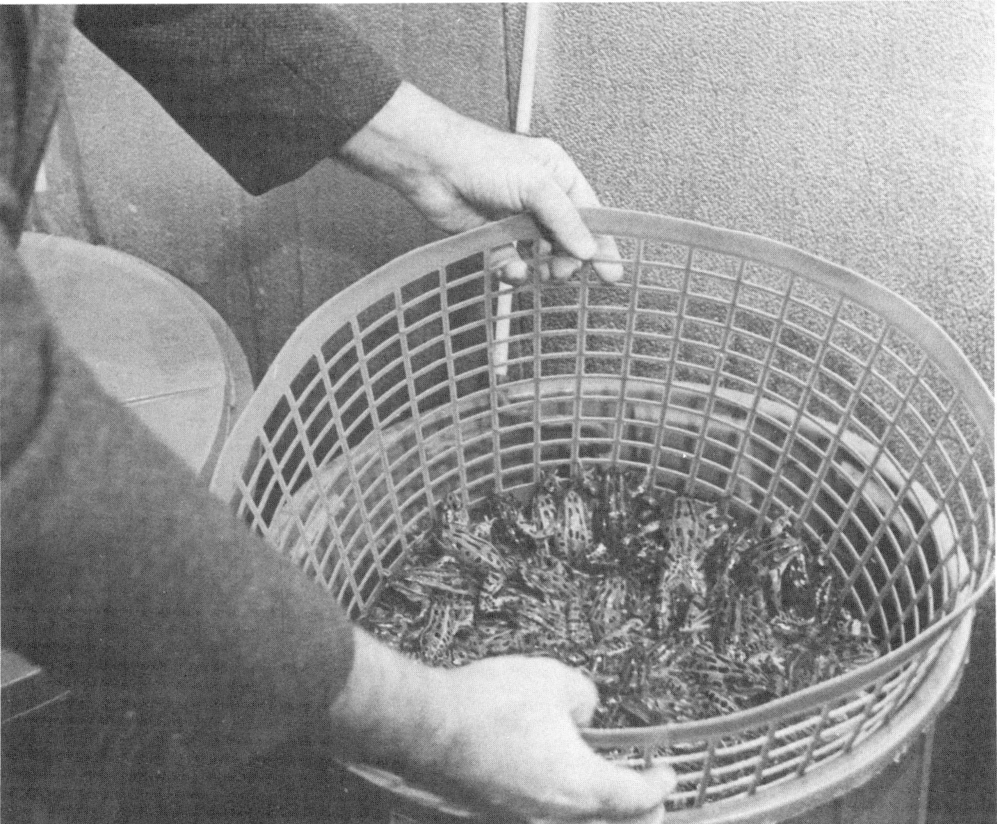

Fig. 2–1. A laboratory hibernaculum placed in a 4°C coldroom and fabricated from a 20-gallon plastic garbage can with an inserted plastic laundry basket. The deep water simulates conditions of the natural hibernaculum, and the volume minimizes temperature fluctuation. The aeration water-cycling system, which consists of a ¾″ acrylic plastic tube through which air is bubbled, does not agitate the frogs, and permits up to 200 animals per can to be kept from October until July with water changes only one or two times a month. (From Gibbs, E.L., Nace, G.W., and Emmons, M.B.: The live frog is almost dead. BioScience *21*:1027–1037, 1971. Reprinted with permission from BioScience, published by the American Institute of Biological Sciences.)

and too much or too little variation in these climatic factors contribute to much of the sickness and death in herpetologic collections. In our present state of ignorance, it is only possible to indicate the nature and complexity of the problem. Solutions will require additional research.

Lighting

Artificial lights that provide a wide spectrum of light are commercially available.* Reptiles are said to thrive better with such lighting than with ordinary incandescent light, and wide spectrum lighting may stimulate the appetite of a reluctant feeder.[58] Alternating periods of light and dark, simulating natural day/night cycles, should be provided for captive herpetofauna.

Caging

Cages should be large enough to permit normal movements, e.g., longer than the length of a snake. Such a large cage may be impractical for the owners of very large snakes. These animals are abnormally cramped in the quarters usually provided for them. Many diurnal reptiles are territorial and crowding may result in fighting, poor feeding, and failure to mate in captivity.

Cages should be of sound construction, without openings for escape or projections such as nails or splinters on which the animals can be injured. Screening should provide adequate ventilation to reduce dampness and odor. Doors, which can be tightly sealed, should provide safe access to the cage for cleaning, feeding, and moving of specimens.

Branches and rocks can be put in the cage for climbing and hiding. These can become fomites, however, e.g., hiding places for mites. If articles in the cage become contaminated, they must be removed and sterilized or discarded.

Hygiene

Adequate sanitation helps to prevent the spread of diseases. Shed skins should be removed promptly from cages, especially since they may harbor mites. Tools used to remove droppings should be dipped in a strong disinfectant, e.g., tamed iodine products, then rinsed with hot water between use in different cages. Cages and water dishes may be disinfected with Clorox®, boiling water, tamed iodine compounds, or benzalkonium chloride (Zephiran, Winthrop Lab). The latter two agents can also be used as topical antiseptics on reptiles. Benzalkonium chloride can support the growth of *Pseudomonas* spp., and, therefore, should be kept in small, tightly sealed containers.[46] Phenol, cresol, and other coal tar derivatives are highly toxic to herpetofauna and should be avoided.

*Vita-lite and the Optima Fluorescent Lamp are available from the Duro-Test Corporation, North Bergen, New Jersey.

It is especially important that water for aquatic species be kept clean, either by circulation and filtration or by frequent changes. It is best to allow tap water to stand for a day before using it for frogs or salamanders, so that the chlorine can evaporate.

Feeding and Nutrition

Certain important principles are involved in feeding herpetofauna. Frogs and toads generally eat moving prey. They should be fed live insects, but can sometimes be induced to eat pieces of meat or liver thrown in their cages and moved teasingly in front of them. Insectivorous lizards can be fed in similar fashion. Frogs and toads have prodigious appetites. Because it is very difficult for the amateur collector to keep them adequately fed, these animals commonly starve to death in captivity. Since it is not practically possible to catch enough insects to feed a collection of amphibians and lizards properly, and since wild insects may not be available at all in the winter, many herpetologists buy mealworms and crickets from commercial sources, such as pet stores, or raise these insects, flies, or cockroaches in order to feed their pets. The obvious drawback with the latter two items is the possibility of escape, which would provide the herpetologist with a never-ending supply of food for his collection within his house. Wingless fruit flies can be raised as food for tree frogs. Insects reared under controlled conditions offer an important advantage as a food source because they are not likely to carry parasites that affect amphibians and reptiles.

I have seen a very elaborate private collection in which the cages were placed at ground level in basement windows. Wide mesh screening on the outdoor sides permitted insects to enter; the indoor sides of the cages were made of glass. Items to attract insects were kept in the cages. Heat lamps protected the reptiles and amphibians from the cold. Thus, the collector was able to confine his specimens indoors while bringing them a natural food supply from outdoors.

All adult amphibians are carnivorous, with the majority being insectivorous. The larger Urodeles (salamander-like amphibians) may include such items as frogs and fish in their diet. The largest frogs can swallow a whole mouse or shrew. Small aquatic salamaders can be raised on the worms and crustaceans sold as live food for tropical fish. I have successfully raised spotted newts *(Notophthalmus [Diemictylus] viridescens)* by feeding them mosquito larvae in water.

Tadpoles, generally, are omnivorous, grazing on organic debris or straining microscopic plant and animal material through their gills. They can be fed small bits of lettuce, ground rabbit, or guinea pig pellets or kibbled dog food, brewer's yeast, and ground raw liver. Small *Xenopus laevis* tadpoles can be fed ground peas or split pea soup powder. As the tadpoles grow, ground rabbit or guinea pig pellets, ground beef mixed with powdered milk, and *Tubifex* worms or *Daphnia* can be added to their diet. Salamander larvae can be fed brine shrimp, *Tubifex*, and *Daphnia* and, when they are large enough, can be fed small earthworms and Purina Trout Chow.[19] The water containing amphibian larvae must be changed frequently to prevent fouling by leftover food.

All snakes are carnivorous, but diet varies with species. Natural food items, such as rats and mice for pilot black snakes *(Elaphe obsoleta)*, fish and frogs for banded water snakes *(Natrix sipedon)*, earthworms and frogs for garter snakes (*Thamnophis* sp.), and other snakes for king snakes (*Lampropeltis* sp.), should be provided whenever possible.

Contrary to common belief, snakes often accept dead food, even strips of meat. This is advantageous because dead food is more easily removed, can be used as a vehicle for drugs, and cannot attack the reptile, as live rats and mice may.

Poisonous snakes kill or paralyze their prey by envenomization prior to eating them, but they may swallow small prey without waiting for the poison to act. Water snakes, garter snakes, racers, and some other snakes simply grasp and swallow their prey. Other snakes, including boas, pythons, king snakes, and pilot black snakes, suffocate their prey in their coils by **constriction**. A very large python or anaconda can kill a man this way.

Snakes always swallow their prey intact and, if two snakes start swallowing an object from opposite ends, the larger snake will continue to eat until he has swallowed the smaller one. Snakes often vomit if disturbed too soon after eating.

Lizards vary greatly in dietary habits. The majority are insectivorous, but some, such as monitors (*Varanus* spp.), are carnivorous, whereas others, such as the chuckwalla *(Sauromalus obesus)* and some of the larger iguanas, are mainly herbivorous. Other lizards, such as the desert iguana *(Dipsosaurus dorsalis)*, are omnivorous.

Aquatic turtles are mainly carnivorous and may be fed insects, worms, slugs, snails, fish, liver, or strips of meat, occasionally supplemented with bits of lettuce or other plant material. A drop of cod liver oil or vitamin concentrate containing vitamins A, D, and E should be put in the food at least once a week. These turtles swallow food items with the head submerged in water, so it is quite useless to offer these animals food on dry land. Commercial turtle food consisting of dried insects is not an adequate diet, but some better balanced rations are now available.

Terrestrial tortoises should be fed on dry land only. The box turtle *(Terrapene carolina)* is omnivorous and can be maintained on lettuce, tomatoes, worms, snails, and cottage cheese. Sea turtles eat invertebrates, fish, and seaweed; the proportions vary with species. Crocodilians should be fed meat, fish, and poultry products in the water. Carnivorous animals should be offered intact prey, e.g., entire fish or mice, or viscera along with strips of meat in order to give a diet well-balanced in vitamins and minerals. Tricks may be necessary to get some reptiles to eat in captivity. Rarely, a lizard or snake will refuse whole mice, but will consume them if they are skinned. Sometimes forced feeding (discussed in the following section) is necessary to maintain nutrition.

Frequency of feeding required by different species varies greatly.

Insectivorous lizards, frogs, and toads, and baby crocodilians and baby turtles should be fed daily, but an occasional day of fasting is acceptable. Larger aquatic turtles should be fed about three times a week. Most snakes can be fed once or twice a week. In general, the larger the reptile, the less frequently it has to be fed, but this is largely dependent on the temperature at which it is kept. Higher temperatures increase metabolic rate and rate of digestion and thus increase the frequency of feeding needed to maintain health. Feeding may occur, but food can remain undigested for a long time at low temperatures.

The chapters by Frye on the care of amphibians and reptiles in the book *Pet Medicine* by R. Caras et al. (McGraw-Hill Co., New York, 1977) provide useful information for the pet owner. Veterinarians can recommend this reading to their clients.

Supportive Therapy

Because very little is known about the dosage and toxicity of drugs in reptiles, the most effective approach to treatment is supportive therapy, including forced feeding and parenteral fluids. Forced feeding may be necessary when a reptile goes on a "hunger strike" as they occasionally do without apparent cause. Giant tortoises and pythons can survive a fast of more than a year, and most snakes can go for several months without eating, even when kept at room temperature. (It is physiologic for them to fast during hibernation, of course.) Many amphibians can survive fasts up to several months. Solid food material such as mice and strips of meat can be gently, but firmly, shoved down a snake's throat after being lubricated, for example, with raw egg. It is even more advantageous to administer some nutritious fluid by stomach tube (page 24), e.g., fish broth for water snakes or meat broth mixed with raw egg, milk, or amino acid and glucose solutions and multiple vitamins for other snakes. The stomach tube can be made of soft polyethylene tubing attached to a large hypodermic syringe (Fig. 2–2). The fluid should not be given too quickly because this may induce regurgitation.

Forced feeding is more difficult in turtles, crocodilians, and lizards and may be a dangerous procedure with the larger specimens. Sometimes these animals can be induced to eat by teasing them with a piece of food dangled from a pole. Large or dangerous reptiles can be anesthetized prior to forced feeding, thus reducing the risk to the handler. Anesthesia also eliminates voluntary regurgitation.[62] The danger of reflex vomiting in an unconscious patient can be reduced by injecting an antiemetic.

Sometimes a fasting reptile will feed when it is brought out of an induced hibernation period of two to three weeks. After the period of "cold storage," bring the animal to room temperature, and offer it food when it becomes active.

Dehydration can result from offering water in inappropriate form. For example, chameleons and some other lizards get water in nature by lapping dew. In captivity they will not drink from a bowl, so water must

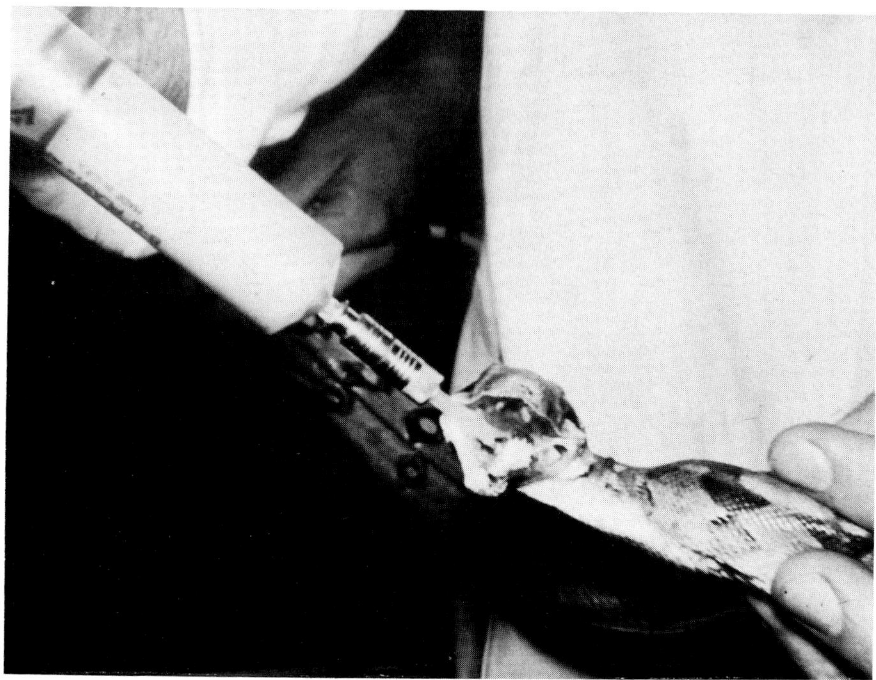

Fig. 2–2. Force-feeding a boa constrictor *(Constrictor constrictor)* liquid nutrients via syringe and polyethylene tubing.

be sprinkled on foliage in their cage. Desert reptiles get most of their moisture from their food. The desert tortoise, for example, can quench its thirst on a succulent cactus leaf. When it is offered water, however, it may drink copious amounts, as, presumably, it may do in the wild during brief rainy seasons.

Ringer's solution of appropriate concentration (page 31), such as that prepared in physiology laboratories, can be given subcutaneously or intraperitoneally to maintain hydration of specimens that refuse to eat or drink. Ambex (Elanco), 4.5 ml per kg, can be given subcutaneously once weekly to snakes;[2] this dosage should be altered according to need and clinical response.

Antibiotic Therapy

Reptiles and amphibians have been treated, often on an arbitrary basis, with most of the common antibiotics. Very little is known about drug toxicity, and most dosages have been established empirically. In general, the same dosage rates used in mammals have been used in reptiles. Recommended doses of various antibiotics in reptiles are listed in the text by Frye.[16] There seems to be a better response to antibiotic therapy if the ambient temperature is maintained at 85° to 90°F. Long-acting antibiotics, such as benzathine penicillin, are useful because the patient need be handled a minimum number of times for treatment.

The excess administration of streptomycin is said to cause vestibular nerve damage in snakes, resulting in incoordination. Affected snakes writhe unnaturally, fall over when trying to climb, and strike erratically at their prey.[54]

Gentamicin, given in doses suitable for mammals, causes damage to proximal renal tubules and causes gout in snakes.[44] A recommended dosage for snakes is 2.5 mg per kg of body weight given subcutaneously every three days and 10 mg per kg, intramuscularly, every two days for turtles.[10,11] A recommended dosage for chloramphenicol in snakes is 40 mg per kg subcutaneously every 24 hours.[10,11]

Physical Examination and Restraint

The specimen should first be examined without restraint. When aroused, the animal should be alert, responsive, and capable of purposeful movement. Unless it is just before shedding, a lizard's or snake's skin should have luster or shine. Reptilian skin is normally dry, whereas the skin of most amphibians, except toads and some salamanders, is moist. The eyes should be bright and clear, except the spectacles of snakes which appear dull and somewhat opaque before shedding (Chap. 1). The general state of nutrition and hydration should be evaluated. Any specimen with dull, sunken eyes, prominent skeleton, loosely folded skin, and apathetic, sluggish behavior is unquestionably ill, probably with far advanced disease.

The safest way to handle a dangerous reptile is to anesthetize it with an inhalant anesthetic in a box having at least one glass side for direct observation (see following section). Anesthesia, best induced parenterally, may be necessary to relax the muscles of turtles enough to permit examination.

Snakes, lizards, and small crocodilians can be captured and restrained with appropriate pinning sticks, nooses, or tongs, available from some herpetologic supply houses. Transparent plastic tubes of various diameters and lengths with removable plugs at either end can be used to restrain snakes and lizards (Fig. 2–3). Holes can be bored in the plastic to permit insertion of hypodermic needles.

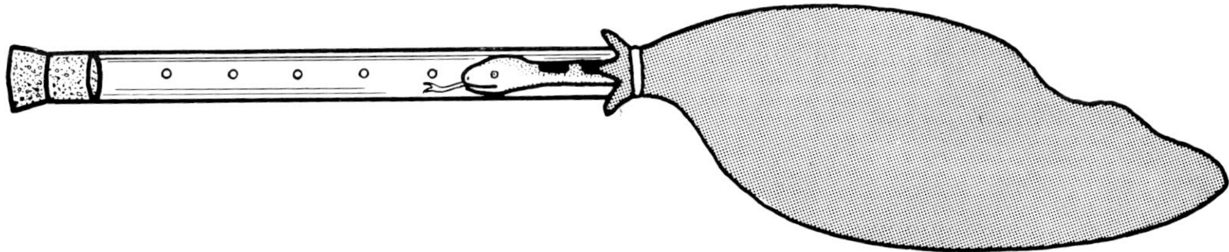

Fig. 2–3. Device for restraint and examination of poisonous snakes. The snake emerges from a bag through an opening whose edges are secured by a tight elastic band around a translucent plastic tube of suitable diameter. The distal end of the plastic tube is closed with a tight-fitting cork or screw cap. Holes can be drilled in the side of the tube to permit access for injections.

Snapping turtles can be lifted by the tail with their belly towards the holder. A turtle's head can reach laterally and dorsally, but is capable of very limited ventral motion.

During the physical examination, a snake should be held firmly, but not too tightly, immediately behind the head, and its body should be supported. If the snake is large, its body can rest on the floor while the person holding the head keeps the tail pinned down with his foot. If held dangling by the neck too long a snake can suffer spinal cord damage or circulatory embarrassment because of an inability to return systemic venous blood to the heart while in a vertical position.

The skin and eyes of snakes should be examined for incomplete shedding. Incompletely shed skin or spectacles can be gently removed with forceps after soaking the animal in lukewarm water. Great care should be taken because the underlying tissue is readily injured and wounds incurred by overzealous peeling readily become infected.

A turtle's shell should be examined for abnormal curvature. Such a deformity may be congenital, but is more commonly caused by improper diet (see p. 178). The shell should also be checked for traumatic lesions. Flaking and necrosis of the shell may result from bacterial infection (see p. 95, Chap. 3), or an overgrowth of algae (see p. 111, Chap. 3).[29]

Besides the obvious danger of being bitten by snakes, large lizards, turtles, or crocodilian species, the veterinarian should be aware that large lizards and crocodilians can deliver hard blows with their tails and that large turtles and lizards can inflict nasty scratches with their claws.

The muscles that close the jaws of these animals are very powerful, but the muscles that open the mouth are relatively weak. One person can keep the jaws of large specimens closed if he has enough help to control the body, legs, and tail of an uncooperative patient.

Anesthesia and Surgery

For minor surgical procedures reptiles and amphibians may be refrigerated at 5°C for approximately two hours[59] or immersed in ice water until they are torpid. Minor surgery can also be done using physical restraint of the specimen and local infiltration with Xylocaine hydrochloride.

The safest, most rapid, and most reliable means of inducing general anesthesia in reptiles is with inhalant anesthetics. These agents also permit relatively rapid recovery after they are withdrawn. Calderwood offers the best available discussion of inhalation anesthesia technique in reptiles.[12] Unfortunately, in his review of parenteral anesthetic agents Calderwood uses the wrong conversion factors (dividing instead of multiplying by 2.2) to change doses from mg/lb to mg/kg. Doses in Table 2–2 of this book are correct.

The best inhalant anesthetics available are halothane (Fluothane, Ayerst Laboratories, Inc.)[25,32] and methoxyflurane (Metofane, Pitman-Moore, Inc.). They have been used alone and in combination with nitrous oxide. During induction with halothane there is an initial excitement phase, which may include violent thrashing activity.

Kraner, Silverstein, and Parshall induced anesthesia in four- to six-foot-long bull snakes *(Pituophis catenifer)* and chicken (Texas rat) snakes *(Elaphe quadrivitata)* by putting them in clear plastic bags from which the air was expressed and then replaced with a mixture of 4% halothane, 72% nitrous oxide, and 24% oxygen.[41] In 20 to 30 minutes the snakes were sufficiently relaxed to be intubated. They were maintained in a state of surgical anesthesia on a mixture of 3% halothane, 49% nitrous oxide, and 48% oxygen. They could be revived quickly by letting them breathe pure oxygen.

Ether has been used on reptiles,[7] but has the disadvantage of being explosive. Ether significantly decreases the coagulation time of turtles, *Chrysemys (Pseudemys) scripta elegans*, during surgical anesthesia and depresses their red cell count and hemoglobin concentration for at least 24 hours after the anesthetic period.[33] Ether can be administered to turtles with a snug-fitting nasal cone. The induction time for *Chrysemys (Pseudemys)* spp. is about one-half hour, and turtles may remain anesthetized for over 10 hours.[34]

The most convenient method of inducing inhalant anesthesia is by spraying the drug or placing gauze soaked with the agent into an enclosed box containing the patient. If a gas heavier than air, e.g., halothane, is used, the box should be shallow so the animal cannot lift its head above the vapor. At least one side of the box should be transparent. The amount of anesthetic agent to use depends on the volume in the box rather than on the size of the patient. Certain species may be more susceptible to specific agents than others, for example, vipers require more halothane and methoxyflurane than elapids (cobras). Anesthetic deaths in cobras have been reported with methoxyflurane.[9]

Using 1 ml of methoxyflurane per approximately 8,400 ml to 190,000 ml (512 to 1160 cubic inches) of cage space (Table 2–3), Gandal has reported induction in 8 to 20 minutes and a state of light to moderate anesthesia lasting 10 to 30 minutes in several species of snakes.[21] The anesthetic is sprayed into the cage and the animal removed when it is immobilized. Then it is easy to intubate the trachea (Figs. 2–4 and 2–5) with polyethylene tubing (anatomy and technique are discussed on page 24 in Chapter 1) and to maintain anesthesia with a closed-circuit inhalation machine. Recovery from anesthesia can be hastened by the use of oxygen.

Turtles have a variable response to inhalation anesthesia because they can hold their breath for a considerable length of time.

Electroanesthesia was used to perform major surgery on green iguanas *(Iguana iguana)*.[45] This anesthetic technique may be applicable to other herpetofauna.

A variety of parenteral drugs has been used to immobilize and/or anesthetize reptiles and amphibians. The use of these agents is summarized in Table 2–2.

Table 2–2. Parenteral Drugs Used to Immobilize and/or Anesthetize Amphibians and Reptiles

SPECIES	DRUG	DOSAGE	ROUTE	EFFECT, COMMENTS	REFERENCE
FROGS					
Leopard frog *(Rana pipiens)*	Pentobarbital Na	60 mg/kg	Dorsal lymph sac	Deep surgical anesthesia obtained in ½ hour, maintained for 9 hours, but poor muscle relaxation.	35
			Intraperitoneal (IP)	Deep surgical anesthesia obtained in 18 minutes, maintained for 9½ hours.	
	Hexobarbital Na	120 mg/kg	Dorsal lymph sac	Deep surgical anesthesia, but muscle relaxation poor. Induction and recovery faster than with pentobarbital.	
Frogs	Paraldehyde	4.2 g/kg	Ventral lymph sac	Narcosis induced in 15 minutes.	34
	Chloral hydrate	10% solution	Dorsal lymph sac		
TURTLES					
Red-eared turtle *(Chrysemys scripta elegans)*	Pentobarbital Na	16 mg/kg	Intracardiac (IC)	The needle is inserted between the neck and forelimb and directed towards the heart. Deep surgical anesthesia. Induction time 30 minutes.	63
			Intraperitoneal (IP)	Induction time 65 minutes, duration >3 hours. Red and white cell counts are lowered more than 20% 24 hours after injection.	33
	Chlorpromazine HCl (Thorazine, Smith, Kline and French, Inc.) and	10 mg/kg and	Intramuscular (IM)	Preanesthetic	
	Pentobarbital Na (given 10 minutes later)	10 mg/kg	IC	Induction time 15 minutes, duration of anesthesia approximately 3 hours.	

Greek tortoise (*Testudo g. graeca*)	Tribromoethanol and Amylene hydrate (Avertin, E.R. Squibb and Sons)	250 mg/kg 125 mg/kg	IP	Induction period 40 to 70 minutes. Deep anesthesia lasts 1 to 2 hours, post-anesthetic depression 12 to 16 hours.	30
	Tribromoethanol and Amylene hydrate	400 mg/kg 200 mg/kg	per rectum	Induction 1 to 2 hrs., deep anesthesia 1 to 1½ hours, postanesthetic depression 6 to 9 hours.	
Turtles (average 1.82 kg)	M-99 (Etorphine M-99, American Cyanamid)	0.5–5 mg (total dose)	IM	Induction in 2 to 20 minutes, immobilization for 30 to 180 minutes.	57
Galapagos tortoises (45–63 kg)		10–15 mg (total dose)	IM	Dosage per unit weight not given in references.	27
				Neither M-99, oxymorphone, nor meperidine HCl was found very effective in various reptile species by Hinsch and Gandal.	
Turtles	Tiletamine HCl and Arylcycloalkylamine (CI-744, Parke-Davis and Co.)	44 mg/kg (20 mg/lb)	IM		10,24
Turtles (*Pseudemys* spp.)	Urethan	2.8 g/kg	Per os (PO)	Average induction time 4.5 hours. Deep anesthesia >10 hours.	34
		2.4 g/kg	Intravenous (IV)	2.25 hours, induction time. Deep anesthesia >10 hours.	
		1.7 g/kg	IC	12 minutes induction time. Deep anesthesia approximately 10 hours.	
		2.8 g/kg	IP	Average induction time 2½ hours. Deep anesthesia >10 hours.	

Table 2–2. Parenteral Drugs Used to Immobilize and/or Anesthetize Amphibians and Reptiles (continued)

SPECIES	DRUG	DOSAGE	ROUTE	EFFECT, COMMENTS	REFERENCE
CROCODILIANS					
American alligator (*Alligator mississippiensis*)	Pentobarbital Na	7.7–8.8 mg/kg (3.5–4.0 mg/lb)	IM (base of tail)	Complete relaxation in 10 minutes. Recovery in 2 to 3 hours.	8
	Nicotine SO_4 (Cap-Chur-Sol, Palmer Chemical and Equipment Co.)	0.51–3.0 mg/kg (0.23–1.38 mg/lb)	IM (base of tail)	Severe spasms, no relaxation. Unsuitable agent.	
American alligator	Phencyclidine HCl (Sernylan, Parke-Davis and Co.)	11–22 mg/kg (5–10 mg/lb)	IM (base of tail)	Relaxed state in 50 to 60 minutes. Recovery in 6 to 7 hours.	8
	Succinylcholine Cl (Anectine, Burroughs Wellcome Co.)	2.99–4.95 mg/kg (1.35–2.25 mg/lb)	IM (base of tail)	Complete relaxation in 4 minutes. Recovery in 7 to 9 hours.	For range of effective doses of succinylcholine in crocodilian species, see Klide and Klein.[40]
American alligator (500–700 g)	Chloral hydrate	1 mg/g	IP	Surgical anesthesia achieved.	1
American alligator (40–68 kg)	M-99 (Etorphine M-99, American Cyanamid)	20 mg dose	IM	Sedated in 20 minutes.	60
Crocodilians (0.23–59 kg)		0.05–20 mg (total dose)	IM	Dosage per unit weight not given in reference. Induction in 2 to 20 minutes, immobilization for 30 to 180 minutes.	57

American alligator	Tricaine methane-sulfonate (MS-222, Sandoz Pharmaceutical Co.)	88–99 mg/kg (40–45 mg/lb)	IM (base of tail)	Complete muscular relaxation in 10 minutes. Recovery in 9 to 10 hours.	8
SNAKES					
Snakes (5 sp.)	Pentobarbital Na	15–30 mg/kg	Intrapleuro-peritoneal (IPP)	Loss of righting reflex in 2 to 29 minutes. Recovery period (regaining righting reflex) from 6 to 54 hours.	37
Water snake *(Natrix rhombifera)*	Pentobarbital Na	30 mg/kg	IPP	Anesthetic concentration 2 to 5 mg/ml. Surgical anesthesia induced in 40 to 60 minutes. Recovery in 30 to 36 hours.	3
	Na-thiamylbarbiturate (Surital, Parke-Davis and Co.)	30 mg/kg	IPP	Anesthetic concentration 2 to 5 mg/ml. Surgical anesthesia in 40 to 60 minutes. Recovery in 18 to 24 hours.	
Water snake *(Natrix taxispilota)* and garter snake *(Thamnophis sirtalis)*	Thiopental Na (Pentothal Na, Abbott Laboratories)	15–25 mg/kg	IPP	Loss of righting reflex in 25 to 45 minutes. Recovery of righting reflex from 1½ to 6 hours.	37
Snakes (3.6–4.5 kg)	Ketamine HCl (Ketalar, Parke-Davis and Co.)	88–110 mg/kg	IM	Effects ranged from tranquilization to deep anesthesia, depending on dosage. Doses greater than 110 mg/kg caused respiratory failure, reversible with intubation and O_2 therapy.	13,23
Snakes (≤0.9 kg)		22–44 mg/kg	IM		
Snakes	Tiletamine HCl and Arylcycloalkylamine (CI-744, Parke-Davis and Co.)	22 mg/kg (10 mg/lb)	IM		10,24

Table 2–2. Parenteral Drugs Used to Immobilize and/or Anesthetize Amphibians and Reptiles (continued)

SPECIES	DRUG	DOSAGE	ROUTE	EFFECT, COMMENTS	REFERENCE
Snakes (4 sp.)	Tricaine methane-sulfonate (MS-222, Sandoz Pharmaceutical Co.)	200–300 mg/kg (0.2–0.3 mg/g)	IPP	Loss of righting reflex in 4 to 50 minutes. Recovery in 2 to 19 minutes.	37
Snakes (various sp.)	M-99 (Etorphine M-99, American Cyanamid)	2.0–15 mg (total dose)	IPP		27

*Table 2–3.** Anesthetizing Snakes in Closed Containers with Methoxyflurane

CONTAINER SIZE	METHOXYFLURANE
22 × 22 × 51 cm (8 × 8 × 12 in)	1.5 ml
23 × 30 × 51 cm (9 × 12 × 20 in)	3.0 ml
30 × 56 × 56 cm (12 × 22 × 22 in)	5.0 ml

*Adapted from Gandel, C.P.: A practical anesthetic technique in snakes, utilizing methoxyflurane. Anim. Hosp., *4*:258–260, 1968.

Intrapleuroperitoneal (IPP) injections in snakes can be given in the ventral midline at approximately the junction of the middle and distal thirds of the body.

Amphibians can be anesthetized by immersion in tricaine methane sulfonate (MS–222), using 0.1% solution for adult leopard frogs *(Rana pipiens)*, 1:2000 to 1:3000 for tadpoles and adults of *Rana temporaria*, and 1:2000 to 1:7500 for the larvae and adults of various salamanders.[34] Adult frogs and newts *(Notophthalmus viridescens)* can be anesthetized by immersion in 0.2% Chloretone. Much more dilute solutions should be used for amphibian larvae.[34] The leopard frog *(Rana pipiens)* can be anesthetized by immersing the frog in 10% ethyl alcohol.[36] A surgical plane of anesthesia is reached in 9½ minutes; this lasts for 19 minutes if the frog is immediately transferred to fresh water. Immersion in 20% ethanol for a few minutes or in 10% ethanol for 20 minutes caused some deaths. In my own experience, putting frogs into ethanol results in too

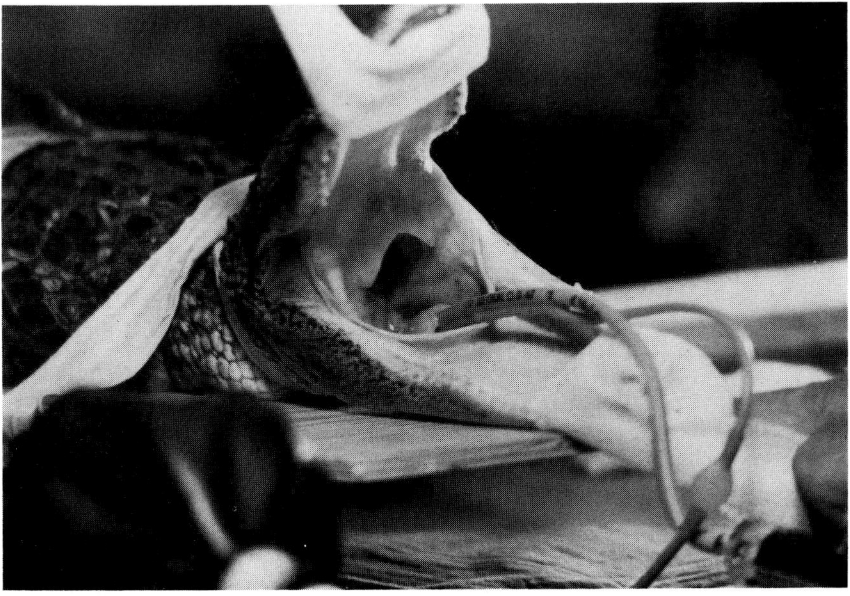

Fig. 2–4. Mouth and larynx of an American alligator demonstrating positioning of an endotracheal tube. Notice the large, well-developed epiglottis, which is capable of completely closing off the pharynx from the mouth cavity. (From Calderwood, H.W.: Anesthesia for reptiles. J. Am. Vet. Med. Assoc., *159*:1618–1625, 1971.)

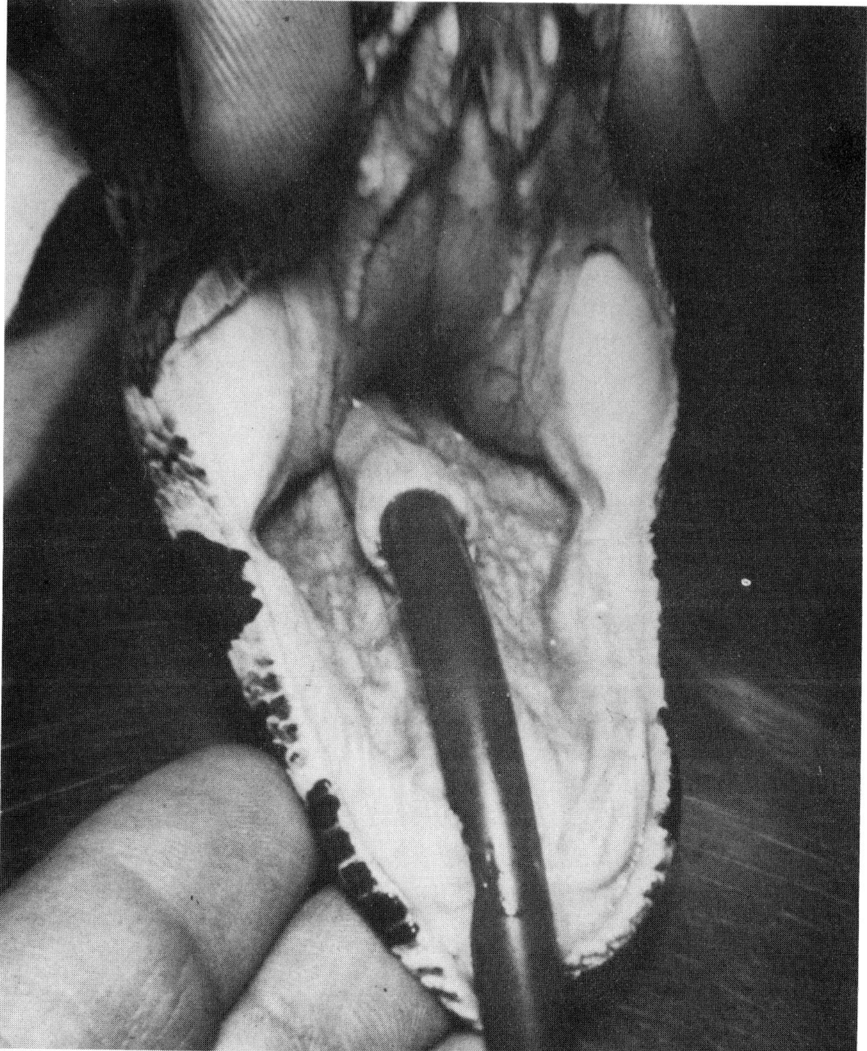

Fig. 2–5. Mouth and larynx of a boa constrictor demonstrating positioning of an endotracheal tube. (From Calderwood, H.W.: Anesthesia for reptiles. J. Am. Vet. Med. Assoc., *159*:1618–1625, 1971.)

much struggling and too little relaxation for clinical application. A 45–gram leopard frog was immobilized for six hours by dropping 0.25 mg of M-99 on its towel-dried abdomen.[60]

First, the righting reflex and then reflex withdrawal from noxious stimuli are lost as a reptile is anesthetized; loss of the latter reflex indicates a surgical plane of anesthesia.

Recovery from anesthesia with parenteral agents such as barbiturates may be hastened by raising the ambient temperature, presumably because it increases the rate of metabolism of these drugs. Conversely, mortality after ether anesthesia is increased by raising the temperature, presumably because heat increases the oxygen demand of the tissues, but is ineffective in increasing ventilation, the principal means of eliminating ether. In addition, heat increases the lipid solubility of ether, which increases its tendency to be bound to brain tissue.

The recovery cage must not contain water in which the animal could drown while coming out of anesthesia. Amphibians, which must be kept moist, can be kept on damp gauze until they are awake and mobile.

A snake, lizard, or small crocodilian can be draped for surgery by pulling a sterile, rolled up stockinette, as used in orthopedic surgery, over the animal's head and unrolling it over the surgical site. Incisions should be made between, rather than across, reptilian scales, whenever possible. Care should be taken to appose (evert) skin edges carefully because inverted scales interfere with healing. Stainless monofilament wire should be used in suturing crocodilian skin,[16] and plastic buttons can be tied into each suture to prevent cutting of the skin by the wire.[26]

Fractures of the Shell and of Bone

Fractures resulting from trauma are common in turtles. To repair the fracture, Wallach recommends debriding and abrading the broken edge with an electric burr, then filling the gap with denture repair material[57] (Tru-Repair, Harry J. Bosworth Co.). A mesh bridge of nylon or stainless steel can be used if the gap is big. A polyester resin (33–031 Polylite (ED524), Reichold Chemicals, Inc.) was used to repair a box turtle's fractured carapace.[64] Hoof Repair Material (H.D. Justi Division, William Gold Refining Co., Inc., Philadelphia) was used to fill a defect in the shell of a Galapagos tortoise.[43] Devco 5 Minute Epoxy (Devon

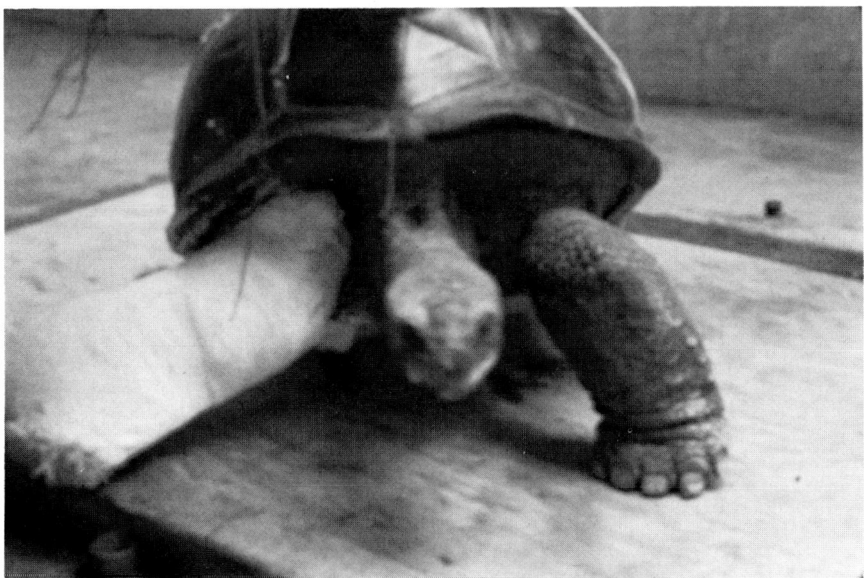

Fig. 2–6. Fractured humerus in a Galapagos tortoise (*Geochelone* [*Testudo*] *elephantopus*) repaired with a plaster of paris cast. Ambulation was made possible by strapping the animal to an auto mechanic's dolly on coasters. (Idea by Thomas Bucci, V.M.D.)

Corp.) is also suitable for repairing turtle shell fractures.[17] After healing has occurred, the repair material should be removed with a rotary burr to permit normal shell growth. The operator should protect himself by wearing goggles and a mask or respirator.[18] Surgical incisions of turtle shell can be done with a rotary electric saw cooled with Ringer's solution.[18]

Fractures of bone often occur in herpetofauna as a result of trauma or secondary to metabolic bone disease (p. 178). Fixation may require some ingenuity (Fig. 2–6). A miniature Thomas splint was used to immobilize fractures of mid to distal thirds of the humerus in iguanas.[50]

Amputations

Limbs should be amputated as high as possible, e.g., at the scapulohumeral joint for the front leg and at the upper one-third of the femur or the coxofemoral joint for the hind leg.[18] Muscles should be transected through their distal tendons. Two curved skin flaps should be apposed over the stump, using nonabsorbable sutures, starting at the center of the flaps and proceeding on alternate sides towards each end, creating a pucker-free closure.[18] The wound should be kept dry for at least two weeks. The animal should have access to drinking water, but immersion should be prevented. Sutures can be removed in three or four weeks.

Surgery on the poison glands of snakes is discussed in Chapter 1 (see p. 28) and gynecological surgery in reptiles in Chapter 3 (see p. 196).

Blood Collection

In most herpetofauna blood collection can be accomplished by cardiac puncture (Fig. 2–7). The position of the heart can be found in crocodilians, snakes, lizards, frogs, and salamanders by holding the animal on its back and observing or palpating the apical pulse. The heart is at the level of the 25th to 30th ventral scute in water snakes *(Natrix sipedon)*, but at scute number 70 to 80 in rattlesnakes.[5] The turtle's heart can be punctured through a hole 1/16 inch in diameter drilled in the plastron ventral to the heart.[18] The site for drilling is through the suture of the

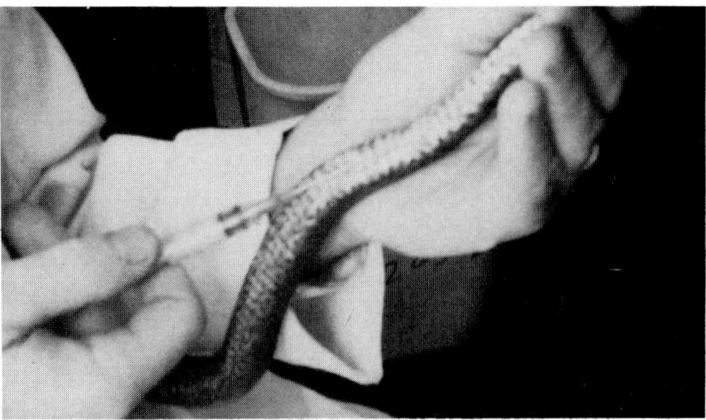

Fig. 2–7. Blood collection from a snake by cardiac puncture. The head of the snake is to the upper right.

plastron on the midline at the junction of the pectoral and abdominal shields. The needle is directed caudodorsally at a 20° angle to the vertical.[20] The hole is sealed with an epoxy resin.

If the reptile is large enough, blood can also be collected from the tail vein by inserting a needle in the ventral midline of the tail with the point directed slightly craniad. Light aspiration of the syringe is done as the needle approaches the vertebrae. Gross anatomy and angiography of the tail veins in lizards are illustrated in the article by Esra, et al.[14a] Blood can also be obtained in turtles from veins in the dorsal and dorsolateral aspects of the tail and from the femoral venous plexus.[53] Crocodilians can be bled from the jugular vein. Snakes can be bled from the palatine veins, which are visible between the maxillary rows of teeth.[47] Small reptiles and amphibia can be bled by inserting and rotating a capillary tube in the medial canthus of the eye, where there is a venous plexus.

Standard anticoagulants can be used to prevent clotting in most herpetofauna, but heparin should be used for turtles because agents that bind calcium (oxalate, citrate, or EDTA) can cause hemolysis.[14]

REFERENCES

1. Akers, T.K.: Some circulatory characteristics of *Alligator mississippiensis*. Copeia, No. 3, 522–555, 1966.
2. Bernstein, J.J.: A clinical view of some reptilian medical problems. J. Zoo Anim. Med., *3*:3–7, 1972.
3. Betz, T.W.: Surgical anesthesia in reptiles with special reference to the water snake, *Natrix rhombifera*. Copeia, No. 2, 284–287, 1962.
4. Bogert, C.M.: How reptiles regulate their body temperature. Sci. Am., *200*:105–120, 1959.
5. Bragdon, D.E.: A contribution to the surgical anatomy of the water snake, *Natrix sipedon sipedon*. The location of the visceral endocrine organs with reference to ventral scutellation. Anat. Rec., *117*:145–161, 1953.
6. Brattstrom, B.H.: Body temperature of reptiles. Am. Midland Naturalist, *73*:376–422, 1965.
7. Brazenor, C.W., and Kaye, G.: Anaesthesia for reptiles. Copeia, No. 3, 165–170, 1953.
8. Brisbin, I. L., Jr.: Reactions of the American alligator to several immobilizing drugs. Copeia, No. 1, 129–130, 1966.
9. Burke, T.J., and Wall, B.E.: Anesthetic deaths in cobras *(Naja naja* and *Ophiophagus hannah)* with methoxyflurane. J. Am. Vet. Med. Assoc., *157*:620–621, 1970.
10. Bush, M.: Reptilian medicine. Am. Assoc. Zoo Veterinanians, Annu. Proc., 68–78, 1974.
11. Bush, M., et al.: Recommendations for antibiotic therapy in reptiles. *In* Reproductive Biology and Diseases of Captive Reptiles. Edited by J.B. Murphy and J.T. Collins. Society for the Study of Amphibians and Reptiles, 1980, pp. 223–226.
12. Calderwood, H.W.: Anesthesia for reptiles. J. Am. Vet. Med. Assoc., *159*:1618–1625, 1971.
13. Cooper, J.E.: Ketamine hydrochloride as an anesthetic for East African reptiles. Vet. Rec., *95*:37–41, 1974.
14. Dessauer, H.C.: Blood chemistry of reptiles: physiological and evolutionary aspects. *In* Biology of the Reptilia. Edited by C. Gans and T.S. Parsons. Academic Press, New York, 1970, Vol. III, pp. 1–72.

14a. Esra, G.N., Benirschke, K., and Griner, L.A.: Blood collecting technique in lizards. J. Am. Vet. Med. Assoc., *167*:555–556, 1975.

15. Frazer, J.F.: Anura (Frogs and Toads). *In* Handbook on the Care and Management of Laboratory Animals. 4th Edition. Edited by UFAW. Williams & Wilkins, Baltimore, 1972, pp. 511–519.
16. Frye, F.L.: Husbandry, Medicine and Surgery in Captive Reptiles. Veterinary Medicine Publishing, Inc., Bonner Springs, Kansas, 1973.

17. Frye, F.L.: Clinical evaluation of a rapid polymerizing epoxy resin for repair of shell defects in tortoises. Vet. Med. Small Anim. Clin., *68*:51–53, 1973.
18. Frye, F.L.: Surgery in captive reptiles. *In* Current Veterinary Therapy V. Edited by R.W. Kirk. W.B. Saunders Co., Philadelphia, 1974, pp. 640–641.
19. Frye, F.L.: General considerations in the care of captive amphibians. *In* Current Veterinary Therapy VI. Edited by R.W. Kirk. W.B. Saunders Co., Philadelphia, 1977, pp. 772–778.
20. Gandal, C.P.: A practical method of obtaining blood from anesthetized turtles by means of a cardiac puncture. Zoologica N.Y., *43*:93–94, 1958.
21. Gandal, C.P.: A practical anesthetic technique in snakes, utilizing methoxyflurane. Anim. Hosp., *4*:258–260, 1968.
22. Gibbs, E.L., Nace, G.W., and Emmons, M.B.: The live frog is almost dead. Bioscience, 1027–1037, 1971.
23. Glenn, J.L., Straight, R., and Snyder, C.C.: Ketamine as an anesthetic for snakes. Am. J. Vet. Res., *33*:1901–1903, 1972.
24. Gray, C.W., Bush, M., and Beck, C.C.: Clinical experience using CI–744 in chemical restraint and anesthesia of exotic specimens. J. Zoo Anim. Med., *5*:12–21, 1974.
25. Hackenbrock, C.R., and Finster, M.: Fluothane: A rapid and safe inhalation anesthetic for poisonous snakes. Copeia, No. 2, 440–441, 1963.
26. Hartman, R.A.: Gastrotomy for removal of foreign bodies in a crocodile. Vet. Med. Small Anim. Clin. *71*:1096–1097, 1976.
27. Hinsch, H., and Gandal, C.P.: The effects of etorphine (M–99), oxymorphone hydrochloride and meperidine hydrochloride in reptiles. Copeia, No. 2, 404–405, 1969.
28. Hirth, H.F.: Weight changes and mortality of three species of snakes during hibernation. Herpetologica, *22*:8–12, 1966.
29. Hunt, T.J.: Influence of environment on necrosis of turtle shells. Herpetologica, *14*:45–46, 1958.
30. Hunt, T.J.: Anaesthesia of the tortoise. *In* Small Animal Anesthesia. Edited by O. Graham-Jones. Pergamon Press, Macmillan Co., New York, 1964, pp. 71–76.
31. Hutchison, V.H., Dowling, H.G., and Vinegar, A.: Thermoregulation in a brooding female Indian python, *Python molurus bivitatus*. Science, *151*:694–696, 1966.
32. Jackson, O.F.: Snake anaesthesia. Br. J. Herp., *4*:172–175, 1970.
33. Kaplan, H.M.: Effects of ether and of sodium pentobarbital upon turtle blood. Lab. Anim. Care, *13*:181–185, 1963.
34. Kaplan, H.M.: Anesthesia in amphibians and reptiles. Fed. Proc., *28*:1541–1546, 1969.
35. Kaplan, H.M., Brewer, N.R., and Kaplan, M.R.: Comparative value of some barbiturates for anesthesia in the frog. Proc. Anim. Care Panel, *12*:141–148, 1962.
36. Kaplan, H.M., and Kaplan, M.: Anesthesia of frogs with ethyl alcohol. Proc. Anim. Care Panel, *11*:31–35, 1961.
37. Karlstrom, E.L., and Cook, S.F.: Notes on snake anesthesia. Copeia, No. 1, 57–58, 1955.
38. Kauffeld, C.: The effect of altitude, ultra-violet light and humidity on captive reptiles. Int. Zoo Yearbook, *9*:8–9, 1969.
39. Kitchell, J.F.: Thermophilic and thermophobic responses of snakes in 2 thermal gradients. Copeia, No. 1, 189–191, 1969.
40. Klide, A.M., and Klein, L.V.: Chemical restraint of three reptilian species. J. Zoo Anim. Med., *4*:8–11, 1973.
41. Kraner, K.L., Silverstein, A.M., and Parshall, C.J., Jr.: Surgical anesthesia in snakes. *In* Experimental Animal Anesthesiology. Edited by D.C. Sawyer. USAF School of Aerospace Medicine, Brooks AFB, Texas, 1965, pp. 374–378.
42. Licht, P.: The relation between preferred body temperatures and testicular heat sensitivity in lizards. Copeia, No. 4, 428–436, 1965.
43. LyVere, D.B.: Repair of the shell of a Galapagos tortoise. Mod. Vet. Pract., *47*:76, 1966.
44. Montali, R.J., Bush, M., and Smeller, J.M.: The pathology of nephrotoxicity of gentamicin in snakes: a model for reptilian gout. Vet. Pathol. *16*:108–115, 1979.
45. Northway, R.B.: Electroanesthesia of green iguanas *(Iguana iguana)*. J. Am. Vet. Med. Assoc., *155*:1034, 1969.
46. Mittleman, M.B.: Letter to the editor. Phila. Herp. Soc. Bull, *10*:9, 1962.
47. Olson, G.A., Hessler, J.R., and Faith, R. E.: Technics for blood collection and intravascular infusion of reptiles. Lab. Anim. Sci., *25*:783–786, 1975.
48. Peaker, M.: Some aspects of the thermal requirements of reptiles in captivity. Int. Zoo Yearbook, *9*:3–8, 1969.

49. Pearson, O.P.: Habits of the lizard, *Liolaemus multiformis multiformis* at high altitudes in southern Peru. Copeia, 111–116, 1954.
50. Redisch, R.I.: Management of leg fractures in the iguana. Vet. Med Small Anim. Clin. *72*:1487, 1977.
51. Regal, P.J.: Thermophilic response following feeding in certain reptiles. Copeia, No. 3, 588–590, 1966.
52. Regal, P.J.: Temperature and light requirements of captive reptiles. *In* Reproductive Biology and Diseases of Captive Reptiles. Edited by J.B. Murphy and J.T. Collins. Society for the Study of Amphibians and Reptiles, 1980, pp. 79–89.
53. Richter, A.G., et al.: Techniques for collecting blood from Galapagos tortoises and box turtles. Vet. Med. Small Anim. Clin., *72*:1376–1378, 1977.
54. Rothman, N., and Rothman, B.: Course and cure of respiratory infection in snakes. Phila. Herp. Soc. Bull., *8*:19–23, 1960.
55. Skoczylas, R.: Influence of temperature on gastric digestion in the grass snake *Natrix natrix* L. Comp. Biochem. Physiol., *33*:793–804, 1970.
56. Vaughn, L.K., Bernheim, H.A., and Kluger, M.J.: Fever in the lizard *Dipsosaurus dorsalis*. Nature, *25*:473–474, 1974.
57. Wallach, J.D.: Medical care of reptiles. J. Am. Vet. Med. Assoc., *155*:1017–1034, 1969.
58. Wallach, J.D.: Environmental and nutritional diseases of captive reptiles. J. Am. Vet. Med. Assoc., *159*:1632–1643, 1971.
59. Wallach, J.D.: Anesthesia of reptiles. *In* Current Veterinary Therapy V. Edited by R. W. Kirk. W.B. Saunders Co., Philadelphia, 1974, pp. 638–640.
60. Wallach, J.D., and Hoessle, C.: M–99 as an immobilizing agent in poikilotherms. Vet. Med. Small Anim. Clin., *65*:163–167, 1970.
61. Wilhoft, D.C.: The effect of temperature on thyroid histology and survival in the lizard *Sceloporus occidentalis*. Copeia, 265–276, 1958.
62. York, W.: Treatment of anorexia in an anaconda. J. Zoo Anim. Med., *5*:11–12, 1974.
63. Young, R., and Kaplan, H.M.: Anesthesia of turtles with chlorpromazine and sodium pentobarbital. Proc. Anim. Care Panel *10*:57–62, 1960.
64. Zeman, W.Z., Falco, F.G., and Falco, J.J.: Repair of the carapace of a box turtle using a polyester resin. Lab. Anim. Care, *17*:424–425, 1967.

3 Specific Diseases of Herpetofauna

Infectious Diseases (Other Than Animal Parasites)

Poor husbandry, malnutrition, and lack of sanitary and hygienic procedures are major causes of disease in captive reptiles and amphibians. These problems predispose to infectious disease, which is a major immediate cause of death in these animals. The infectious diseases of reptiles have been reviewed by Marcus,[195] and a guide to the laboratory identification of bacterial pathogens in herpetofauna, fish, and molluscs has been published by Glorioso.[112]

Bacterial Infections

The most important group of pathogens, causing the highest morbidity and mortality, are the gram-negative bacilli. Among these, *Aeromonas hydrophila (Proteus hydrophilus)* is the organism that has received the greatest attention. It is a motile, nonsporulating gram-negative rod in the family Pseudomonadaceae. The two medically important genera in this family are *Pseudomonas*, which metabolizes glucose oxidatively, and *Aeromonas*, which ferments glucose, producing H_2 and CO_2.[46] It is interesting that *A. hydrophila* and *A. liquefaciens*, pathogens of cold-blooded animals, grow best at 37°C in vitro.[46] Herpetofauna can form agglutinating antibodies to *A. hydrophila*, which may provide some protective immunity.[29,281]

Aeromonas hydrophila has been incriminated as a causative organism in ulcerative stomatitis and pneumonia in snakes and in septicemia in a variety of reptiles.[125] It is also known to infect man. Human infections have included cases of enteritis, osteomyelitis, and fatal septicemias.[188,255] Human infections are rare, however, and are most likely to occur in patients whose resistance is lowered by immunosuppressive therapy or intercurrent disease. Experimentally, the organism is pathogenic for mice, guinea pigs, and rabbits.

Ulcerative Stomatitis. Also known as **"canker-mouth"** or **"mouth-rot,"** ulcerative stomatitis is an infectious disease of the oral mucosa characterized by ulceration and caseous exudate. It is very common in captive snakes and is less frequently seen in lizards.

Page isolated *Aeromonas hydrophila* from naturally occurring ulcerative stomatitis in snakes and reproduced the disease with this organism.[221,222] Heywood described ulcerative stomatitis as a manifestation of chronic infection with *A. hydrophila.*[125] *Aeromonas hydrophila* is markedly proteolytic at room temperature, which contributes to its necrotizing properties in poikilotherms.

Pseudomonas aeruginosa was isolated from cases of ulcerative stomatitis,[118] but the disease was not reproduced experimentally with the organism, so its etiologic role was not proven. However, *P. aeruginosa* was repeatedly isolated from a recurrent infection in the head and mouth of a reticulated python *(Python reticulatus)* and there was favorable response to supportive treatment plus gentamicin sulphate, to which the bacteria were sensitive in vitro. During the last recurrence the infection was treated without antibiotics, using a bacterin prepared from the *Pseudomonas* culture with apparent cure.[4] A study of enzootic septicemia and mouthrot at a snake farm revealed that 18% of cases were associated with *Pseudomonas* infection and 63% with *Aeromonas* spp.[65]

Gray, Davis, and McCarten ascribed "necrotic enteritis," most commonly involving the posterior one-third of the gut, to intestinal infection by *Pseudomonas aeruginosa* acquired by swallowing the exudate from mouthrot lesions.[118] Zwart has also observed that necrotizing enteritis may be associated with ulcerative stomatitis.[313] However, similar enteric lesions are found in amebiasis (see p. 116), enzootic in the Washington Zoo where the study by Gray, et al. was done, and they did not indicate that this was specifically ruled out.[118]

Wallach suggests that malnutrition, especially lack of vitamin C, may predispose to ulcerative stomatitis.[285] Another predisposing factor is thought to be injury to the mouth, as may occur during force-feeding or when snakes are teased into striking against the glass sides of their cage. Some snakes have a habit of rubbing their heads against wire screening in the cage, especially while being acclimatized to captivity. This frictional damage causes ulceration which may heal with excess granulation tissue (Fig. 3–1). If infected with the appropriate organisms, such a lesion might progress to ulcerative stomatitis.

In the typical case, ulceration of the oral mucosa is covered by abundant caseous exudate (Fig. 3–2). The disease may progress to involve tooth sockets and jawbones with resultant loss of teeth and osteomyelitis.

Untreated, snakes usually die from complications. For example, aspiration of the exudate may cause pneumonia or the organism may invade the bloodstream, resulting in septicemia. The oral ulcerations interfere with eating, resulting in anorexia and starvation. If lesions in the palate extend to involve the organ of Jacobson (p. 44), exudate may block the lacrimal duct, resulting in obstruction of flow from the

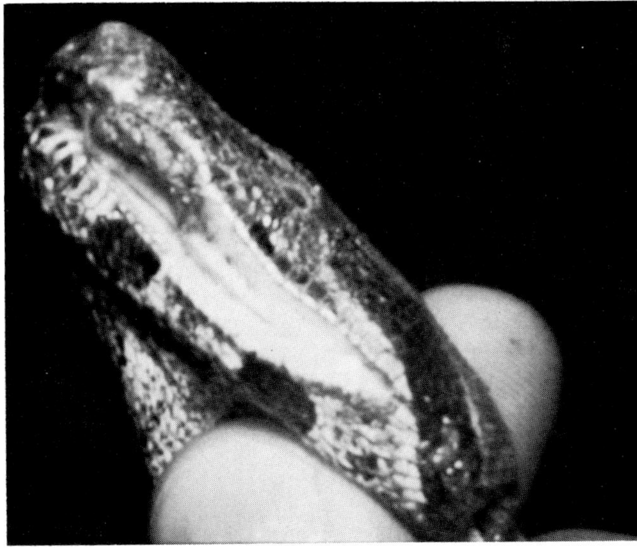

Fig. 3–1. Traumatic lesion with eschar in a boa constrictor *(Constrictor constrictor)* resulting from rubbing the head on a wire cage. Such lesions may initiate ulcerative stomatitis.

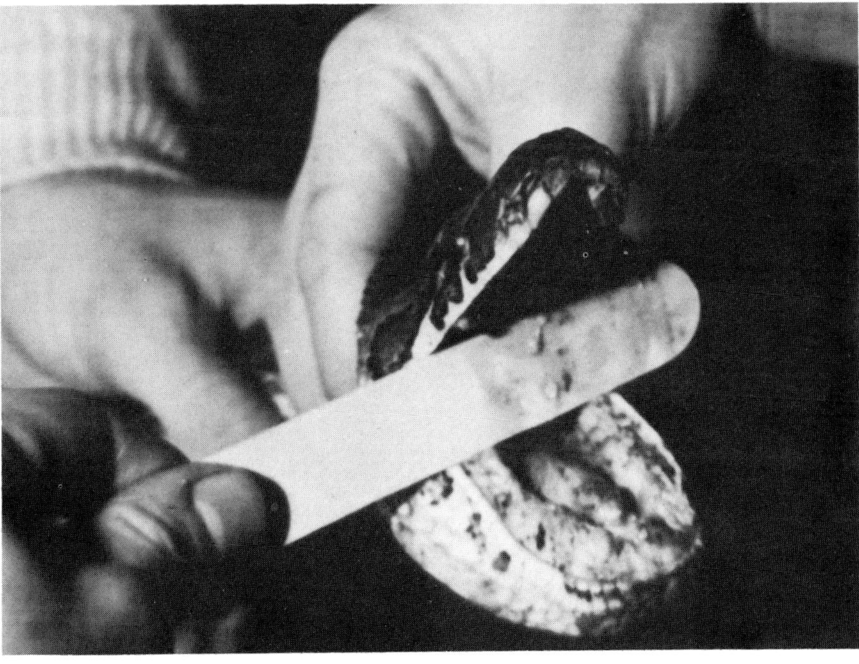

Fig. 3–2. Severe case of ulcerative stomatitis in a reticulated python *(Python reticulatus)*. The tissues of the lower jaw are markedly swollen. Some of the caseous exudate in the mouth is adherent to the tongue blade. (Courtesy of Dr. Robert Altman.)

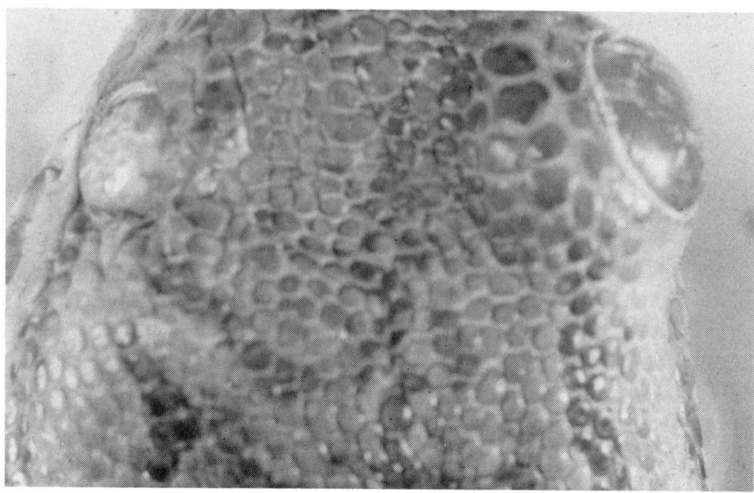

Fig. 3–3. Dorsal view, head of a boa constrictor *(Constrictor constrictor)*. There is swelling of the corneo-spectacular space bilaterally because the duct of the harderian gland is obstructed by the exudate of ulcerative stomatitis. (Armed Forces Institute of Pathology negative.)

harderian gland (p. 44) and distention of the space between cornea and spectacle (Figs. 3–3, 3–4, 3–5, and 3–6), a condition I call corneo-spectacular swelling. It is also known as pseudobuphthalmos.[32] This fluid may also become infected, resulting in opacity and blindness (Fig. 3–7).

The clinical features of ulcerative stomatitis are fairly distinctive. The only entity I have seen that mimicked this condition was a case of mycotic stomatitis in an anaconda (see p. 112).

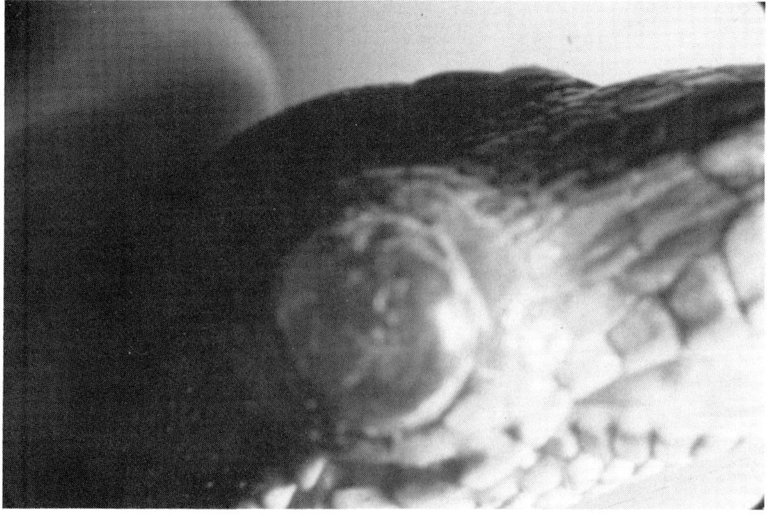

Fig. 3–4. Lateral view, right eye of the boa constrictor shown in Figure 3–3. (Armed Forces Institute of Pathology negative.)

Prevention of "mouthrot" depends on the maintenance of sanitary conditions in the cages and an adequate nutritional state in the animals. Affected snakes should be quarantined while being treated, and contaminated quarters should be disinfected with products that are nontoxic to reptiles, such as benzalkonium chloride (Zephiran) or diluted sodium hypochlorite solution (Clorox).

Treatment of ulcerative stomatitis consists of debridement of necrotic tissue and the topical application of 25% sulfamethazine (questionable value), mafenide acetate,[92a] or mild antiseptics such as thimerosal (Merthiolate), benzalkonium chloride, or 3% hydrogen peroxide. Tetracycline should be given by mouth (p.o.) using 25 to 50 mg/kg twice a day (b.i.d.) until at least two days beyond clinical recovery. Alternatively, ampicillin can be given intramuscularly (IM) or subcutaneously 3 to 6 mg/kg until at least two days beyond clinical recovery.[96] Wallach recommends the use of ascorbic acid with an initial dose of 50 mg given parenterally followed by 10 to 30 mg p.o. daily for 10 days.[285] Supportive

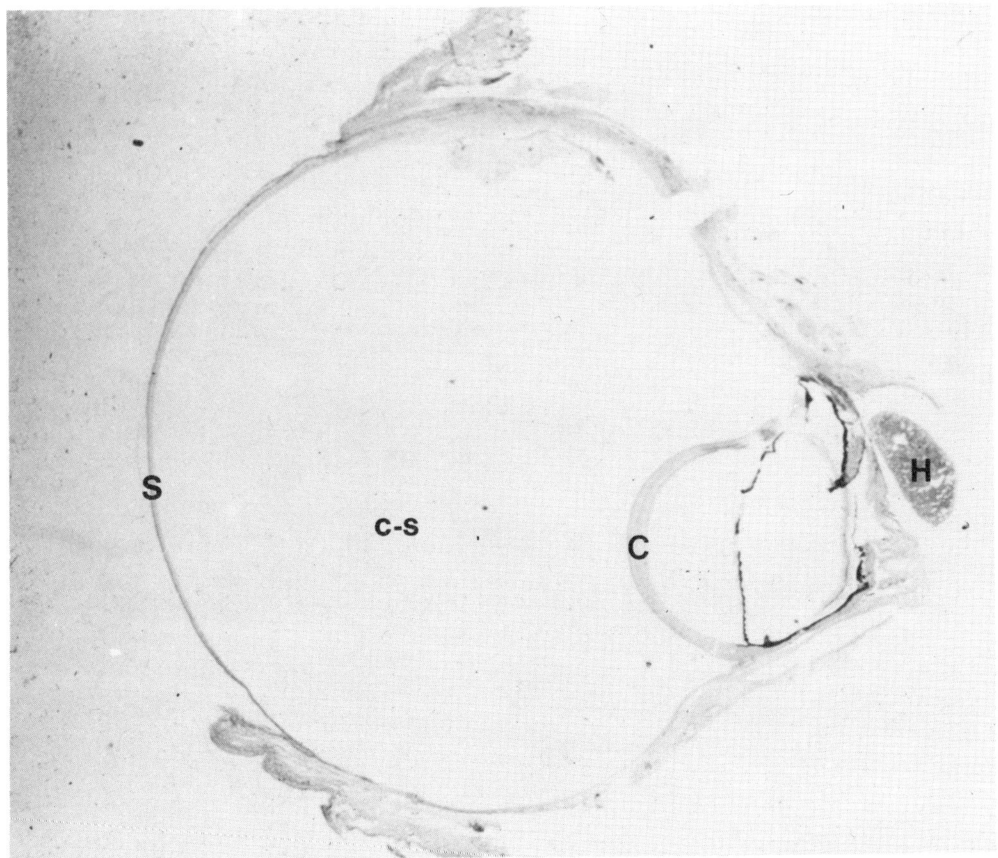

Fig. 3–5. Off-center section through the right eye of the boa constrictor shown in Figures 3–3 and 3–4. Spectacle **(s)**; cornea **(c)**; corneo-spectacular space **(c–s)**; harderian gland **(H)**. 2½×. (Armed Forces Institute of Pathology negative.)

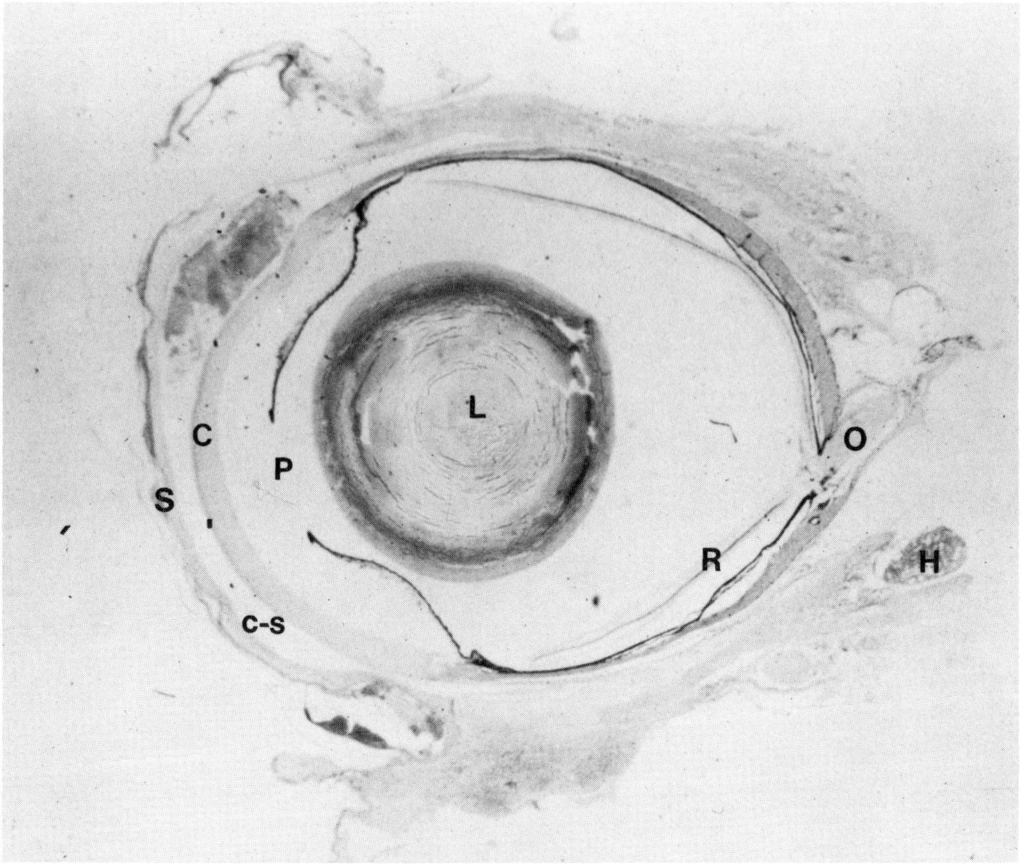

Fig. 3–6. Section through pupil **(P)** and optic nerve **(O)** of left eye of boa constrictor shown in Figure 3–3. Lens **(L)**; retina **(R)**; spectacle **(s)**; cornea **(c)**; corneo-spectacular space **(c–s)**; harderian gland **(H)**. 3½×. (Armed Forces Institute of Pathology negative.)

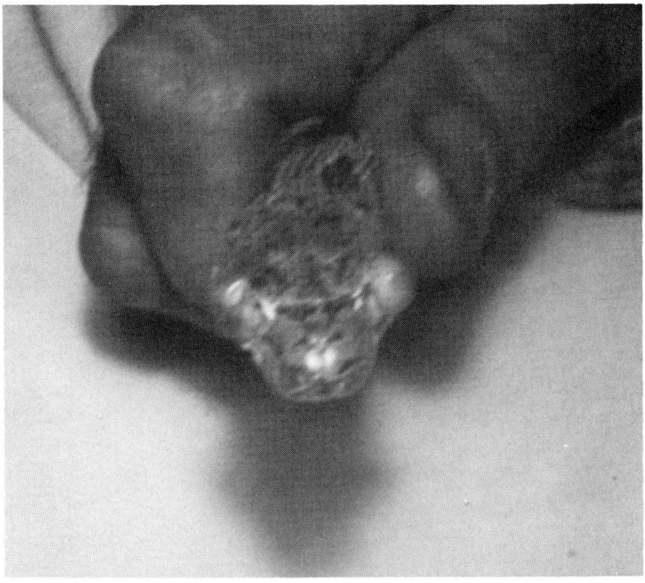

Fig. 3–7. Corneo-spectacular swelling with infection and opacification of the harderian gland fluid in a grey rat snake *(Elaphe obsoleta spiloides)*.

therapy with intubated feedings and parenteral fluids may be necessary in debilitated animals.

Corneospectacular swelling may clear up by curing the stomatitis and with shedding of the spectacle during ecdysis. Severe corneospectacular swelling should be treated by making a semicircular flap from 3 to 9 o'clock around the ventral border of the eye, washing the corneospectacular space with an ophthalmic solution, and installing an antibiotic ophthalmic ointment.

Pneumonia. Common in reptiles, pneumonia is responsible for considerable morbidity and mortality in collections. A variety of microorganisms may cause pulmonary infection. The immediate discussion is limited to pneumonia in snakes caused by *Aeromonas hydrophila.* Like ulcerative stomatitis, pneumonia is considered one manifestation of *A. hydrophila* infection in snakes by Heywood.[125]

The principal means of infection is transmission by the snake mite, *Ophionyssus natricis*.[237] Transmission by aerosol or direct contact would seem likely, but has not been proven. Sudden changes in ambient temperature, especially sudden chilling, inanition, and debility owing to parasitism or other disease are thought to predispose to pneumonia.

Signs of pneumonia include nasal discharge, gaping of the mouth, intercostal retractions, bubbly and wheezing respiratory sounds, listlessness, and anorexia. The nasal discharge is probably the result of intercurrent rhinitis, rather than drainage from the lung. Sometimes pneumonia can kill reptiles without producing obvious signs, as occurred in a group of tokay geckos *(Gecko gecko)* with pulmonary *Klebsiella pneumoniae* infection.[32a] Differential diagnosis of pneumonia caused by *A. hydrophila* includes other bacterial, mycobacterial (see p. 104), mycotic (see p. 112), and verminous (see p. 158) pneumonia and oral trematodiasis, which may also cause gaping (see p. 141). Most untreated cases of *A. hydrophilia* pneumonia terminate fatally within two weeks of onset.

Postmortem examination reveals congestion and fibrinopurulent or caseous exudate in the lungs (Fig. 3–8). Direct smears of infected lung tissue may reveal numerous gram-negative bacilli.[190]

Diagnosis and specific therapy can be established by culture and sensitivity studies of exudate obtained by tracheal aspiration. Direct smears stained appropriately can be examined for mycobacteria and fungi. Pending the results of culture and sensitivity studies, treatment can be started with tetracycline, using at least 50 mg/kg twice a day. Doses of 50 mg for "small" snakes and 100 mg for "large" snakes per day have been recommended in the herpetology literature. It is important to keep the snakes at an ambient temperature above 72°F. Failure of tetracycline at doses up to 125 mg/kg to cure pneumonia in snakes has been reported.[214] Tylosin, 25 mg/kg, given IM or p.o. once daily for seven days was found effective and safe.[214]

Prevention of pneumonia depends on eradication of the mite vector. Once an outbreak has occurred, sick animals should be isolated and cages and other fomites should be disinfected.

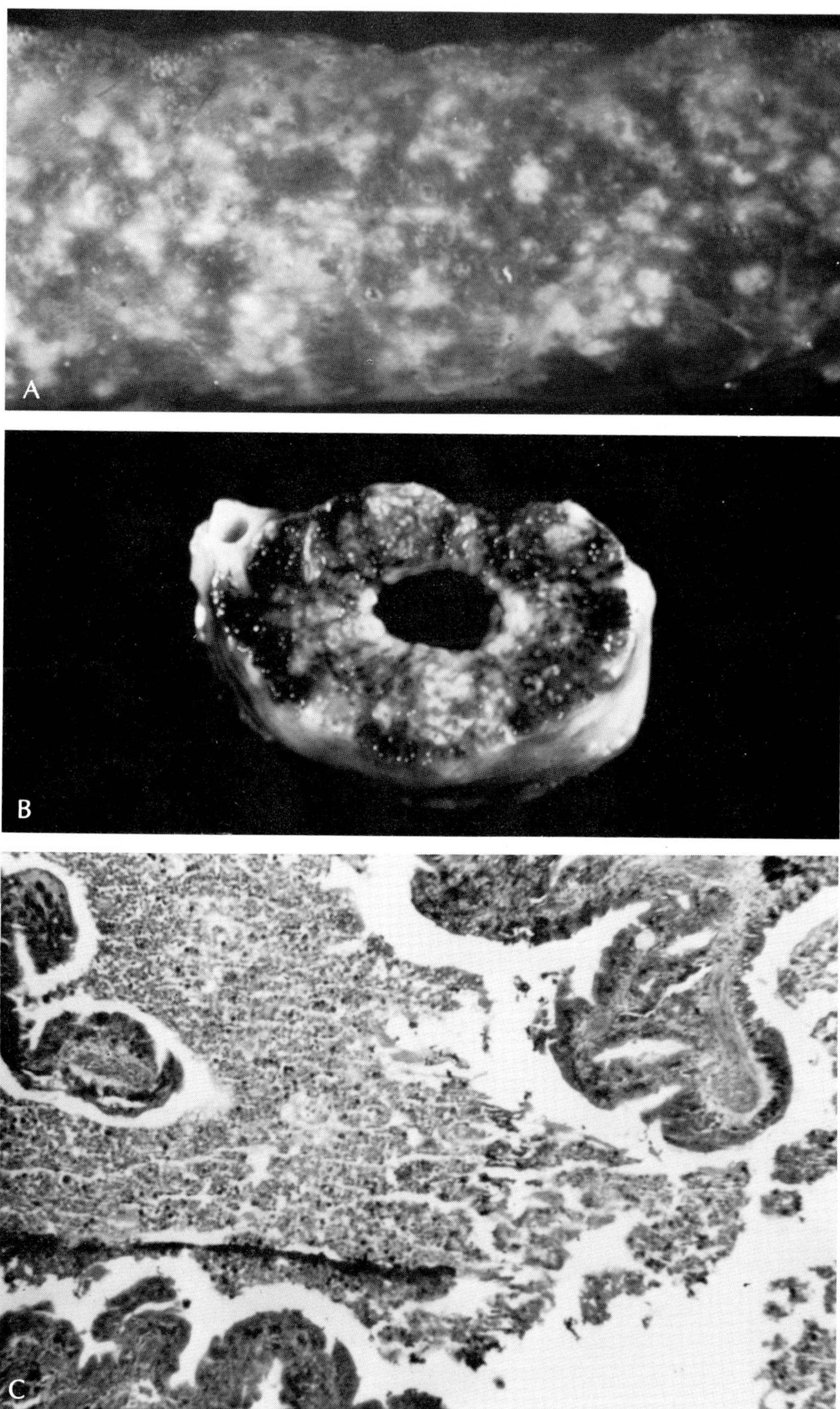

Fig. 3–8. Pneumonia in a Jamaican boa *(Epicrates subflavus)*, caused by *Arizona* sp. **A.** Pleural surface of lung. **B.** Cut surface. (A and B courtesy of Dr. Marilyn Anderson and the Ohio State University, Department of Veterinary Pathobiology.) **C.** Pneumonia in a timber rattlesnake *(Crotalus horridus)* Purulent exudate fills the air space. 20×.

Septicemia. In reptiles and amphibians, septicemia, a common, major disease problem, is most commonly caused by gram-negative bacilli. *Aeromonas hydrophila* is often incriminated.

Aeromonas hydrophila may be transmitted by contact with infected water, as is probably the usual situation in frogs and aquatic reptiles, or it may be transmitted by the mite *Ophionyssus natricis* in snakes[51] and, probably, in lizards. Direct contact of contaminated soil and water with wounds in the skin and oral mucosa was the probable source of enzootic *Aeromonas* and *Pseudomonas* infections in an African snake farm.[65]

It many cases, preceding illness is not noticed, and the septicemic patient is presented in a terminal state, twitching, convulsing, or comatose. A cardinal sign of septicemia is hemorrhage, usually petechial, on skin and on mucosal and serosal surfaces. History and physical examination or necropsy will often reveal the underlying cause and source of infection, for example, ulcerative stomatitis, cutaneous lesions, mite infestation, or pneumonia.

Heywood described three syndromes in *Aeromonas hydrophila* infections in snakes: acute septicemia, pneumonia, and chronic infection.[125] The acute, septicemic form was mainly seen in younger snakes and was clinically manifested by sluggishness, weakness, and terminal convulsions, with death occurring within 24 hours of onset. Postmortem findings included bloody fluid in the body cavity and lungs, enlarged mottled liver, enteritis, and epicardial and endocardial hemorrhages. In the respiratory (pneumonic) syndrome, clinical signs were lethargy, anorexia, and nasal discharge, which was serous initially but became purulent by the third day. Deaths generally occurred on the fifth day of illness and catarrhal pneumonia was demonstrable at postmortem. A chronic form of the infection was found in larger snakes that suffered from ulcerative stomatitis, respiratory distress, and nasal discharge. Deaths occurred five to six weeks after onset, and the pathologic findings included ulceration of the mouth and trachea, and consolidation and necrosis in the lungs. Snake mites (*Ophionyssus natricis*) were found on all affected snakes in Heywood's report, and he indicates that control and prevention of the infection are dependent on eradication of the mite (see p. 169). *Aeromonas hydrophila* isolated from the sick snakes was sensitive to tetracycline, streptomycin, neomycin, and chloramphenicol, and resistant to ampicillin in vitro.

Redleg is the term commonly applied to septicemia in frogs. It is usually caused by *Aeromonas hydrophila* but *Mima* species can often be isolated from blood and viscera concurrently.[110] Clinical signs of redleg include weight loss, dull skin color, decreased activity, loss of coordination in movement, cutaneous hemorrhages and ulceration, and terminal hemoptysis and convulsions (Figs. 3–9 and 3–10). "Redleg" refers to the hemorrhagic lesions usually seen on the skin of the hind legs of affected frogs.

In the author's experience, the first sign of septicemia in frogs is anorexia. A healthy frog should immediately gulp down a moving insect within its reach, assuming its stomach is not already filled to

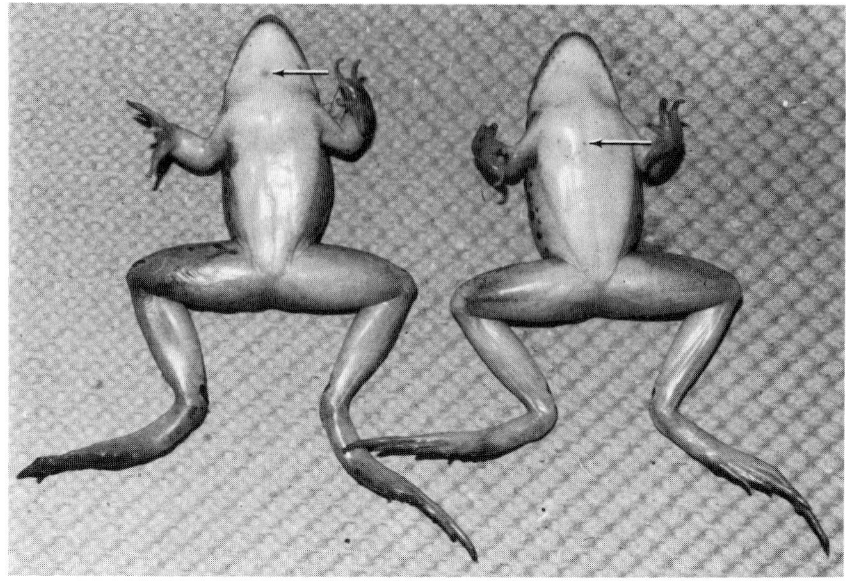

Fig. 3–9 Ecchymoses on the hind legs and petechiae (arrows) on the intermandibular and thoracic areas of leopard frogs *(Rana pipiens)* with redleg disease.

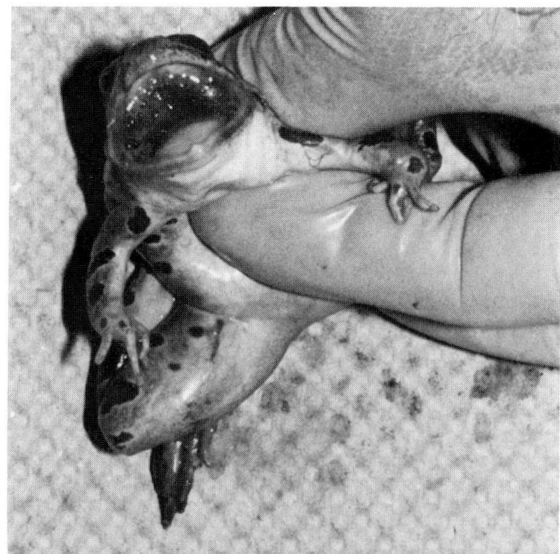

Fig. 3–10. Frothy hemorrhagic exudate from the mouth of a leopard frog *(R. pipiens)* in terminal stage of redleg disease.

capacity and the ambient temperature is in the range for normal activity. Any frog that does not feed immediately when offered appropriate food is probably sick. Because of its prevalence and high morbidity and case fatality rate, redleg is the first disease that should be considered and ruled in or out. Frogs with redleg have macrocytic anemia, leukopenia, and thrombocytopenia. Clotting time and erythrocyte sedimentation rate increase, and there is anisocytosis and poikilocytosis. Total protein decreases significantly (from 2.5 to 1.7 g/dl), especially the globulins, so the A/G ratio increases from a mean normal of 1.38 to 1.5.[109]

Aeromonas hydrophila was incriminated as the cause of an epizootic of septicemia in a colony of Mexican axolotls *(Ambystoma [Siredon] mexicanum).*[40] The disease was characterized by sluggishness, anorexia, generalized edema and congestion, and cutaneous petechiae or ecchymoses. *A. hydrophila* was isolated in pure culture from hemorrhagic lesions in the skin, heart blood, peritoneal fluid, liver, and spleen, and the disease was reproduced by inoculation of the organism into apparently healthy animals. The mortality rate was 5%, with 150 animals in a colony of 3,000 dying of the disease, and there was a 90% case fatality rate among those animals that showed clinical signs.

The outbreak was controlled by improved sanitation with daily cleaning of cages and washing of hands after handling each animal. The disease did not occur in healthy stock removed from the colony and refrigerated at 4° to 5°C for two weeks. Some diseased axolotls recovered with treatment by cold storage; treatment of other sick animals with tetracycline resulted in recovery in most cases (no statistics given).

Necropsy of septicemic reptiles and amphibians reveals widespread congestion and hemorrhages in muscle, thoracic and abdominal viscera, and on serosal and mucosal membranes (Fig. 3–11).

Definitive etiologic diagnosis of septicemia is made by blood culture. Treatment of affected and exposed animals should be started immediately, pending results of sensitivity tests. Redleg in frogs should be treated with 5 mg of tetracycline in 0.2 ml of distilled water via stomach tube (dose for a 30-gram *Rana pipiens)* twice a day for five to seven days.[110] This is equivalent to 1 mg per 6 g of body weight. Reptiles should be treated with at least 50 mg of tetracycline per kg twice a day for at least one week. In an uncontrolled study, chloramphenicol apparently halted an epizootic and cured early symptomatic cases of redleg in toads (*Bufo marinus*) with an initial dosage of 5 mg per 100 g of body weight followed by 3 mg per 100 g twice a day for five days.[259]

Prevention of septicemia depends on eradication of mite vectors, isolation or elimination of sick animals, and disinfection of quarters. *Aeromonas hydrophila (Proteus hydrophilus)* was found in the gallbladders of three frogs that appeared healthy, so it is possible that some frogs could be asymptomatic carriers.[174] Unfortunately, chemicals that effectively inhibit *A. hydrophila* are also toxic to frogs during prolonged contact, so it is not practical to leave frogs in disinfectant baths.[162]

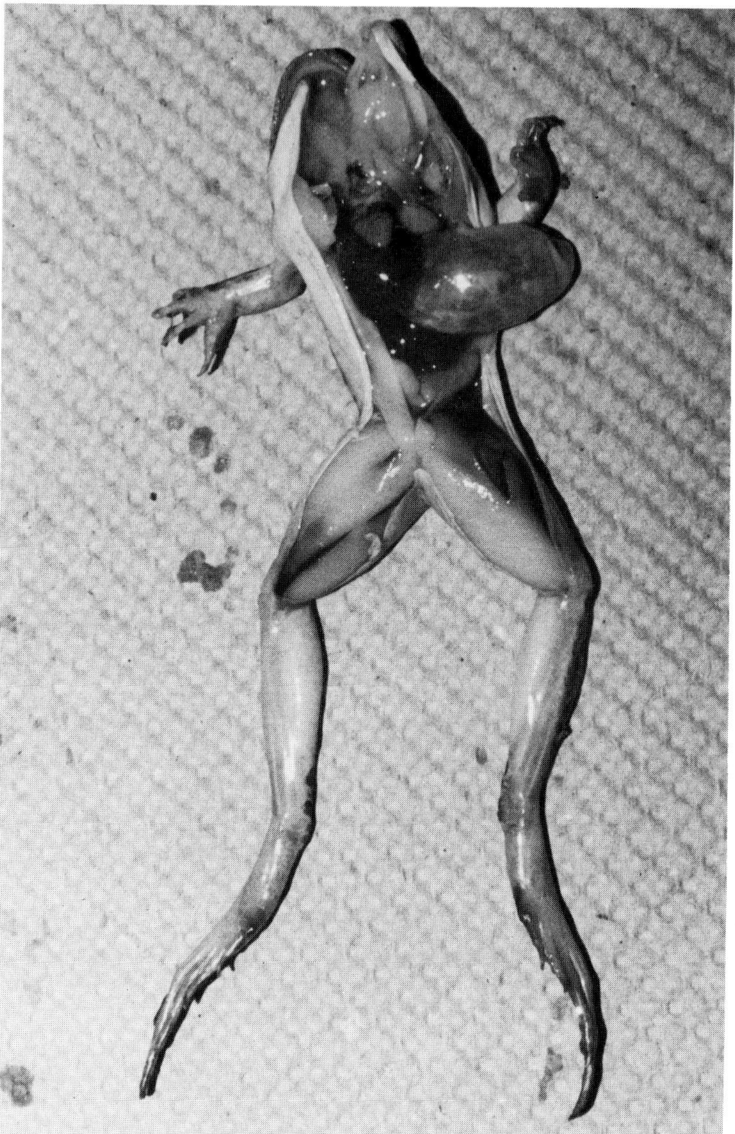

Fig. 3–11. Ecchymoses of the skin on the hind feet, in the thigh muscles, and in the stomach in a leopard frog *(R. pipiens)* with redleg disease.

Without offering any specific supporting data, Kulp and Borden claimed they could protect frogs against redleg by immunizing them with a killed bacterial vaccine.[174] They also cited earlier work in which a "60 to 100 per cent successful immunization" was achieved.

In June, 1971 the American news media brought national attention to a situation in Lake Apopka, Florida in which thousands of animals, including fish, alligators, snakes, turtles, and birds were found dead in a short period of time. This epizootic was found to be due to infection with *Aeromonas hydrophila* and *A. shigelloides,* which, in turn, was blamed on pollution of the lake by fertilizers, sewage, and other organic pollutants.[257]

Pseudomonas reptilivora is another gram-negative rod pathogenic for herpetofauna. It causes a disease in the mudpuppy *(Necturus maculosus)* similar to redleg in frogs. According to Kaplan and Glaczenski,

> "a cutaneous hyperemia is particularly evident in the unpigmented ventral surface. The gills turn pale gray and degenerate from a feathery appearance to stubs on the gill arches. The red blood cells become vacuolated. In untreated cases all animals succumb. The destruction of the gills, resulting primarily from overwhelming infection, apparently contributes greatly to death in that the animals are not able to obtain sufficient oxygen."[161]

Kaplan and Glaczenski treated *Pseudomonas reptilivora* infections by sprinkling approximately 0.2 g of Furacin Soluble Powder (Eaton Laboratories) on the gills daily for 10 days.[161] The gills appeared improved within a few days and eventually regained their normal appearance. The authors also recommend giving chloramphenicol (Chloromycetin, Parke, Davis and Co.) by stomach tube in an initial dose of 8 mg in 2 ml of water followed by 4 mg in 1 ml of water daily for 6 days and then 4 mg once a week until clinical cure is achieved.

Pseudomonas reptilivorus was found to be pathogenic for the Mexican beaded lizard *(Heloderma suspectum)*, chuckwalla *(Sauromalus ater)*, and horned toad *(Phrynosoma solare)*, causing fatal septicemia in these lizards.[50]

Septicemic Cutaneous Ulcerative Disease of Turtles. This disease was originally described by Kaplan in 1957.[156] The causative organism was originally named *Escherichia freundii*, and, therefore, Kaplan renamed the disease escherichiosis.[157] The organism has since been reclassified as *Citrobacter freundii*,[79] so it may be advisable to return to the original, more cumbersome name. We can refer to it by its acronym, SCUD.

Citrobacter freundii is a gram-negative rod normally found in soil and water and in the intestinal tract of various animals, including man. Turtles are thought to become infected through skin abrasion while in contaminated water.

Clinical signs in turtles include lethargy, reduced muscle tone, paralysis of limbs, loss of claws or digits, and cutaneous vasodilatation, hemorrhage, and ulceration. Erythrocytes may be vacuolated and may contain numerous bacteria. Hemolysis and multiple foci of necrosis are found in internal organs. The bacteria are readily cultured on eosin-methylene blue agar from cutaneous sores, blood, and visceral necrotic foci. Most untreated turtles die, but some recover spontaneously. The disease is naturally transmissible to frogs which also develop superficial ulcers and fatal septicemia.

An epizootic in turtles with clinical features similar, if not identical, to SCUD was associated with other gram-negative bacteria, e.g., *Serratia* sp. alone or with *Citrobacter* sp.[143]

SCUD reportedly responds to therapy with chloramphenicol. The initial dosage is 8 mg per 100 g of body weight followed by 4 mg per 100 g of body weight twice a day for 7 days, given intramuscularly (IM) or intraperitoneally (IP) to turtles, or injected in the dorsal lymph sac of frogs.

Ulcerative Shell Disease (shell rot, spot disease, rust). Ulcerative shell disease of turtles is a contagious, chronic condition characterized by blotchy darkening, loosening, and shedding of the keratinized shell plates of the plastron and carapace, caused by a gram-negative bacillus, *Beneckea chitinovora*. The condition has been described in several species of freshwater turtles.[287a,287b] The affected plates slough, leaving a raw ulcer and brownish yellow pseudomembrane from which the causative organism can be cultured. Differential diagnoses include SCUD (above) and algal infection (see p. 111).

Untreated, most cases heal spontaneously, leaving a permanently pitted or pocked shell. Death may result from secondary infections.

To prevent the introduction of *B. chitinovora* in a turtle colony, newly acquired turtles should be quarantined for two weeks and affected animals should be removed. Overcrowding should be avoided. *B. chitinovora* also infects crayfish, lobsters, and crabs, so these crustaceans should not be fed to, or housed with, turtles.[287a,287b]

Recommended treatment consists of giving chloramphenicol, 40 mg/kg parenterally, local curettage,[287b] and topical antiseptics.

Abscesses. Abscesses, very common in reptiles, usually are subcutaneous (Fig. 3–12), but internal organs may also be involved (Fig. 3–13). The lesions are usually discrete, round, and encapsulated by fibrous connective tissue. The consistency of the exudate varies from thick, brown, liquid pus to dense, consolidated, laminated material

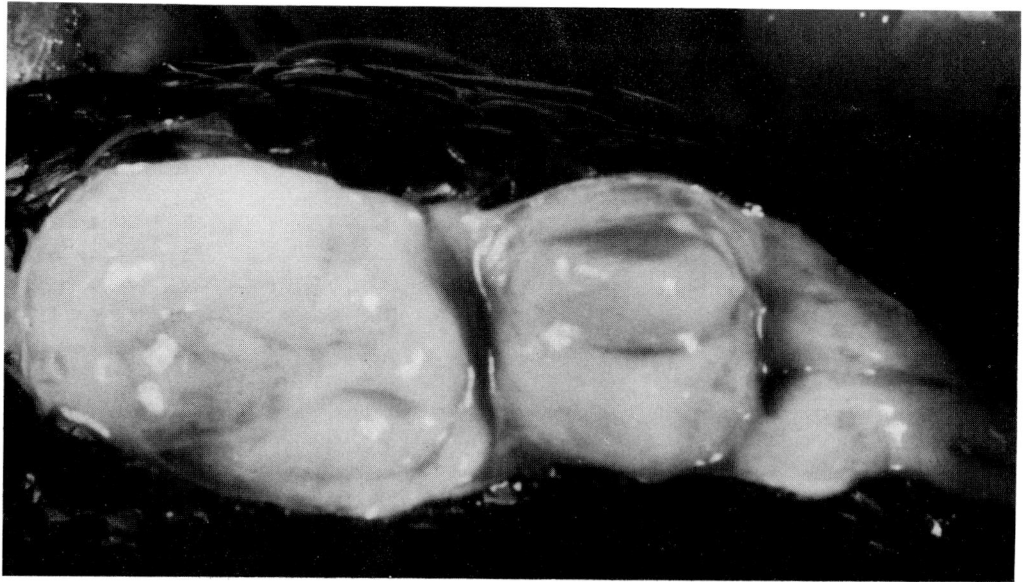

Fig. 3–12. Three contiguous subcutaneous abscesses in a cottonmouth moccasin *(Agkistrodon piscivorus)*. The skin overlying the three abscesses has been incised, as has the fibrous capsule over the middle abscess, revealing the firm, inspissated material in the center. (Armed Forces Institute of Pathology Accession No. 1058160.)

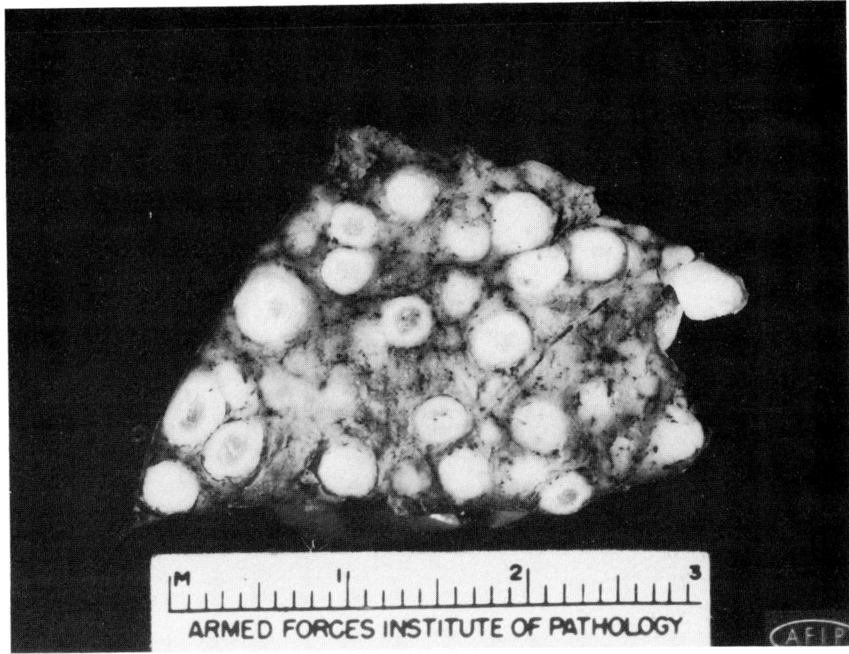

Fig. 3–13. Multiple hepatic abscesses in a sidenecked turtle. (Armed Forces Institute of Pathology Negative No. 63–2190).

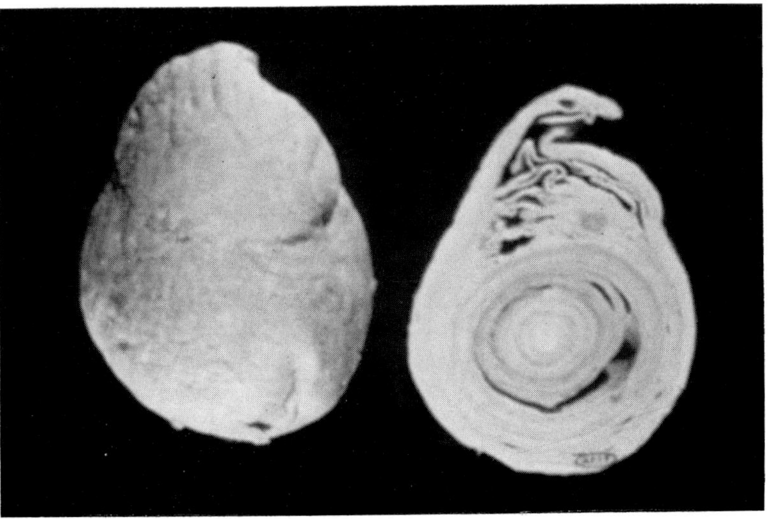

Fig. 3–14. Formalin fixed exudate surgically removed from a subcutaneous abscess in a boa constrictor *(Constrictor constrictor)*. The specimen is 3 cm wide. Concentric, laminated structure is apparent on the cut surface (right). (Armed Forces Institute of Pathology Negative No. 63–5120).

resembling the exudate of caseous lymphadenitis in sheep and goats (Fig. 3–14).[194] In the latter situation, microscopic examination may reveal concentric laminar deposits of an eosinophilic material that is surprisingly acellular (Fig. 3–15).

Various bacteria have been isolated from these abscesses. *Serratia anolium* was isolated from "a contagious tumor-like condition" in the anole lizard, *Anolis equestris*,[58] and *Bacterium sauromali* was isolated from abscesses in the chuckwalla, *Sauromalus varius*.[61] Micrococci, *Salmonella marina*, and *Serratia marcescens* have been individually isolated from subcutaneous abscesses in iguanid lizards.[31]

A mixed flora of gram-negative rods was isolated from an abscess that presented as a unilateral swelling on the lateral aspect of the neck of a box turtle *(Terrapene carolina)*[144] (Fig. 3–16). I have seen three box turtles with an identical clinical appearance. Jackson, et al. suggest pathogens may enter the area via pharyngeal trauma.[144] The box turtles probably had otitis, as described in the tortoise *Testudo graeca*[117,312] (Fig. 3–17).

Factors that may predispose reptiles to having abscesses include local trauma from ectoparasites or tan bark bedding, excess dampness, excess contact with droppings, and malnutrition, the latter presumably causing a catabolic state and impaired integrity of tissue. Recommendations to prevent abscesses include maintaining clean, dry quarters, eliminating ectoparasites and improper bedding, and maintaining optimal nutrition.

Differential diagnosis includes mycobacterial infections (p. 104), dermatophilosis (p. 109), cutaneous geotrichosis (p. 112), sparganosis (p. 139), cutaneous filariasis (p. 160), cutaneous myiasis (p. 175), parasitic and mycotic granulomas, and neoplasms such as squamous cell carcinoma (p. 206). The presence of laminated exudate rules

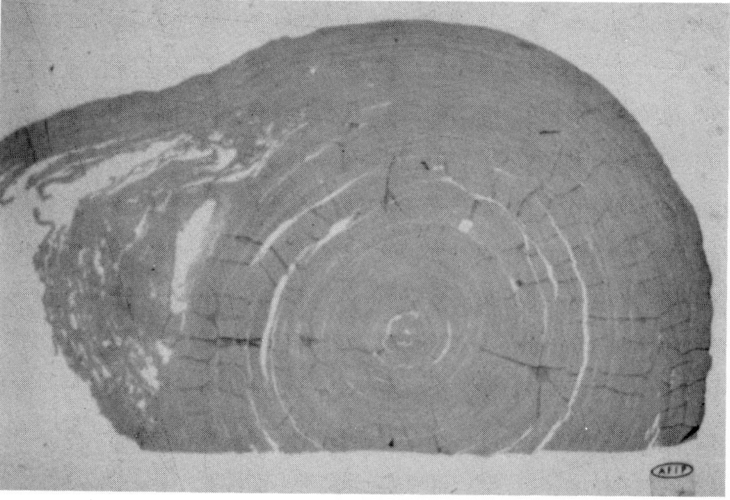

Fig. 3–15. Laminated exudate from subcutaneous abscess in a boa constrictor *(Constrictor constrictor)*. The eosinophilic lamellae were virtually acellular and no microorganisms were seen with special stains. This lesion was not cultured. 1.7×. (Armed Forces Institute of Pathology Negative No. 63–5120.)

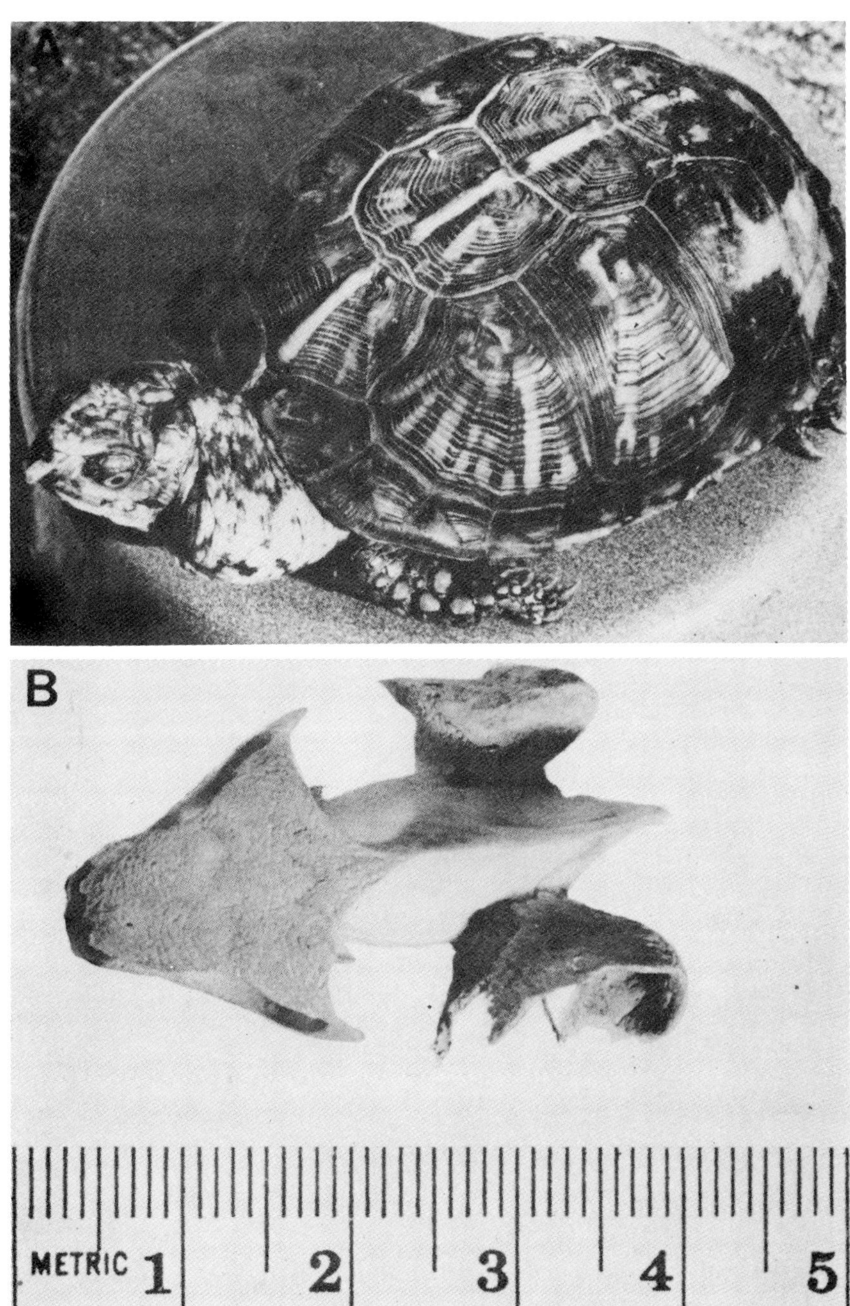

Fig. 3–16. Massive bacterial infection of a box turtle. **A**, Living animal exhibiting large swelling on lateral aspect of neck. **B**, Dorsal view of skull showing greatly enlarged and eroded left squamosal bone. (From Jackson, C.G., MacDonald, F., and Jackson, M.M.: Cranial asymmetry with massive infection in a box turtle. J. Wildl. Dis., *8*:275, 1972.)

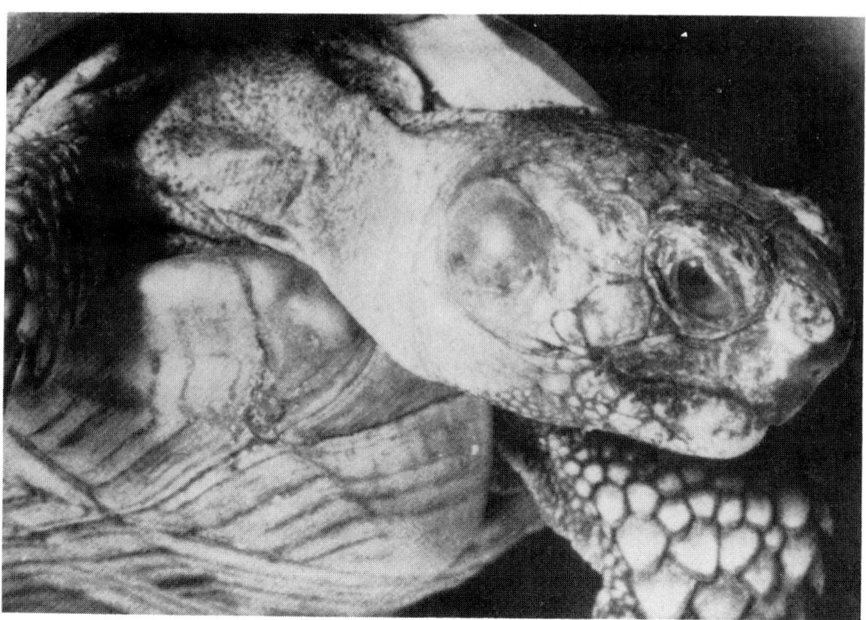

Fig. 3–17. Greek tortoise *(Testudo graeca)* with otitis media. Note the bulging cutaneous membrane over the ear. (From Zwart, P.: Ziekten van reptielen II: aandoeningen van de ogen, de oren, de mondholte en de longen. Lacerta, *30*:72–79, 1972a.)

out these other diagnoses. Differential diagnosis is usually clarified on gross examination of the cut specimen, but a definitive diagnosis sometimes must await culture and histopathologic examination.

Treatment must include surgical drainage if there is liquid pus, or, if the exudate is solid, it should be shelled out of its fibrous capsule like a pea from a pod. Culture and sensitivity studies should be done on the exudate. The surgical site should be irrigated with an antiseptic or antibiotic solution, or mafenide acetate can be instilled in the cavity. Benzalkonium chloride, 1:1000 (Zephiran, Winthrop Labs), may be effective as an irrigant and for treating superficial sores,[211] but its usefulness is limited by its capacity to support the growth of *Pseudomonas*.[7] Postoperatively, the wound can be infused with a proteolytic enzyme (Kymar Ointment, Armour-Baldwin Laboratories), and the animal should be given systemic antibiotics, as indicated by culture and sensitivity testing.

Salmonellosis (or, hazards of the shell game). Limerick lovers will recall the classic lines:

There once was a lady named Myrtle
Who had an affair with a turtle
But dimensions phenomenal
Around her abdominal
Proved to Myrtle
The turtle was fertile.

It is now apparent that we have more to fear from these reptiles than unwanted pregnancies.

Salmonellosis is the major zoonosis associated with reptiles. More than 200 serotypes of *Salmonella* and the *Arizona* group of Enterobacteriaceae have been isolated from their intestinal flora.[169]

Boycott, et al.[39] reported that 10 out of 11 tortoises *(Testudo graeca)*, a species imported by the hundreds of thousands from Morocco to England as pets, had *Salmonella* representing 17 different serotypes in their stool. Jackson and Jackson[145] isolated six *Salmonella* and one *Arizona* serotype from cloacal swabs of 15 of 124 turtles from nine zoos in the United States, giving an apparent rate of infection of 12.1%. In a later study, 37 of 127 zoo turtles (29%) were found to carry intestinal *Salmonella*.[220]

Many anole lizards *(Anolis carolinensis)* in my laboratory harbored *Salmonella*, and geckos in zoos have also been shown to be carriers.[232,240] Snakes commonly carry *Salmonella*.[127] Kennedy found *Salmonella* and *Arizona* in various snakes, especially constrictors kept on display at a Canadian museum.[171] These bacteria were isolated with high frequency from the terminal colon and occasionally from other viscera of snakes captured in India.[170] Although turtles have been incriminated more often than other herpetofauna as a source of human salmonellosis, all reptiles should be considered possible reservoirs.

Most of the turtles kept as pets in the United States (the most common species being the red-eared turtle, *Chrysemys (Pseudemys scripta elegans)* are raised on farms in the South.[16,168] Original stock animals, caught in the wild, may be naturally infected with *Salmonella*. They are then raised in crowded conditions in ponds where the water is often stagnant. The turtles on many of these farms are fed uncooked meat scraps and offal from local abattoirs, feed which is often heavily contaminated with enteric pathogens. Soil in the banks of the ponds, where the turtles nest, is often heavily contaminated, and since *Salmonella* can penetrate turtle eggs,[86] baby turtles can emerge from the eggs already infected.[168] The combination of crowding, stagnant water, and contaminated feed is conducive to dissemination of *Salmonella*, and the problem is compounded when the animals are packed together for shipment and later kept in a common display case in a pet shop. It is not unusual for 25 to 50% of turtles in a pet shop to harbor *Salmonella* and *Arizona* bacteria.

Salmonellosis is usually asymptomatic in reptiles, with the animal acting as a carrier. Turtles may carry the infection asymptomatically for at least 12 months.[167] Occult *Salmonella* and *Arizona* infections in turtles can be made patent by stress, e.g., dehydration.[79a]

Rarely, reptiles suffer enteritis or septicemia with pneumonia (see Fig. 3–8 A and B) and necrotic foci in the liver and other viscera. (For example, see the report on *Arizona* septicemia in boa constrictors by Boever.[31a]) Sick animals might have diarrhea, anorexia, and listlessness. Differential diagnosis includes amebiasis, gastrointestinal helminthiasis, chemical intoxication, and septicemia by *Aeromonas hydrophila*. Specific diagnosis of salmonellosis in the individual live animal is only possible on the basis of positive cultures from stool, cloacal swab, or blood. On postmortem, cultures should be taken of lesions, blood, bile, intestinal contents, and the female reproductive tract. To determine the presence of *Salmonella* in a group of animals kept together, water from their enclosure should be sampled.

There are few reports of *Salmonella* in amphibians. *S. enteritidis* was found in the tank water and focal necrotic lesions of the liver of leopard frogs *(Rana pipiens)* which suffered high mortality after an average of seven to 10 days of illness.[262] Reichenbach-Klinke and Elkan cite one case of salmonellosis causing paralysis and cutaneous ecchymosis in an edible frog *(Rana esculenta)*.[233] Eighteen of 129 frogs (14%) caught in and around Hissar, India were found to harbor *Salmonella*,[254] so it is possible that amphibians are significant reservoirs of infection in some areas.

Because the organisms are so common and the public health hazard so great, it is prudent to culture the stool of any reptilian pet to determine if it is a *Salmonella* carrier. A single culture may fail to reveal the organisms. *Salmonella* excretion rate is variable, and a turtle that is a heavy shedder one time may later have a negative stool culture.[167] Therefore, sanitary precautions, outlined in the following section, must be maintained in caring for reptiles. Although there is considerable variation in pathogenicity of different serotypes for different host species, any *Salmonella* or *Arizona* serotype found should be considered a potential human pathogen.

Definitive, controlled studies on the efficacy of antibiotic treatment of *Salmonella* infections in reptiles are lacking. In a limited study, 200 mg of neomycin sulfate per five gallons of tank water kept at 29.5°C (85°F) for four days seemingly eliminated enteric *Salmonella* in three asymptomatic turtles. Two other turtles whose water temperature was not controlled required four more days with twice the above concentration of neomycin to eliminate the infection.[276] In another study, apparent elimination of *Salmonella* from the gut (on the basis of three successive negative stool cultures) was achieved in tortoises by treating them with 50 mg of oxytetracycline per os daily for six days.[297]

In man cholecystectomy may be required to eliminate the carrier state for *S. typhi* because typhoid organisms residing in the gallbladder may not be susceptible to chemotherapy. *Salmonella* have been isolated from the biliary tract of turtles,[169] but it is self-evident that cholecystectomy in these animals is not a practical approach to the problem. Unless one were prepared to do very carefully controlled studies with adequate precautions guarding human health, it would seem more advisable to kill rather than treat infected reptiles. If any attempt is made to treat salmonellosis in pet reptiles, the veterinarian is obligated to warn the owner of the hazard to human health, and to advise him on proper isolation of the animal and the hygienic precautions to be taken, including sanitary disposal of feces, disinfecting potential fomites, and thorough washing of hands after handling the animal or its cage. Small children should not be permitted to handle reptiles, their cages, or items contaminated with their stool unless their hands can be washed by an adult immediately afterwards. Herpetofauna and their containers should neither be held nor washed in the kitchen sink or otherwise brought into contact with areas where human food is kept.

Based on data available on other species, chloramphenicol or ampicillin are the drugs of choice for systemic (extraintestinal) salmonellosis. In man, antibiotic treatment for enteric salmonellosis prolongs the shedding of organisms in the stool. Therefore, human *Salmonella* enteritis is usually treated symptomatically, e.g., with fluid therapy. If reptile carriers are treated with antibiotics, several stool cultures should be taken, at least up to several weeks after cessation of treatment, to be sure that the infection is eliminated. As explained previously, one negative stool culture cannot be considered definitive.

Reinfection can occur via food items, such as rats and mice fed to snakes. Packaged turtle foods, commonly found in pet stores, have not been found to contain *Salmonella*.

Numerous case reports and epidemiologic studies have proven that reptiles, particularly baby freshwater turtles, are a major source of human salmonellosis, especially in children.[5] It was estimated that 14%, or 280,000 of the approximately 2,000,000 human cases of salmonellosis occurring yearly (1970, 1971) in the United States, were contracted from turtles.[180] Attempts to control the problem by testing turtles for *Salmonella* failed, and numerous human infections were traced to turtles certified as "*Salmonella*-free." Therefore, the Food and Drug Administration has ruled that it is illegal to sell viable turtle eggs or live turtles with a carapace length less than four inches in the United States.[8] (Marine turtles are excepted from this law because they have not been demonstrated to be a significant reservoir of *Salmonella*. Sale of these sea animals should be restricted, however, because they are endangered species which do not reproduce in captivity. Viable turtle eggs and baby turtles sold for "bona fide scientific, educational, or exhibitional purposes" are also exempted from this law.) Restricting turtle sales has resulted in a marked decrease in turtle-associated human salmonellosis.[60a]

An appropriate, updated limerick might be:

There once was a maiden named Nelly
Who developed a pain in her belly.
Some bacilli she caught
From a turtle she bought
Turned her stool into cranberry jelly.

Besides *Salmonella* and *Arizona* spp., the enteric flora of herpetofauna can include other bacteria potentially pathogenic for man. *Aeromonas, Enterobacter, Klebsiella, Pseudomonas, Citrobacter, Serratia,* and *Proteus* are found in the feces of turtles.[201] *Edwardsiella tarda* has been found in the stool of American alligators[300] and in turtles.[148] *Yersinia enterocolitica* and related bacteria were isolated from the feces of frogs.[36] *Listeria monocytogenes* was isolated from the feces of frogs (*Rana p. pipiens* and *R. catesbeiana*) and a painted turtle (*Chrysemys picta*),[37] but these poikilotherms may have passively carried this organism from a polluted environment. No evidence of multiplication of *L. monocytogenes* in frogs was found after oral inoculation.[35]

Mycobacterial Infections. In captive reptiles and amphibians, mycobacterial infections are fairly common. They cause multifocal granulomatous lesions in the skin and internal organs, resulting in disease which is usually chronic, debilitating, and eventually fatal. Mycobacterial infections of cold-blooded vertebrates are reviewed by Vogel,[283] and their pathology is described by Ippen.[141]

Most mycobacteria causally associated with disease in herpetofauna are rapid growers in Group IV of Runyon's classification of acid-fast bacilli.[153,219] Valid species include *M. ranae (fortuitum)* first isolated from frogs by Kuester in 1905, *M. xenopi,* a non-chromogen, in Runyon's Group III, first isolated from the South African clawed toad, *Xenopus laevis*, by Schwabacher in 1959,[249] *M. thamnopheos*, first isolated from garter snakes *(Thamnophis sirtalis*) by Aronson in 1929,[12] and *M. chelonei (friedmanii, runyoni, abscessus, borstalense)* originally isolated from turtles by Friedmann in 1903. *M. marinum (balnei)* has been isolated from lymphosarcoma lesions in *Xenopus laevis* (see p. 205). Speciation is of more than academic interest because some Mycobacteria found in herpetofauna, e.g., *M. ranae, M. chelonei, M. marinum,* and *M. xenopi,* have been recognized as pathogens in man (see p. 108).

Various herpetofauna are suitable laboratory hosts for *M. ulcerans,* the cause of a severe necrotizing panniculitis and dermatitis of man in certain tropical and subtropical countries.[197] It is hypothesized that reptiles or amphibians could harbor this organism in nature and could possibly be a reservoir of infection for man.[198]

It has also been claimed that leprosy is transmissible experimentally to reptiles.[176,177] If confirmed, this could lead to major breakthroughs in leprosy research.

Saprophytic mycobacteria are commonly found in aquaria and in water tanks containing reptiles and amphibians. Thus, the isolation of acid-fast bacilli from lesions, especially on the skin, is not enough to prove the pathogenic role of the organism. Koch's postulates must be fulfilled to prove the pathogenicity of a given organism. Short of this, acid-fast bacilli must at least be demonstrated histologically associated with lesions to give credence to their pathogenic role and to prove that organisms found in culture are not just contaminants.

Reichenbach-Klinke and Elkan report that animals that are debilitated owing to injury, malnutrition, or other disease are most susceptible to mycobacterial infection and that the presence of the bacteria alone is not sufficient to induce disease.[233] This parallels the situation with tuberculosis in man.

Cutaneous mycobacterial infections in amphibians may produce granulomatous ulcers that may be fungating, or there may be a diffuse tuberculous dermatitis (Fig. 3–18). Diagnosis is readily confirmed by culture, direct smear, and biopsy of the lesion. If the disease is limited to internal organs, clinical diagnosis is much more difficult. There may be progressive wasting before the animal dies. Granulomas in internal

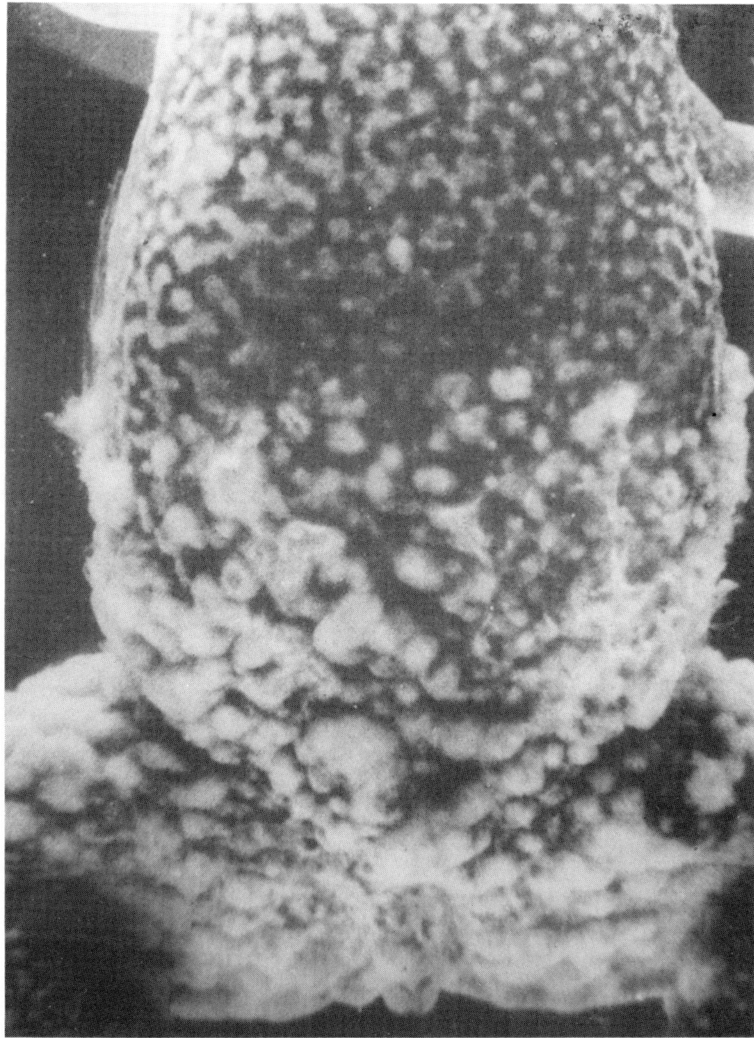

Fig. 3–18. African clawed frog *(Xenopus laevis)* with diffuse mycobacterial dermatitis. (From Reichenbach-Klinke, H. and Elkan, E.: The Principal Diseases of Lower Vertebrates. New York, Academic Press, 1965. Photograph courtesy of Dr. E. Elkan.)

organs may be miliary (Fig. 3–19). Large granulomas may be palpable, cause urinary, alimentary, or respiratory obstruction (Fig. 3–20), or displace a vital organ.

At necropsy, the skin of the affected amphibians should be examined by transillumination to demonstrate the "moth-eaten" appearance caused by diffuse tuberculous dermatitis. Reichenbach-Klinke and Elkan found the liver, spleen, kidney, and testes to be involved most commonly in systemic disease.[233] Tubercles tend to be expansile rather than invasive. Thus, a frog's lung might be completely consolidated, but the disease process might not extend beyond the pleura.

Histologically, mycobacterial infections in herpetofauna are charac-

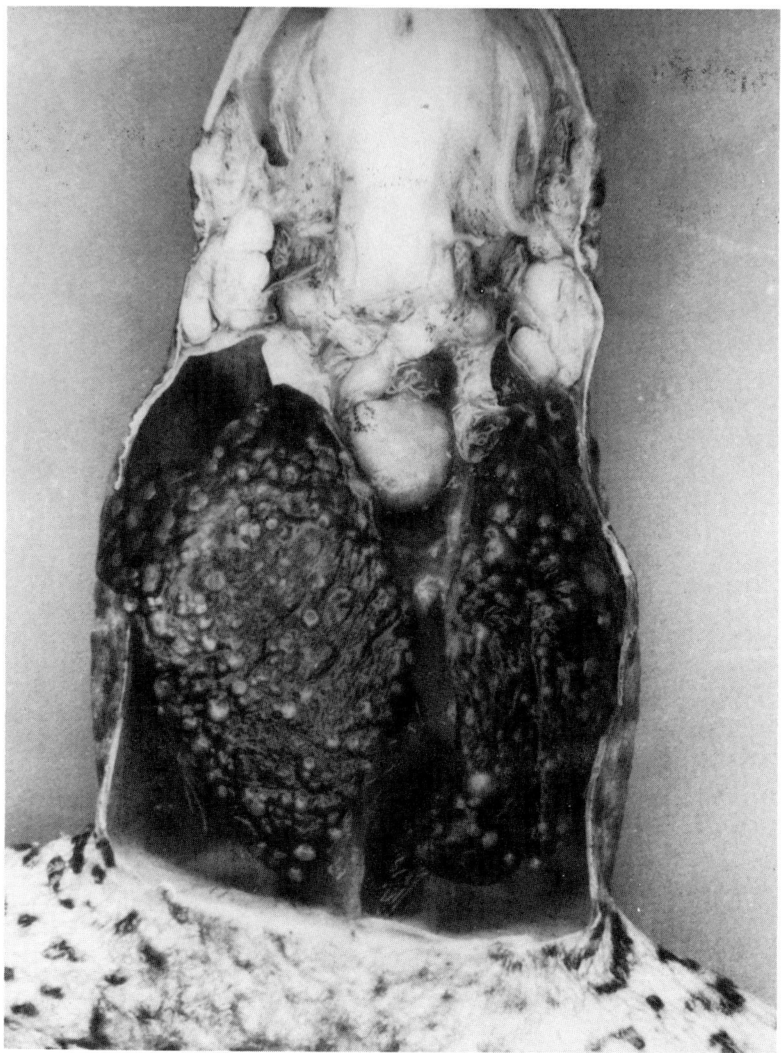

Fig. 3–19. Multiple disseminated mycobacterial granulomas in the liver of a toad *(Bufo bufo)*. (From Reichenbach-Klinke, H. and Elkan, E.: The Principal Diseases of Lower Vertebrates. New York, Academic Press, 1965. Photograph courtesy of Elizabeth Canning.)

terized by a granulomatous response, either diffuse or focally discrete, in which acid-fast bacilli can be demonstrated (Fig. 3–21). Central caseous necrosis may be present in reptilian tubercles, but is not prominent in amphibian lesions. Calcification is very rarely seen in amphibian or reptilian tubercles. Multinucleated giant cells are found occasionally. In cases where the liver is extensively destroyed, melanin, a normal constituent of amphibian and reptilian hepatic tissue, may be released into the blood and concentrated in the kidney where it is demonstrable as dark pigment granules in tubular epithelium.

Machicao and LaPlaca found a 19.6% prevalence rate of granulomatous disease due to an unidentified *Mycobacterium* in wild Bolivian frogs

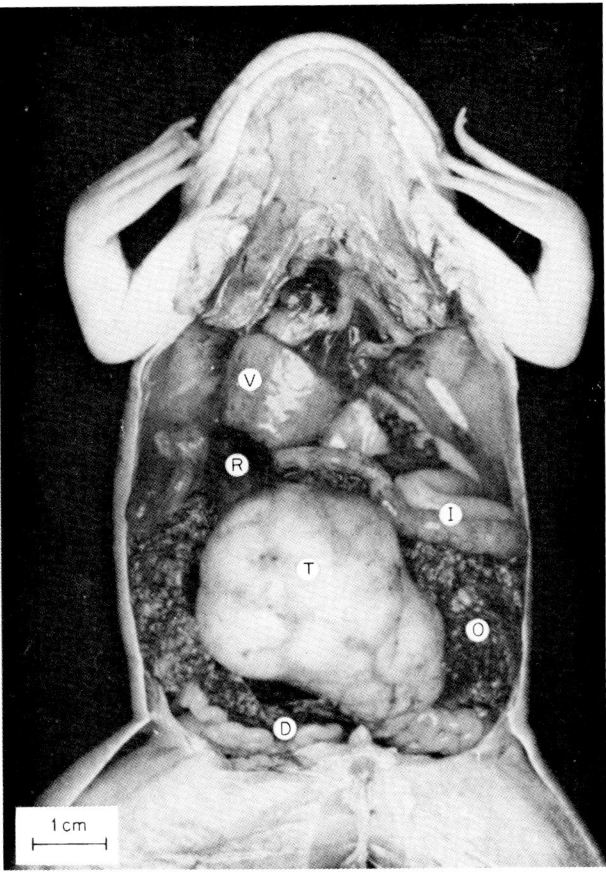

Fig. 3–20. Massive mycobacterial granuloma obstructing the rectum in an adult female African clawed frog *(Xenopus laevis)*. **D**, oviduct; **I**, small intestine; **O**, ovary; **R**, ileorectal junction distended by fecal matter; **T**, mycobacterial granuloma obstructing rectum; **V**, ventricle. (From Reichenbach-Klinke, H. and Elkan, E.: The Principal Diseases of Lower Vertebrates. New York, Academic Press, 1965. Photograph courtesy of Dr. E. Elkan.)

(Pleurodema cinerea and *P. mormoratus)*.[191] The skin and liver were most often involved, but lesions were also seen in the gastrointestinal tract and mesentery and, less often, in the kidney, spleen, lungs, trachea, and bronchi. Acid-fast bacilli (AFB) were seen among chitinous remains in the frogs' guts and within the intestinal tract of certain insects commonly eaten by these frogs. The mycobacteria could not be cultured from the frog lesions on a variety of media held at 18°, 25°, or 37°C. No bacteriologic studies were reported on the AFB found in the insects, but the authors suggest these may have been the source of the amphibian disease. Because peripheral nerves were commonly involved in the infection, and because macrophages often appeared crammed with AFB (such cells are called globi in human leprosy), and because the organisms could not grow in vitro, Machicao and LaPlaca referred to the lesions as "lepra-like granulomas."

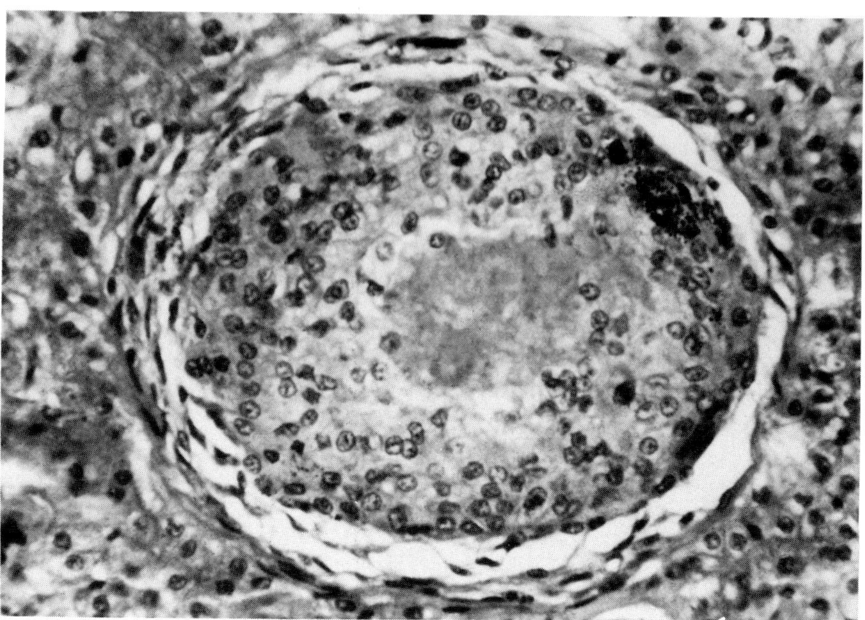

Fig. 3–21. Mycobacterial granuloma in the liver of a python *(Python spilotes)*. A zone of caseous necrosis is surrounded concentrically by mononuclear inflammatory cells and a thin fibrous capsule. 200×. (From Ippen, R.: Vergleichende pathologische Untersuchungen über die spontane und experimentelle Tuberkulose der Kaltblüter. Abh. Deutsch. Akad. Wiss. Berlin Klass Med. *1*:1–90, 1964. Photograph courtesy of Dr. Rudolf Ippen.)

Chemotherapy of amphibian and reptilian mycobacterial disease has not been investigated. It would seem more practical to eliminate infected animals from a colony and to disinfect contaminated quarters. I am not aware of the usefulness of tuberculin testing in herpetofauna to detect infected animals.

Various *Mycobacterium* species that are pathogenic in herpetofauna can also cause disease in man. *M. xenopi* has been isolated from cases of human pulmonary disease.[224] *M. ranae (fortuitum)* is occasionally found as a saprophyte in sputum, but it has also been isolated from abscesses, pulmonary infections, and a case of endocarditis in man.[224] *M. cheloni (abscessus)* was associated with an outbreak of injection abscesses in people, apparently due to contamination of a batch of histamine.[140] *M. marinum* causes a granulomatous dermatitis that may ulcerate, which is known as swimming pool granuloma or Daphne sore. Some human infections with *M. marinum* have been traced to contaminated fish tanks.[3,124]

The role of herpetofauna as reservoirs of atypical mycobacterial infection in man has not been investigated. It is probable that man and cold-blooded animals usually get infected from environmental sources rather than by interspecies transmission. It would appear advisable, however, to regard mycobacteria isolated from amphibians and reptiles as potential human pathogens and to deal with infected material accordingly.

Leptospirosis. In frogs, turtles,[113] and snakes leptospirosis occurs spontaneously. In nature, it is most likely that reptiles acquire infection by contact with infected water or by eating infected prey such as rodents.[6]

Abdulla and Karstad infected snakes and turtles with *Leptospira pomona* by direct inoculation and demonstrated that snakes could transmit the infection among themselves by direct contact.[1] Leptospires were demonstrable in snake kidneys 6½ months after inoculation, and infections were shown to persist after a 70-day period of induced hibernation. One snake infected with leptospirosis was found to have interstitial nephritis, but most infected reptiles did not have any associated lesions. In one field study, agglutinins to several serotypes, including *ballum, icterohemorrhagiae,* and *pomona* were found in snake sera, but no leptospires were cultured from the kidneys or livers.[299] A high prevalence of infection by *L. interrogans* serotype *tarrasovi* was found in turtles from settling ponds in Georgia. The organisms were isolated from the turtles' kidneys and cloacae by inoculation of hamsters.[113] Reptiles might be a reservoir for leptospirosis, and this might be especially significant over the winter months. Evaluation of this awaits the gathering of more field data.

Miscellaneous Bacterial Infections. *Erysipelothrix insidiosa* was isolated from the liver and spleen of a 6- to 8-week-old caiman *(Caiman crocodilus)* and as part of mixed bacterial flora from cutaneous lesions of an old crocodile *(Crocodilus acutus).* Evidence in this report suggests that *E. insidiosa* was the primary cause of disease in the two crocodilians.[152]

Pasteurella pseudotuberculosis was isolated from hepatic lesions in a Greek tortoise *(Testudo graeca)*[89] and *Serratia marcescens* was isolated from an inflamed stifle joint of a teju (tegu) lizard *(Tupinambis teguixin).*[2]

Clostridium novyi can cause fatal septicemia in turtles; the signs are anorexia and lethargy. A vaccine was prepared that was effective in preventing the infection.[79] *Clostridium welchii* was in a mixed bacterial flora associated with post-traumatic gangrene of the legs and septicemia in iguanas.[87]

The actinomycete, *Dermatophilus congolensis,* was the apparent cause of hyperkeratotic nodules on the skin of the legs and trunk of two marble lizards *(Calotes mystaceus).*[9] *D. congolensis* was found in a subcutaneous abscess and in superficial nodular skin lesions in bearded dragon lizards *(Amphibolurus barbatus).*[213,258]

Staphylococcus epidermis was isolated from purulent infections of the legs of frogs *(Rana pipiens),* but this was much less common than infection by *Aeromonas hydrophila.*[110] Like the latter infection, staphylococcal cellulitis responds to tetracycline. (The treatment of redleg disease is discussed earlier in this chapter.)

Other bacterial infections in amphibians cited by Reichenbach-Klinke and Elkan include a septicemia of *Rana temporaria* caused by a gram-negative rod, *Bacterium ranicida,* and an epidemic in frogs characterized by enteritis, edema, and hemorrhages caused by a gram-negative diplobacillus, *Diplobacterium ranarum.*[233]

VIRAL INFECTIONS

The only significant attention given to viral infections of herpetofauna has been relevant to oncogenesis and to a possible reservoir of arbovirus infections. Volume 126 of the Annals of the New York Academy of Sciences (August 19, 1965) is entitled "Viral Diseases of Poikilothermic Vertebrates," but in 46 papers and 680 pages it has nothing on viral diseases of reptiles. Two entities in amphibians are covered in some detail—lymphosarcoma in *Xenopus laevis*, the South African clawed toad, and Lucké's renal adenocarcinoma in the leopard frog, *Rana pipiens* (see pp. 199 to 205). Studies on viruses associated with reptilian tumors are reviewed by Jacobson.[149b]

Polyhedral Cytoplasmic Amphibian Virus (PCAV). This virus has been isolated from normal appearing tissue of leopard frogs *(Rana pipiens)*, bullfrogs *(R. catesbeiana)*, and newts *(Notophthalmus viridescens)* and, apparently as an incidental finding, in Lucké tumors of leopard frogs. PCAV is not known to cause lesions or illness in these natural hosts, but it causes death with multiple visceral lesions when inoculated into Fowler's toad *(Bufo woodhousei fowleri)*.[56]

Tadpole Edema Virus (TEV). This type of PCAV can cause a fatal illness in bullfrog tadpoles up to two months old. Infection can be induced by putting the virus in the tadpoles' water, and it is likely that the infection spreads this way in nature. Death occurs in five to 13 days after infection. Lesions include edema and necrosis of the liver, kidneys, gastrointestinal tract, and skeletal muscle.[307]

Viral Encephalitis. Eastern (EE), western (WE), St. Louis (SLE), and Japanese B (JBE) encephalitis viruses have been isolated from snakes captured in the wild. EE, WE, SLE, and two other arboviruses that can infect man, Powassan (POW) and Bunyamwera, have been isolated from turtles captured in the wild.[40a,130] There is serologic evidence that snakes can be naturally infected with POW and vesicular stomatitis virus (VSV), turtles with VSV, lizards with EE and tick-borne encephalitis (TBE), and American alligators with EE.[130]

Reptiles often respond to EE or WE infection with a rise in neutralizing antibody titer, but they are not known to become clinically ill. Congenital infection of snakes with WE and transmission of virus to mosquitoes feeding on infected snakes has been demonstrated.[106] Reptiles might be a significant reservoir of infection for eastern and western encephalitis, especially over the winter months, and the same may be true of Japanese B encephalitis. In unpublished data, Detels reported that JBE virus has been isolated from water snakes, frogs, and toads caught in Taiwan. Immunologic evidence exists that cobras *(Naja naja)* in China are hosts for this virus.[256] JBE was isolated from two rat snakes *(Elaphe rufodorsata)* among 747 snakes surveyed in Korea.[149b] However, in a survey of Japanese snakes, JBE virus could not be isolated from any of 305 serpents representing six species, and only six out of 270 snakes had low levels of specific antibody. It was also very difficult to experimentally infect Japanese snakes with JBE. It was concluded that in Japan snakes do not play a significant role as a reservoir of this infection.[266]

Herpes Viruses. A herpes-like virus has been isolated from iguanas.[56a] (References for cultivation of cell lines from poikilotherms are in the bibliography of the article by Clark and Karzon.[56a]) A similar virus was associated with a disease in iguanas characterized by anorexia, lethargy, lymphocytosis, lymphoid hyperplasia in the spleen, and mononuclear cell infiltration of liver, myocardium, and bone marrow.[102c]

Herpesvirus-like infection in two Pacific pond turtles *(Clemmys marmorata)* was associated with sudden onset of lethargy, anorexia, and weakness. Cowdry type A intranuclear inclusion bodies and herpes-like virions were demonstrable in the liver and spleen.[102c]

A herpes virus causes grey patch disease, a cutaneous infection, in two- to three-month-old green sea turtles *(Chelonia mydas)*. Epidermal cells contain basophilic intranuclear inclusion bodies.[149b]

Other Viral Diseases. A pox-like virus was associated with a dermatitis in spectacled caimans *(Caiman sclerops)*.[149b] Grey-white circular lesions were scattered over the body. Epidermal cells contained large eosinophilic intracytoplasmic inclusion bodies.

A paramyxovirus was isolated from the lungs of fer-de-lances *(Bothrops atrox)* that died in an epizootic at a snake farm. There was loss of muscle tone and terminal gaping of the mouth with discharge of exudate from the glottis.[149b]

Some intraerythrocytic pathogens, formerly thought to be protozoan, are now thought to be viral (*Pirhaemocyton* sp.) or rickettsial *(Haemobartonella* and *Grahamella* sp.). These pathogens are discussed on page 132. Q fever, a rickettsial infection, is discussed in the section on acariasis (pp. 173 to 175).

Algal and Mycotic Infections

No mycoses of major epizootiological importance affect captive herpetofauna. Fungal infections may occur opportunistically, e.g., secondary to malnutrition, dampness, cold, or debilitating illness. The skin and respiratory system are the sites most commonly involved.[149a]

Algae. The shells of aquatic turtles are commonly covered with algae. Such growth might be symbiotic, providing camouflage for the turtle in its native habitat.[137] In captivity, however, if water contaminated with leftover food is allowed to stagnate, algae may become deposited in layers on the shell, lifting up the margin of the shields (large scales on the shell) and causing their desquamation. Eventually, the malpighian layer and underlying bone are eroded and the turtle may die a couple of weeks later.[137] Some infections of the shell thought to be caused by algae may have been ulcerative shell disease caused by *Beneckea chitinovora* (see p. 96).

Infection of the chelonian shell by algae is prevented by adequate sanitation. Treatment consists of washing the shell with Lugol's solution or 1% copper sulfate.[137]

In the study of the epizoophytic algae of North American turtles, Edgren, et al. found that the amount and distribution of algae on the shell varied according to the habits of the host species, especially the relative amounts of time spent in the water or basking in the sun.[80] They considered the relationship between turtles and algae in the wild to be commensal, and they made no mention of pathologic findings.

Mycotic Pneumonia. This infection is occasionally found in turtles. *Aspergillus* can cause consolidation and gangrene of the lungs, terrestrial tortoises being affected more often than aquatic turtles.[136] *Beauvaria bassiana* caused fatal infections of the lung in two giant tortoises at the Chicago Zoological Park, and pulmonary infection was experimentally induced in a box turtle by direct inoculation of the fungus into the lung.[108] (*Beauvaria bassiana* is the first microbial organism found to cause a disease. Bassi described it as a pathogen in silkworms in 1835.) A third tortoise at the Chicago Zoo died of mycotic pneumonia caused by *Paecilomyces fumoso-roseus.*

Basidiobolus ranarum. This saprophytic fungus is found in the gut of salamanders, frogs, toads, turtles, lizards, and snakes in various parts of the world. It has been found in the gut of herpetofauna in Arkansas and Missouri.[217] It was found in a granulomatous lesion in the mouth of an Aldabra tortoise *(Testudo gigantea elephantina).*[149a] *B. ranarum* is a cause of subcutaneous phycomycosis in people in Indonesia and Africa.[187,303] The importance of the reptilian and amphibian hosts in maintaining the fungus in nature is not known.

Miscellaneous Mycoses. *Geotrichum candidum* has been isolated from caseous subcutaneous nodules in a banded watersnake *(Natrix sipedon)* and from cutaneous pustules in a garter snake *(Thamnophis* sp.*)* and in carpet snakes *(Morelia spilotes variegata).* A continuously damp environment is thought to predispose to cutaneous geotrichosis in snakes.[222] The infection starts between the scales and spreads to cause necrosis of contiguous scales.[203] Differential diagnoses include abscesses (p. 96) and scale rot (p. 195).

An adult anaconda *(Eunectes murinus)* autopsied by the author at the National Zoological Park in Washington, D.C. had an infection of the mouth that looked like ulcerative stomatitis (see p. 84), with hyperemia, ulceration, and caseous necrosis of the oral mucosa. The disease process extended into the mandible. Microscopic examination revealed a mycotic stomatitis and osteomyelitis. The fungal elements were pigmented and were histologically identified as belonging to the genus *Cladosporium* (Fig. 3–22). A fungus with similar morphology was found in a granuloma in the lumbar muscles of a captive tiger salamander *(Ambystoma tigrinum mavortium).*[210]

Saprolegnia, an aquatic mold, frequently infects cold-blooded animals, *S. parasitica* being the most common pathogen in the genus. It can infect tadpoles,[41] fish, turtles, and salamanders[277] and is a common disease problem in colonies of the mudpuppy *(Necturus maculosus).*[161] The mold produces a white mycelial growth on the skin starting at the cephalic end. The disease is highly contagious, probably through direct contact. Affected animals can be treated by dipping them for 15 seconds in a 1:15,000 solution of malachite green (0.2 g malachite green in 3 liters of distilled water). Immersion in the dye solution for much longer than 15 seconds causes massive epidermal exfoliation. Treatment should be repeated once daily for two or three days.

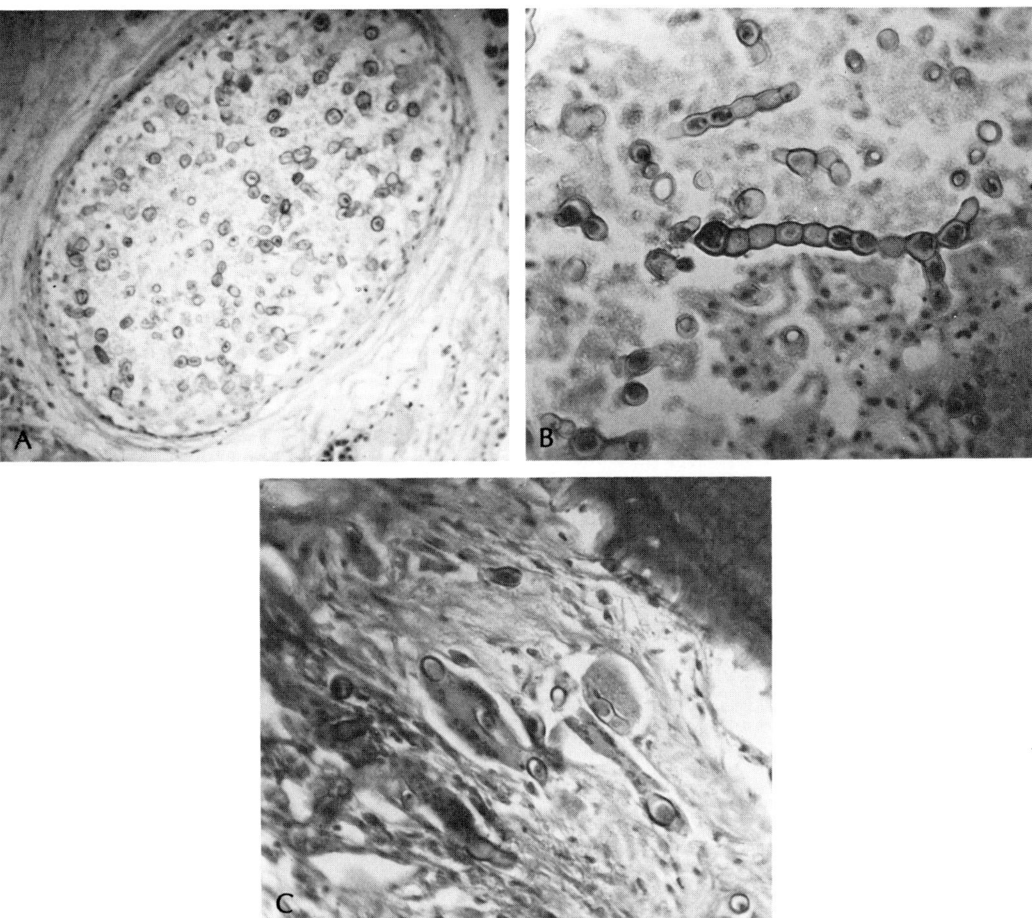

Fig. 3–22. Mycotic (*Cladosporium* sp.) stomatitis in an anaconda *(Eunectes murinus)*. Phagocytosis of fungal elements by giant cells is seen in C. The dark tissue in the upper right corner of C is bone (mandible). **A**, 125×. **B** and **C**, 250×.

An alternative, but less efficient treatment for *Saprolegnia* infection in mudpuppies is immersion for two minutes in a 1:2000 solution of copper sulfate. This treatment must be repeated daily for at least five days and then continued once a week until there is a clinical cure.

Cutaneous mycotic infections in axolotls *(Ambystoma mexicanum)* can be treated with baths of 0.001% chloramine (paratoluol sodium sulphonchloramide).[34] Mercurochrome, 0.002 to 0.004%, is also said to be an effective fungicidal bath.[34]

Cephalosporium sp. was found in a swelling in the gut of a grass snake *(Tropidonotus natrix)* and in necrotic lesions of the liver and lungs of three caimans *(Caiman sclerops)*.[279] Hyphae invaded the walls of thrombosed blood vessels. The crocodilians had been on an experimental vitamin E deficient diet which may have increased their susceptibility to cephalosporiosis.

Fusarium solani was isolated from ulcers on the eyes, skin, and shell and from normal-appearing skin and gut of baby loggerhead turtles *(Caretta caretta)*. Fusariosis was associated with high mortality during their first six months after hatching.[231] *Fusarium* sp. has been found in cutaneous infections in tortoises, a caiman, and a python and has been associated with corneal ulceration in a rainbow boa *(Epicrates cenchris)*.[149a]

A septate fungus of undetermined species caused cutaneous nodules up to 2 cm in diameter in 46% of Malayan toads *(Bufo melanostictus)* caught in or around Kuala Lumpur. One third of the toads with skin lesions also had visceral granulomas, usually involving the liver and kidney and occasionally the spleen, ovary, heart, or lungs.[75]

Phycomycosis was found in an intussuscepted colon of a Jackson's chameleon *(Chameleo jacksoni)*.[253]

Mycotic lesions are occasionally submitted to the Registry of Tumors in Lower Animals (see p. 209). Included in the Registry are two cases of adiaspiromycosis in red-spotted newts *(Notophthalmus viridescens)*.

Parasitic Diseases

Reptiles and amphibians harbor a huge variety of protozoan and metazoan parasites. The parastic burden is often heavy, and every body surface and organ may be invaded by some kind of larval or adult parasite. Indeed, parasitism is so common that it is often difficult to determine its clinical significance.

In general, the parasites that are most successful in propagating themselves are the ones that do the least harm to their hosts, the most successful relationships being commensal or symbiotic. Captivity-caused stress, e.g., crowding or altered diet, may change the host-parasite relationships and result in disease. In general, it is those parasites with a direct life cycle that can increase disproportionately in captive specimens and become pathogenic. Parasites with indirect life cycles are less likely to increase in numbers or be transmitted in a collection because of the nonavailability of suitable intermediate hosts.

In the following discussion, emphasis will be placed on those parasites that are most common and that have known pathogenic significance. Many of the references cited contain bibliographies that will enable the interested reader to pursue the subject further. An extensive list and bibliography of the parasites of Amphibia has been published by Walton,[292,293,294] and surveys of the endoparasites of some South African and North American snakes have been published by Fantham and Porter.[84,85] The parasitic diseases of reptiles have also been reviewed by Marcus[196] and Telford,[273] and an informative review of parasitism in laboratory reptiles and amphibians was written by Kaplan.[159]

Protozoan Diseases

Amebiasis. Reichenbach-Klinke and Elkan list half a dozen amebae found in amphibians, but ascribe pathogenicity only to one, *Entamoeba ranarum*, which is found in the gut and liver of tadpoles.[233]

Many different species of amebae are found in reptiles, but the one that has been recognized as a pathogen and has received the most attention is *Entamoeba invadens*. This organism causes high morbidity and mortality among captive snakes and, to a lesser degree, in captive (especially carnivorous) lizards.

Amebiasis is contracted by ingestion of infective cysts passed in the stool. The amebae develop in the gut into motile trophozoites which multiply by binary fission. Trophozoites phagocytize particulate matter and can invade tissue. Some trophozoites are transformed into cysts which are passed in the stool, and the life cycle is completed when another suitable host ingests these cysts. Trophozoites are also passed in the stool, but they probably are not infective.

E. invadens occasionally is pathogenic in turtles, but these animals usually harbor this intestinal parasite without apparent ill effects. It is possible that turtles may act as a reservoir of infection for snakes and lizards. Meerovitch suggests that the commensal relationship in turtles may be due to the higher proportion of plant material in their diet, which provides starch needed by the amebae for encystment, whereas in snakes, which are strictly carnivorous, the trophozoite form is favored.[207,208] In humans the trophozoites of *Entamoeba histolytica* are associated with tissue damage. People who chronically pass cysts rather than trophozoites in their stools are often asymptomatic. The same relationship between stage of parasite and pathogenicity probably applies in reptiles.

Definitive diagnosis of amebiasis is made by demonstrating the protozoa in the stool, or in impression smears of the liver or other infected tissues. In wet preparations, trophozoites may be observed to move rapidly in one direction by extension of pseudopodia. They ingest leucocytes, liver cells, cellular debris, bacteria, and starch grains, but have not been observed to ingest erythrocytes.[107] The range and average dimensions of the trophozoites are given in Table 3–1. Cysts are 11.0 to 20.2μ in diameter (average 13.88 μ) and have four nuclei when mature.

Reptiles that become ill with *Entamoeba invadens* suffer ulcerative gastritis and colitis, the latter usually being more severe than the former. The small intestine is less frequently and less severely involved. The classic study of the pathogenesis and pathology of amebiasis in

*Table 3–1.** Size of Trophozoites, *Entamoeba invadens* (Average Dimensions in Parentheses)

	FROM INTESTINE	FROM LIVER
Length (μ)	10–34 (15.68)	9.2–38.6 (18.8)
Width (μ)	8–30 (13.29)	9.2–27.6 (16.0)
Nuclear diameter (μ)	3.5–7.3 (4.57)	3.6–7.3 (5.0)
Ratio, nuclear diameter: Trophozoite diameter	0.28–0.34 (0.31)	0.26–0.30 (0.28)

*Adapted from Geiman, Q.M. and Ratcliffe, H.L.: Morphology and life cycle of an amoeba producing amoebiasis in reptiles. Parasitology, *28*:208–228, 1936.

snakes was published by Ratcliffe and Geiman in 1938.[230] My observations of naturally occurring cases confirm their findings. They found that snakes suffered at least a two-week period of anorexia after they ingested infective cysts. Progressive listlessness and weight loss occur, and droppings may contain blood and mucus. The case fatality rate approaches 100%. In experimental infections death occurs between 13 and 77 days after inoculation, survival time being inversely proportional to the size of the inoculum. In a spontaneous epizootic the disease can spread rapidly through a collection, and every snake may become ill and die.

Postmortem findings include ulcerative gastritis, enteritis, and colitis. Lesions begin as small ulcers that coalesce until extensive necrosis of a large segment of bowel is apparent. Lesions are most common and most severe in the colon, in which extensive hemorrhage may be evident (Fig. 3–23), or there may be severe caseous necrosis of the mucosa (Fig. 3–24), and the serosa may appear cyanotic and injected (Fig. 3–25). Destruction of the bowel wall may be so extensive that propulsion of gut contents cannot occur. When asked about a snake's bowel function in such a case, the owner, who may not have noticed earlier blood and mucus in the droppings, might only be aware of the snake's failure to pass stool during the last few days of life.

The organisms are spread hematogenously to other organs where they can be demonstrated histologically, often without accompanying reaction or necrosis. Hepatic abscesses, portal thrombosis, and hepatic infarcts are common, however, and occasionally one sees a diffuse inflammatory response in the liver associated with amebae in the hepatic parenchyma (amebic hepatitis) (Fig. 3–26). Grossly, the liver may be swollen, mottled, or friable, and may contain discrete necrotic

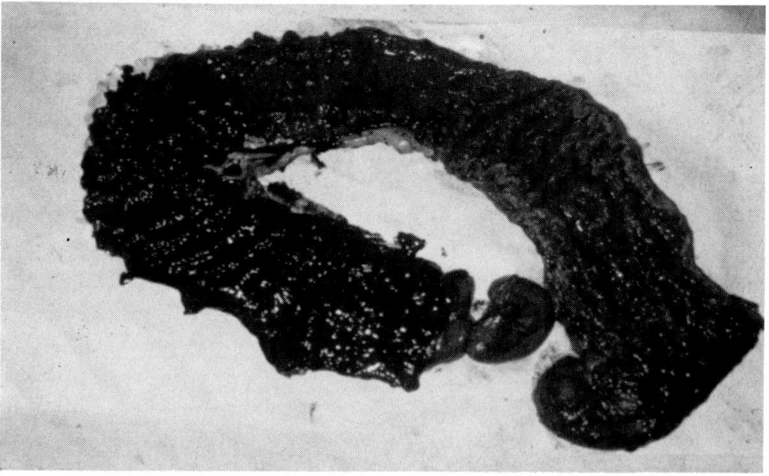

Fig. 3–23. Diffuse hemorrhagic colitis in a Komodo dragon (*Varanus komodoensis*) due to *Entamoeba invadens*. Thickened mucosal folds are in the proximal portion (top and right). Profuse melena is in the rectum (left and bottom). (Armed Forces Institute of Pathology Accession No. 1134021.)

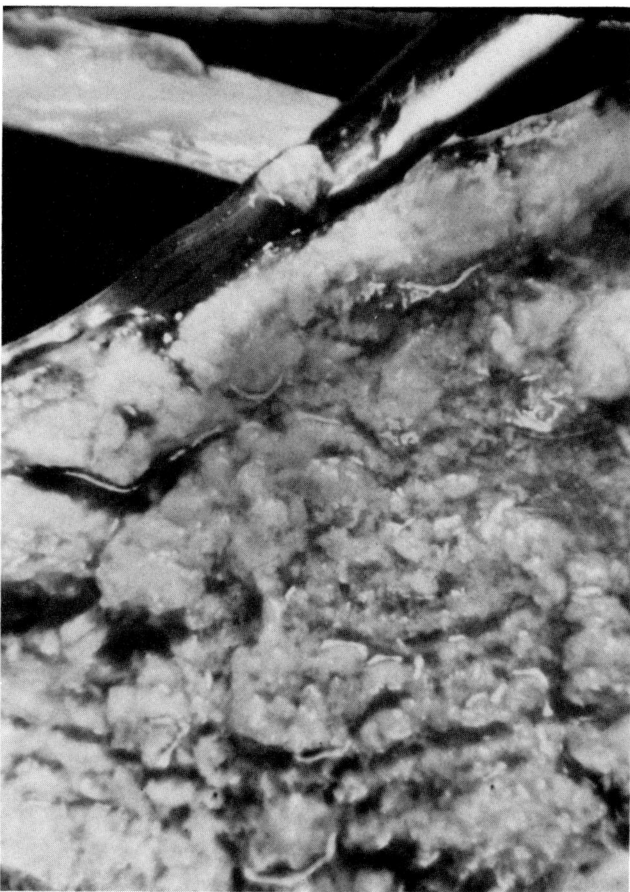

Fig. 3–24. Amebiasis in a Formosan (Taiwan) rat snake *(Zaocys dhumnades)*. Caseous necrosis of the colonic mucosa. (Armed Forces Institute of Pathology Accession No. 1058269.)

foci. Amebae can often be demonstrated in the kidneys, where they may be associated with focal necrosis.[309]

Bacteria always accompany amebae in enteric lesions and may also be associated with amebic lesions in other organs. Defining the relative importance of bacteria and amebae in causing pathologic change is problematic, but it is likely that both contribute significantly to the disease.[306] Amebiasis is often associated with thrombosis of vessels in the gut and liver, so tissue destruction results from infarction as well as from direct action of amebae and bacteria (Figs. 3–27, 3–28).

Diagnosis of amebiasis is made by demonstration of the cysts and/or trophozoites in the stool. It is best to examine that part of a stool containing blood and mucus. The chances of finding the amebae will be significantly increased if the stool is cultured on appropriate media.[76,199] Differential diagnosis includes salmonellosis and intestinal nematodiasis, but neither of these causes as high a morbidity or mortality, and both can be ruled out by appropriate stool examination and culture. It is possible that certain poisons might cause a hemor-

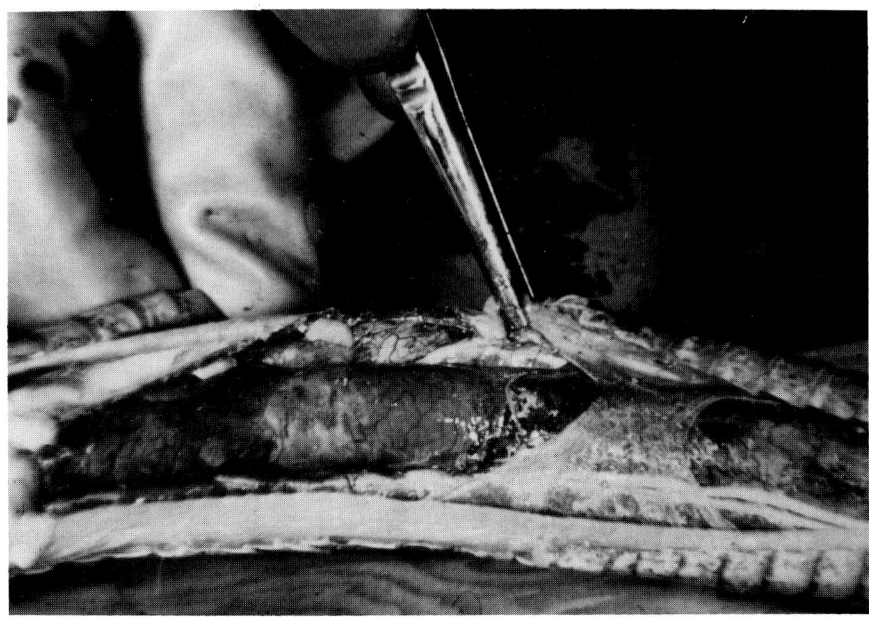

Fig. 3–25. Amebiasis in a Formosan (Taiwan) rat snake *(Zaocys dhumnades)*. The colon is markedly cyanotic and friable, the serosal vessels are injected, and there is fibrinopurulent peritonitis. (Armed Forces Institute of Pathology Accession No. 1058269.)

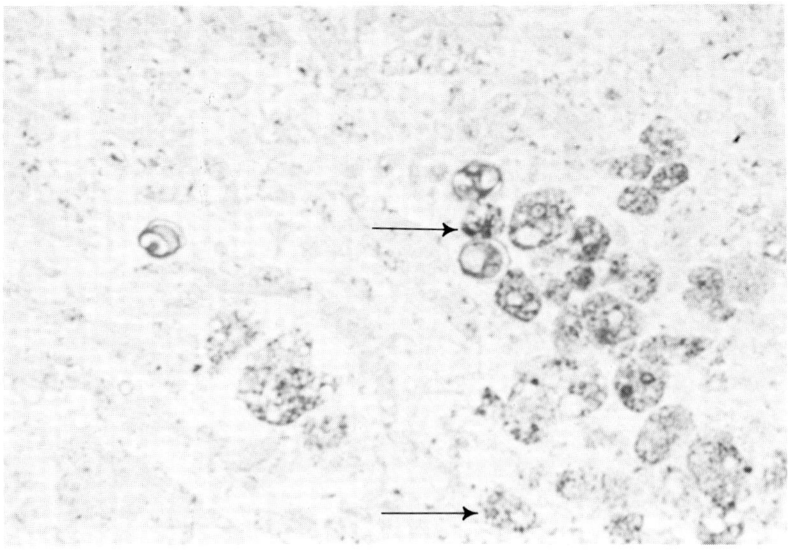

Fig. 3–26. Amoebae (arrows) in the liver of a Komodo dragon *(Varanus komodoensis)*. 250×. (Armed Forces Institute of Pathology Accession No. 1058270.)

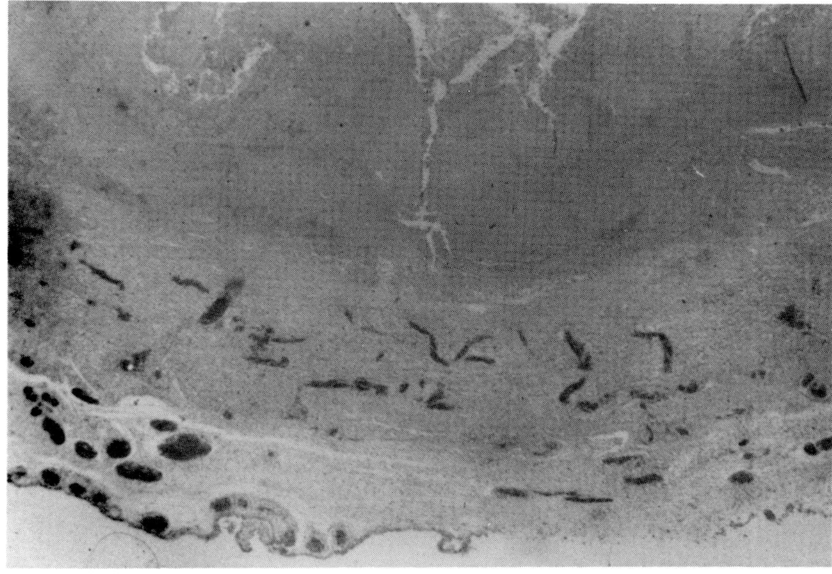

Fig. 3–27. Amebiasis in the colon of a lesser Indian rat snake *(Elaphe carinata)*. There is diffuse caseous necrosis of the mucosa (top) and submucosa and congestion and thrombosis of blood vessels in the muscularis and serosa. The serosa (bottom) is edematous. 8×. (Armed Forces Institute of Pathology Accession No. 1058270.)

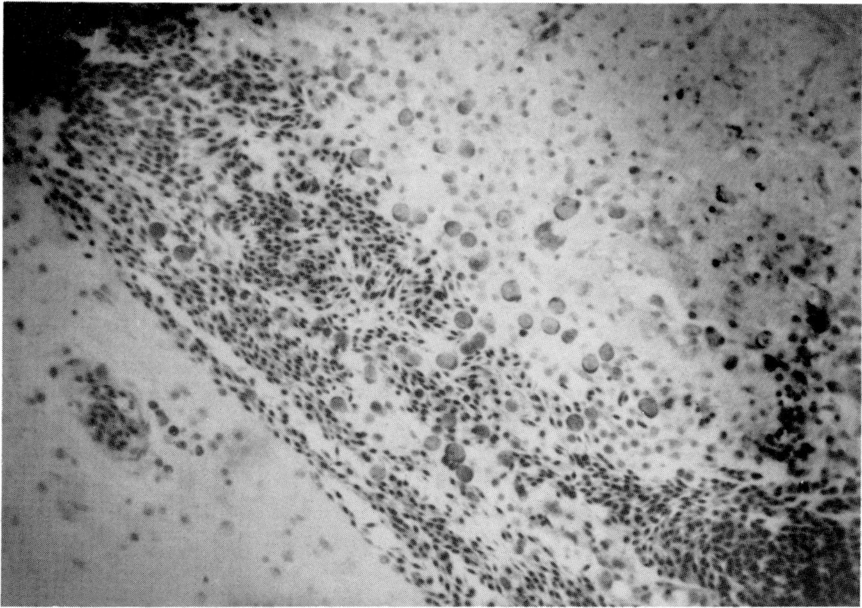

Fig. 3–28. Amebiasis in a lesser Indian rat snake *(Elaphe carinata)*. Serosa of the colon contains numerous amebae (large round cells) and cellular reaction. A thrombosed blood vessel is to the lower left. Giemsa stain, 125×. (Armed Forces Institute of Pathology Accession No. 1058270.)

rhagic or necrotizing enteritis, but history and laboratory tests should be definitive. (See also "necrotic enteritis," p. 84.)

Prevention of amebiasis depends on adequate quarantine and sanitation. Telford reports that *E. invadens* may be found as a commensal organism in snakes of the southeastern United States, but when amebic strains from one geographic area are permitted to infect hosts from another area, disease with invasion of tissues can occur.[273] Therefore, an adequate quarantine program includes examination of stools for parasites, keeping susceptible reptiles from different geographic areas caged separately and avoiding contact between carrier turtles and susceptible snakes and lizards. Separate tools for cleaning each cage should be kept, or instruments should be disinfected between use in each cage, and items such as water bowls or perches should be disinfected before being transferred from one cage to another. Prophylactic treatment of exposed snakes at the start of an epizootic may reduce losses.[78a]

Temperature has a marked effect on the outcome of amebiasis in reptiles. Barrow and Stockton found that snakes experimentally infected with *E. invadens* and then kept at 13° to 14°C (55° to 57°F) did not develop gross lesions even though amebae could be cultured from their intestines.[25] Other snakes, similarly inoculated and kept at 25°C (77°F), developed classic amebic lesions of gut and liver. Similar lesions were seen in snakes kept at 13°C for two weeks after inoculation and then transferred to 25°C. In a small group of snakes kept at 30°C (86°F) after inoculation, enteric and hepatic lesions developed, but the authors thought there was evidence of healing of intestinal lesions in one of these snakes. Photographic or descriptive documentation of this healing process was lacking. The therapeutic value of elevated temperature was more convincingly demonstrated by Meerovitch who found a lower rate and severity of infection in snakes kept at 35°C (98°F) than 25°C after infecting them with *E. invadens*.[209] If therapeutic trials of amebacides are done in reptiles, temperature must be controlled. If amebiasis in reptiles is treated by elevating the temperature, the patients should be observed for evidence of dehydration, which can occur quickly in overheated quarters.

Reptilian amebiasis has been treated successfully with amebacides used in human medicine. Success has been reported with the administration of diloxanide (Entamide) at a dosage of 500 mg per kg of body weight p.o.[88] Diloxanide furoate has been reported to be more effective than diloxanide in treating experimental amebiasis in rats and may be worth therapeutic trials in reptiles. Treatment with iodochlorhydroxyquin (Entero-Vioform, Ciba Pharmaceutical Co.) and the oral tetracyclines has also been recommended, but I am not familiar with the efficacy of these products in reptiles. Tetracycline hydrochloride, 400 to 800 mg per meter of body length, was not effective in curing or preventing amebiasis in snakes at a zoo.[78a] Paromomycin (Humatin, Parke-Davis Co.) is another amebacide; recommended dosage varies from 33 to 55 mg/kg (15 to 25 mg/lb)[27] to 110 mg/kg (50 mg/lb).[73] Schweinfurth found 25 to 100 mg per kg of paromomycin daily for four weeks cured amebiasis in snakes.[250] Bernstein recommends giving two doses of paromomycin one week apart for "necrotic enterohepatitis,"[27] which I presume is caused by amebiasis. All of the above drugs are suitable for intestinal amebiasis.

Amebiasis in a 125-pound Komodo dragon *(Varanus komodoensis)* was apparently cured by daily retention enemas for 14 days with 650 mg of diiodohydroxyquin (Diodoquin, Searle and Co.) in 150 ml of 0.9% saline followed by seven daily intramuscular injections of 65 mg of emetine hydrochloride.[119] Intramuscular emetine hydrochloride used to be the treatment of choice for extraintestinal amebiasis in man, but it has now been replaced by oral metronidazole (Flagyl, Searle and Co.), which is also considered to be the best therapeutic agent for severe intestinal amebiasis in man.[206a] The recommended dosage for metronidazole in reptiles is 275 mg/kg (125 mg/lb).[73] One such dose of metronidazole reportedly cured a symptomatic boa constrictor with amebae in its stool.[78a]

Entamoeba invadens is not known to be pathogenic for man or other mammals, but there are many similarities to *Entamoeba histolytica* in its biology and clinicopathologic manifestations,[199] so amebiasis in reptiles is a useful model for the study of human amebiasis.

Telford has reported that reptiles may harbor certain free-living Acanthamoebae in their gut.[267] I am not aware of any reports linking these forms with infection by free-living amebae *(Naegleria, Acanthamoeba,* and *Hartmannella* spp.) in the brain and lungs of man and lower mammals,[200,235] but the question of a reptilian reservoir of this disease may be worthy of study. *Acanthamoeba* spp. isolated from the intestines of snakes and lizards and injected into white rats caused widely disseminated infection.[304a]

Coccidiosis. Many species of Coccidia (most in the genus *Eimeria*) have been described in reptiles, and a few have been found in amphibians.[38,233] The life cycle of these obligate intracellular parasites may be direct,* with development (gametogony) occurring in epithelial cells of the host. Oocysts are released to the external environment where further development (sporogony) occurs. The cycle is completed when infective sporozoites are ingested by the host. Most coccidia of reptiles are highly host-specific. Most reptilian coccidia invade the intestine (Fig. 3–29), but a few are found in the biliary tract (Fig. 3–30). Oocysts are passed in the stool. *Isospora lieberkühni* has been found in the kidney of the edible frog, *Rana esculenta*, and renal coccidiosis, caused by *Klossiella boae*, has been described in a boa constrictor.[310]

Coccidiosis in wild reptiles is usually self-limiting, but under unsanitary conditions in captivity it may become severe enough to produce illness.[273] Wallach suggests that coccidiosis may cause enteritis, which may be hemorrhagic, in snakes and lizards.[285] Coccidiosis causes anorexia and restlessness in Old World chameleons (*Chameleo* spp.),[30] and may cause intestinal intussusception in these lizards.[314] The pathogenic role of coccidia can be evaluated clinically by therapeutic response, correlating symptomatology with oocyst count before and after treatment.

*Indirect life cycles of reptilian coccidia (*Sarcocystis* spp.) have recently been described, with reptiles as definitive hosts and prey such as rodents as intermediate hosts.[213a,213b]

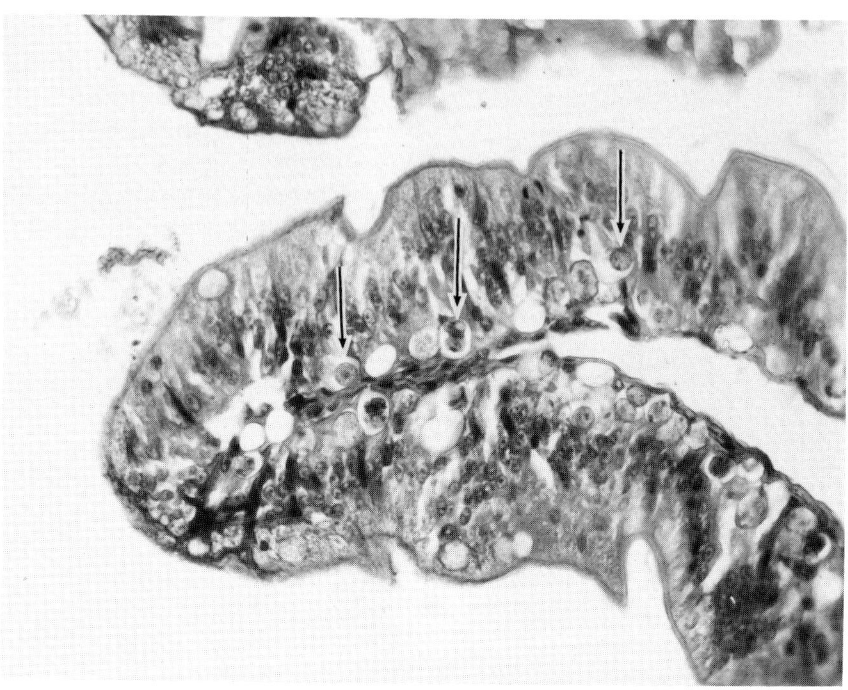

Fig. 3–29. Coccidiosis in the small intestine of a rattlesnake *(Crotalus* sp.). Developmental stages of the parasite are in the epithelium (arrows) without an inflammatory response. 375×. (Armed Forces Institute of Pathology Negative No. 72–4807.)

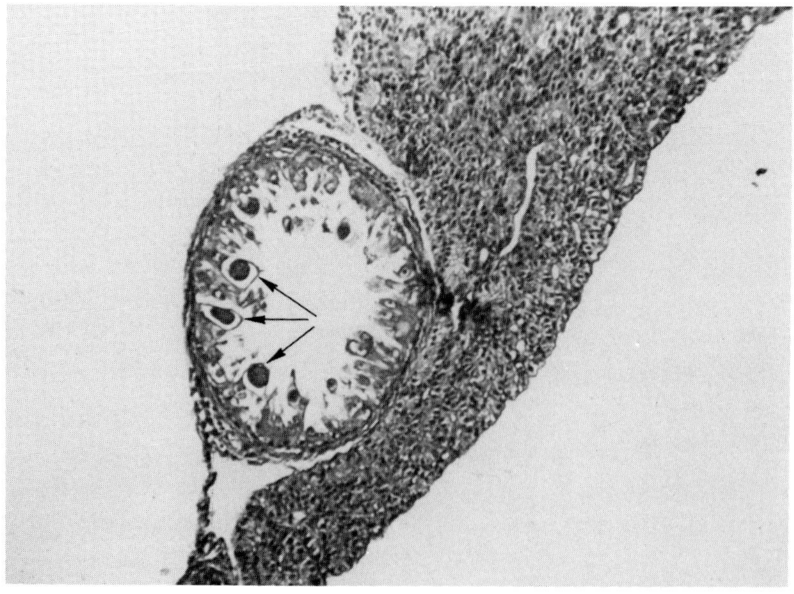

Fig. 3–30. Cholecystic coccidiosis in an anole lizard *(Anolis carolinensis)*. The protozoa (arrows) have caused little damage to the gallbladder and there is little inflammation. 160×.

Coccidia of the genus *Cryptosporidium* cause a chronic hypertrophic gastritis in snakes. The clinical course lasts for weeks or months and is characterized by persistent postprandial regurgitation, weight loss, and firm midbody swelling. Mortality is high. The stomach wall is grossly thickened, and the lumen contains excess mucus. There is hyperplasia of mucous neck cells, atrophy of granular cells, cyst formation, and focal necrosis of the gastric mucosa. Many *Cryptosporidium* are found on the microvillar surfaces. Affected snakes have a pale, tan, fatty liver. Clinical diagnosis is established by demonstration of oocysts in stained fecal smears (they may not be demonstrable by flotation or direct smear).[42a]

Differential diagnosis of enteritis in herpetofauna should include coccidiosis, other intestinal parasites, salmonellosis, and *Pseudomonas* infection. Specific diagnosis of coccidiosis is made by finding the oocysts in the droppings (Fig. 3–31). Postmortem diagnosis can be made by demonstrating oocysts in gut contents or other stages of the parasite in histologic sections. The pathologist's report should include a description of the inflammatory response to the organism.

Wallach suggests treating coccidiosis in reptiles with one ounce of sodium sulfamethazine per gallon of drinking water for 10 days.[285] Deakins recommends a dosage of 75 mg/kg for seven days,[73] but Zwart has not found this very effective.[314] ESB3, a poultry coccidiostat used in the drinking water in a concentration of 1 g per liter for three days, effectively treats coccidiosis in chameleons.[30]

Reptiles occasionally harbor intestinal (sexual) and intramuscular (asexual) stages of *Sarcocystis* or related organisms.[213a,213b]

Other Intestinal Protozoa. Many ciliate and flagellate species inhabit the amphibian and reptilian gut, but none is known to be pathogenic.

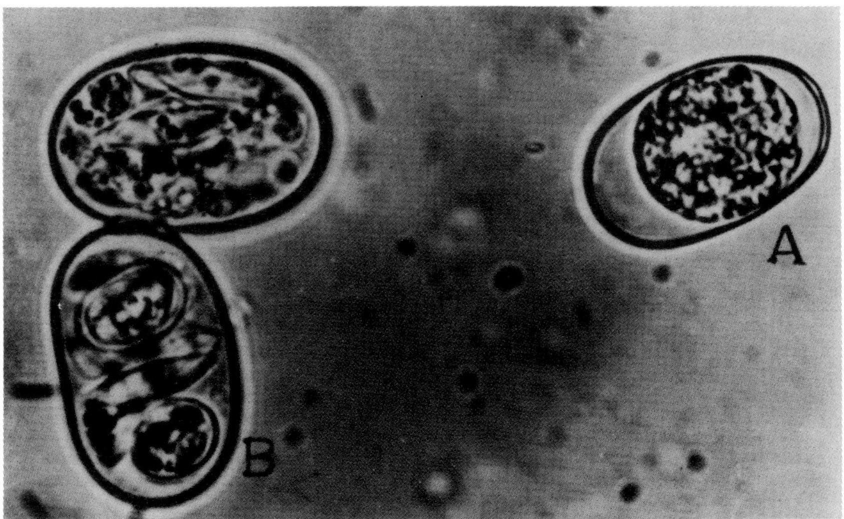

Fig. 3–31. Coccidia in the stool of a chameleon (*Chameleo* sp.). **A.** Freshly passed (immature) oocyst. **B.** Sporulated oocyst. 1,500×. (From Blok, J.: Eetlustvermindering bij Kameleons. Lacerta, *29*:87–88, 1971.)

The clinician should be aware of their benign nature and their frequent appearance on routine stool examinations. Occasionally they have even been seen in the blood, but without apparent ill effect. A list and description of these ciliates and flagellates can be obtained in the publications and bibliographies of Walton,[292,293,294] Reichenbach-Klinke and Elkan,[233] Telford,[267,271,273] Fantham and Porter,[84,85] and Kaplan.[159]

Hemoflagellates (Trypanosomiasis). Trypanosomes are often seen in the blood of amphibians and reptiles (Fig. 3–32), but most species are not associated with obvious disease. *Trypanosoma inopinatum,* however, causes an infection that is usually fatal in its acute form in Old World anurans and *T. diemictyli* causes a fatal illness in American newts. *T. pipientis* causes splenomegaly and infection with low mortality in leopard frogs *(Rana pipiens)*.[159]

Trypanosomes are transmitted to reptiles and amphibians by invertebrate intermediate hosts. Leeches act as vectors for many aquatic animals, e.g., turtles and frogs.[77,233] *Trypanosoma rotatorium* is transmitted to tadpoles by the leech *Hemiclepsis marginata*, and the hemoflagellate persists in the blood of the adult frog.[202] Various blood-sucking insects transmit trypanosomes to terrestrial and other aquatic reptiles and amphibians. In Africa, tsetse flies (*Glossina* spp.) transmit trypanosomiasis to some reptiles. For example, Hoare[128,129] demonstrated that *Glossina palpalis* can transmit *T. grayi (kochi)* to the Nile crocodile *(Crocodylus niloticus)* by deposition of the protozoa in the reptile's mouth. Crocodiles commonly bask with their mouths open and tsetse flies can be observed entering the mouth to feed on the richly vascularized oral epithelium. Infective stages are deposited in the crocodile's mouth when the fly defecates (the trypanosomes occupy a posterior station in the fly's gut) or are released when the crocodile snaps its jaws shut on the unlucky insect. This fecal deposition of trypanosomes differs from the transmission pattern seen in African (human) sleeping sickness and nagana of cattle in which infection occurs via the bite of the tsetse fly. It is not clear what role, if any, African reptiles play as reservoirs for trypanosomiasis in man and

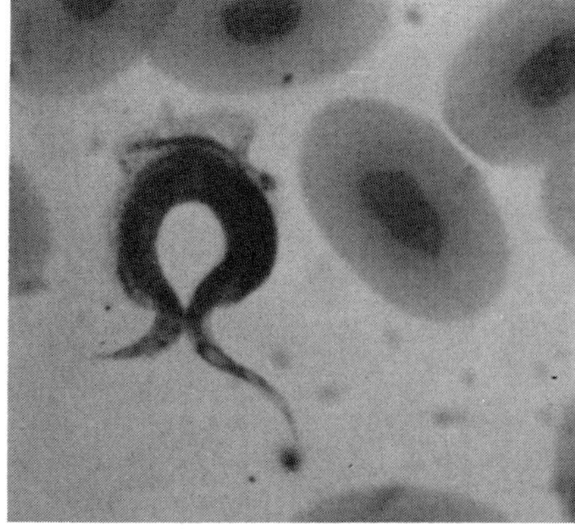

Fig. 3–32. Trypanosome in the blood of a banded water snake *(Natrix sipedon)* from New York State. The snake appeared healthy. 900×.

domestic animals,[308] but reptilian blood is a food item in the diet of certain tsetse flies and this may be significant in maintaining these insects in certain areas.

The alligator lizard *(Gerrhonotus multicarinatus webbii)* was shown to be a suitable laboratory host for *Trypanosoma cruzi*, the causative agent of Chagas' disease (South American trypanosomiasis).[239] The vectors of Chagas' disease are blood-sucking reduviid bugs. Some of these bugs are known to feed on lizards, but the dietary tables are frequently turned and a bug comes to dinner, not where he eats, but where he is eaten, as was the fate of Polonius[252a] (Shakespeare, W., 1604). Infective trypanosomes are transmitted in bug feces, and lizards can become infected by eating the bugs. The possibility of this cycle occurring in nature would seem to be very worthy of study, for bugs and lizards often cohabit the huts of people who suffer from Chagas' disease, which is a major cause of human morbidity and mortality in Latin America. If lizards were a significant reservoir of this disease, its control would be greatly complicated.

Protozoa in the genera *Leptomonas* and *Leishmania* infect herpetofauna, but little is known about their pathogenicity.

Nothing has been published on chemotherapy of trypanosomiasis in herpetofauna, nor does treatment seem to be indicated in the vast majority of cases. An extensive monograph on the trypanosomes of anurans was written by Diamond.[77]

Blood-Borne Sporozoa

Reptiles and amphibians harbor a bewildering variety of intracellular (mostly intraerythrocytic) parasites in their blood. Most of these protozoa are in the order *Eucoccidia*, which is characterized by schizogony and the presence of sexual and asexual phases. They require an invertebrate intermediate host, although the specific life cycle for many of these parasites is unknown. Most of the studies published on these Sporozoa deal with their morphology and life cycle. Little is known about their pathogenicity, but my own experience and available reports indicate that most cases of infection with these parasites are not associated with overt clinical illness.

The major genera parasitizing herpetofauna and a brief description of their life cycles are as follows:* [192,202,225]

Schellackia. Schizogony and sporogony occur in the intestines of a vertebrate (e.g., lizards); sporozoites usually enter red blood cells (a few

*Recent advances in protozoology modify or challenge some aspects of the descriptions of life cycles offered here. See Frenkel for a review of these concepts and for references on other genera of reptilian blood or tissue protozoa i.e., *Parahaemoproteus, Simondia, Lainsonia* and *Fallisia*.[94] In addition, see Lainson, Shaw, and Landau for descriptions of *Fallisia* spp., which undergoes schizogony and gametogony in leucocytes and thrombocytes, and of *Garnia multiformis*, which has early schizogony and gametogony in immature red blood cells.[178]

Saurocytozoon is closely related to *Leucocytozoon*, often found in birds. Gametocytes develop in lymphocytes, monocytes, or immature erythrocytes. No asexual stages are seen in peripheral blood. *S. tupinambi* was found in a teiid lizard, *Tupinambus nigropunctatus*.[177b] *S. mabuyi* was found in a Brazilian skink, *Mabuya mabouya*.[177a]

enter leucocytes); bloodsucking mites or mosquitoes ingest infected red cells. No further development of the parasite occurs until the infected arthropod is ingested by a lizard. Sporozoites enter the vertebrate's intestinal epithelium to complete the cycle.[179]

Lankesterella. Schizogony and sporogony occur in the endothelium of blood vessels; sporozoites enter erythrocytes; a leech ingests infected red cells. No further development of the parasite occurs until sporozoites are inoculated into another vertebrate host when the leech feeds again. Sporozoites enter vascular endothelium completing the life cycle. Examples in this genus are *L. minima* in the edible frog, *Rana esculenta,* and *L. canadensis* in the bullfrog, *R. catesbeiana.*

In the next five genera *(Haemogregarina, Hepatozoon, Karyolysus, Plasmodium,* and *Haemoproteus),* blood cells of the vertebrate host contain gametocytes which are ingested by a bloodsucking invertebrate. In this invertebrate sexual development occurs with the formation of oocysts from which sporozoites are released. The sporozoites are transferred to the reptile or amphibian via the invertebrate host (either when the invertebrate is eaten by the reptile or amphibian or when it takes its next blood meal).

Haemogregarina. Schizonts and gametocytes occur in red blood cells of snakes and turtles. In the invertebrate host (e.g., a leech), an oocyst develops containing free sporozoites which are transferred to the vertebrate when the leech feeds again. The best known member of the genus is *H. stepanowi,* transmitted to various freshwater turtles by the leech, *Placobdella catenigera* (Fig. 3–33).

Hepatozoon. Schizogony occurs in internal organs, usually in endothelium of blood vessels; in different species schizogony tends to occur in specific organs, e.g., liver or lung.[186] Gametocytes enter red or white blood cells and are ingested by an invertebrate host (e.g., tick, mite, fly, or mosquito) in which oocysts develop containing sporocysts, which, in turn, contain sporozoites. *Hepatozoon* spp. are not very host-specific and can be transferred from one species of reptile to another using mosquito vectors.[33,54]

Karyolysus. Schizogony occurs in endothelium of blood vessels. Gametocytes develop in red blood cells that are ingested by the invertebrate host (e.g., a mite) in which oocysts containing sporoblasts develop; motile sporokinetes escape from the oocyst and enter the egg of the mite. Sporocysts develop in the intestinal epithelium of the larval mites and sporozoites are passed in their stool. Lizards become infected by ingesting the sporozoites either in the mites or in their stool. The species that has been studied most carefully is *Karyolysus lacertarum,* which is transmitted by the mite *Neoliponyssus saurarum* to the wall lizard *Lacerta muralis.*[233]

The genera *Haemogregarina, Hepatozoon,* and *Karyolysus* are included in the parasites referred to as **hemogregarines.** They are very common endoglobular parasites of reptiles. It would be most unusual to examine blood from any large, diverse collection of snakes, lizards, turtles, and crocodilians and not find cases of infection with these protozoa. Hemogregarines are usually seen as intraerythrocytic banana-shaped

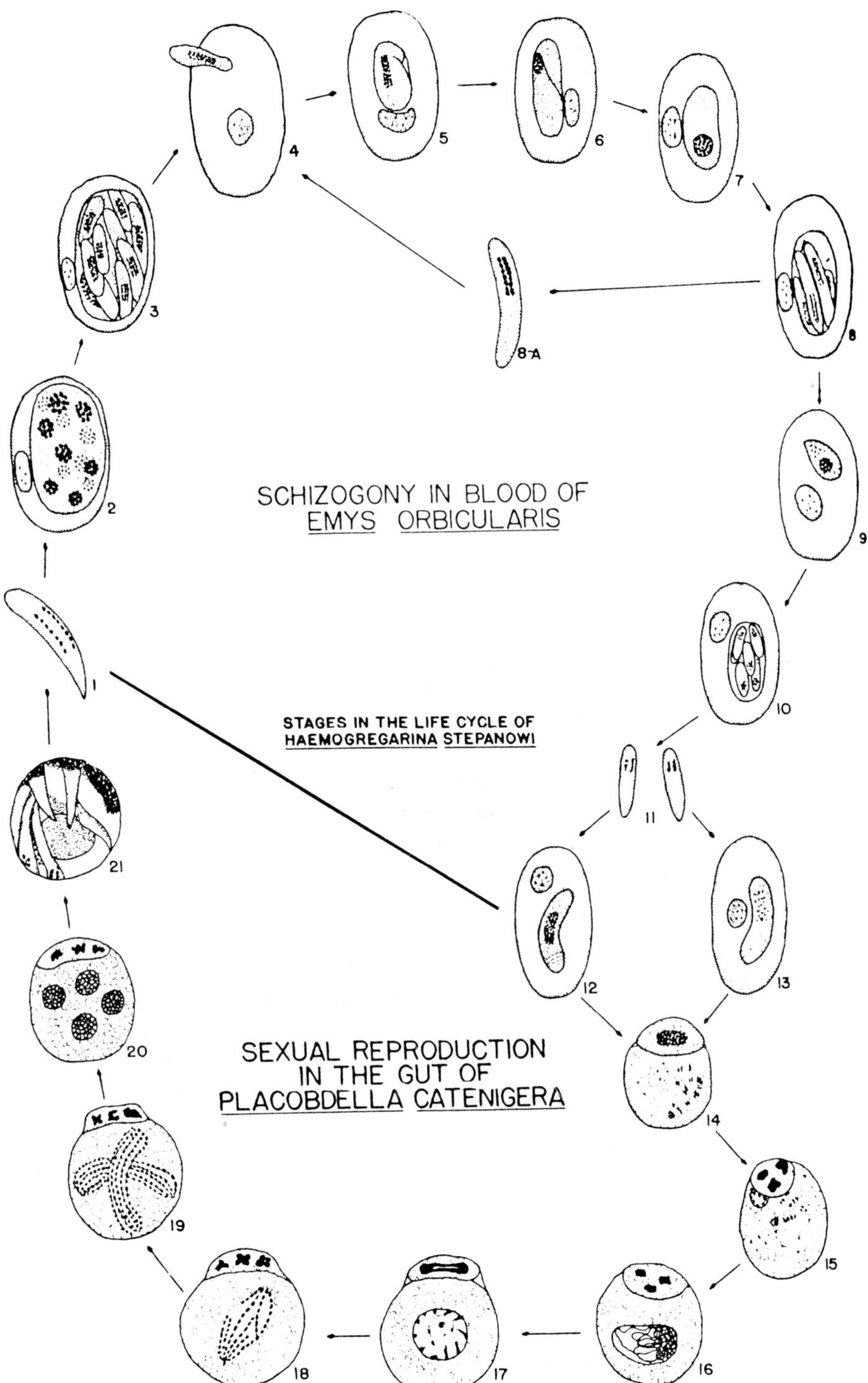

Fig. 3–33. Stages in the life cycle of *Haemogregarina stepanowi*, a coccidian parasite of the turtle *Emys orbicularis* and the leech *Placobdella catenigera*. **1**, A single sporozoite. **2–8**, Schizogonic stages. **8 A**, A single merozoite reinfecting an erythrocyte of vertebrate host, thus repeating the schizogonic phase of the cycle. **9** and **10**, Stages in gametocyte formation. **11**, Young macro- and microgametocytes. **12**, Mature microgametocyte. **13**, Mature macrogametocyte. **14** and **15**, Association of gametocytes. **16**, Fertilization taking place in gut of leech host. **17–21**, Division of the zygotic nucleus to form eight sporozoites. (All figures redrawn and modified after Reichenow, 1919.) (From Cheng, T.C.: The Biology of Animal Parasites. Philadelphia, W.B. Saunders Co., 1964.)

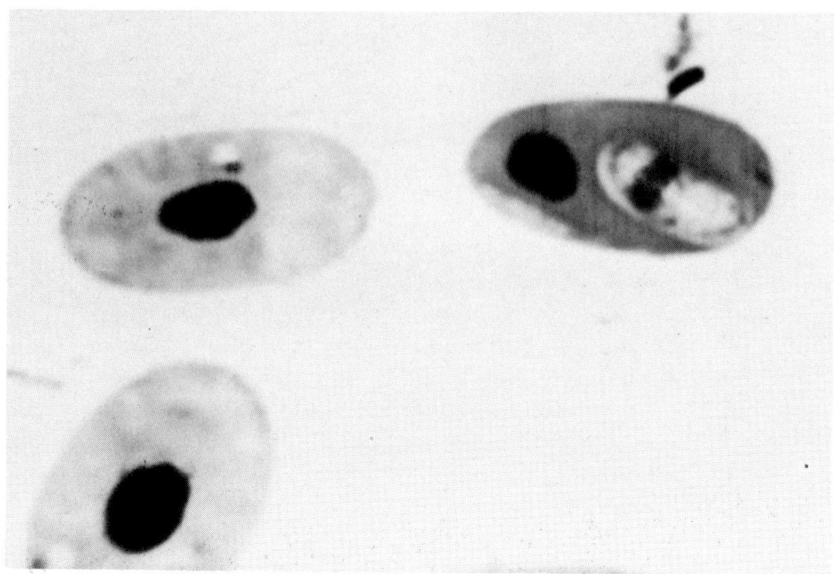

Fig. 3–34. Hemogregarine in a red blood cell in an American alligator *(Alligator mississippiensis)* (upper right). The oval, slightly crescentic parasite is pushing the host nucleus to the left. Giemsa stain, 450X.

organisms lacking associated pigment (Fig. 3–34). Infected cells may be greatly altered in size and shape[19] and their nucleus is displaced to one side by the parasite. Most of the intraerythrocytic forms are probably gametocytes, but some of them may be trophozoites; identification of these forms is controversial.[18,134] Occasionally extracellular forms are seen in blood films.

As a group, hemogregarines are less host-specific than are the Plasmodia, both in regard to invertebrate and vertebrate hosts. Hemogregarines were formerly given specific names according to the host from which the parasite was isolated. This is of questionable taxonomic validity. Proper identification of species should depend on the very tedious process of comparing all phases of the life cycle including developmental forms in invertebrate hosts and experimental transmission of the parasite to various hosts.[18,270]

It probably suffices for the veterinary practitioner that he should recognize hemogregarines as such when they are seen in a blood film. He should be aware that they are common, that they are transmitted by bloodsucking arthropods or leeches, and that they may alter the morphology of cells that they parasitize, but are not known to cause significant illness in herpetofauna.[123a] There is equivocal evidence that they may contribute to anemia and inanition in snakes.[87] Little is known about chemotherapy of hemogregarine infection. Pyrimethamine (Daraprim, Burroughs Wellcome Co.) reportedly has no effect on heavy infections.[87] Treatment probably is not indicated in the great majority of cases.

Plasmodium (Fig. 3–35). Asexual cycles (schizogony) occur both in tissue (usually liver) and blood cells of the vertebrate host; gametocytes

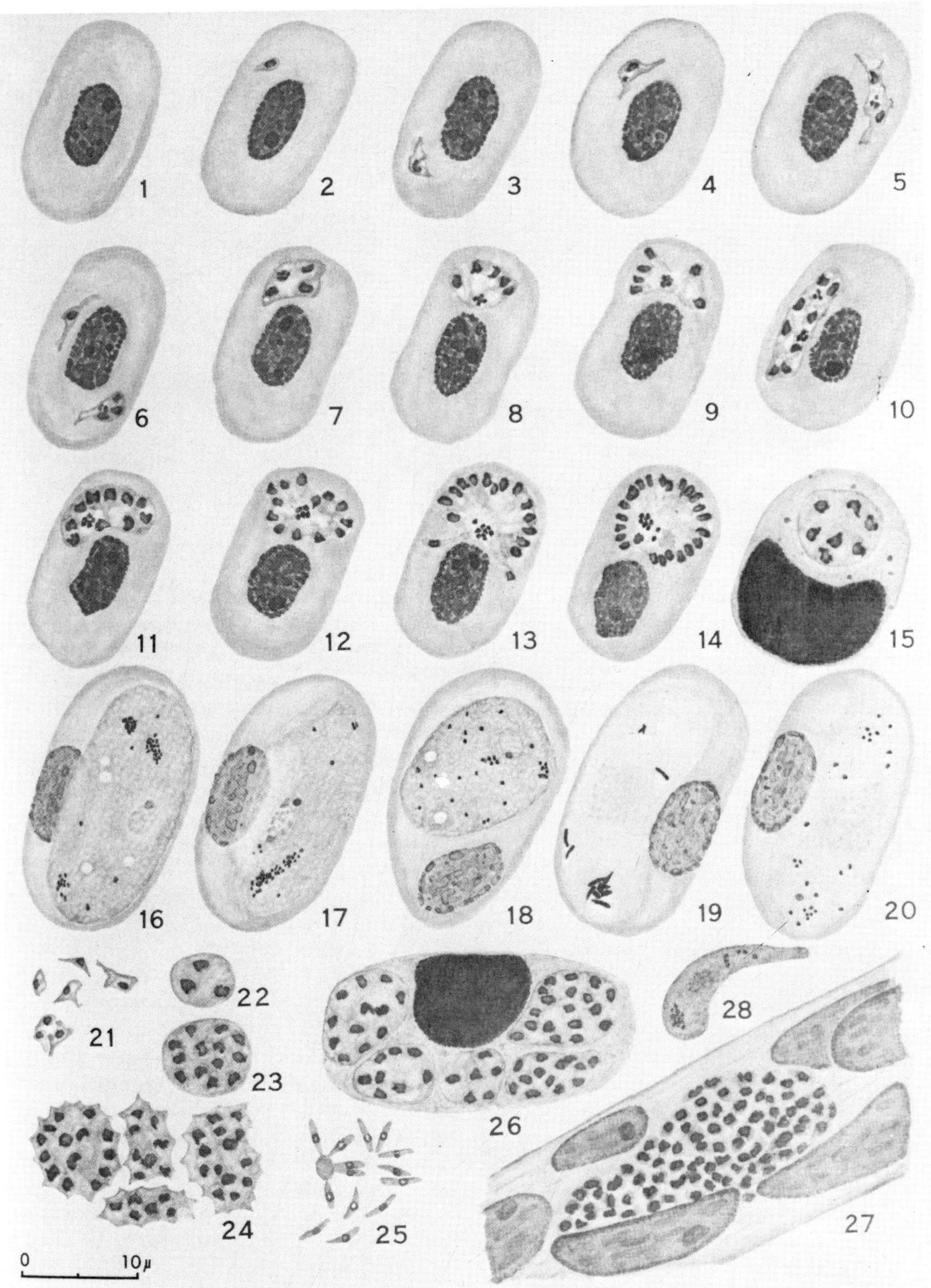

Fig. 3–35. The California strain of *Plasmodium mexicanum*. **1**, Uninfected erythrocyte. **2–4**, Trophozoites. **5–11**, Schizonts. **12–14**, Segmenters. **15**, Exoerythrocytic schizont in medium-sized leukocyte. **16–18**, Mature macrogametocytes. **19–20**, Mature microgametocytes. **21–25**, Free exoerythrocytic forms in peripheral blood, trophozoites, schizonts, and merozoites. **26**, Exoerythrocytic schizonts in large leukocyte, liver. **27**, Exoerythrocytic schizont in vascular endothelial cell, brain. **28**, Ookinete in 12-hour blood meal of *Lutzomyia* (= *Phlebotomus*) *vexatrix occidentis*. (From Ayala, S.C.: A new strain of *Plasmodium mexicanum* from California lizards. J. Parasitol., *56*:417–425, 1970.)

are found in red blood cells; a sexual cycle (gametogeny and sporogony) occurs in insects (almost always mosquitoes). As an exception to the rule that the sexual cycle can only occur in mosquitoes, sporozoites of a lizard parasite, *P. mexicanum,* were shown to develop in two species of Phlebotomine sandflies,[15] although actual transmission of saurian malaria by these insects was not demonstrated. Another exception to taxonomic rules was found by Telford who described gametocytes of three *Plasmodium* species in the thrombocytes and lymphocytes of six species of Central American lizards.[271]

Another characteristic of *Plasmodium* spp. is the presence of Prussian blue negative, birefringent malarial pigment in cells infected with certain stages of the parasite. Telford described two malarial parasites, *P. gonatodi* and *P. morulum*, in Panamanian lizards in which the typical malarial pigment could not be found.[272]

Thirty-two species of *Plasmodium* have been described in reptiles, the overwhelming majority of these being in lizards. In some lizard populations the prevalence of malaria is extremely high, and in individual lizards more than half the circulating red cells may be parasitized. There may be seasonal variation of levels of parasitemia. Most transmission of *P. mexicanum* occurs in late spring and early summer in western fence lizards *(Sceloporus occidentalis)* in California.[14] These lizards suffer seasonal relapse of infection in the spring when maximal numbers of asexual forms are found in their blood. During the rest of the year, gametocytes predominate (Fig. 3–36). Despite the heavy concentration of parasites in individuals and in populations,

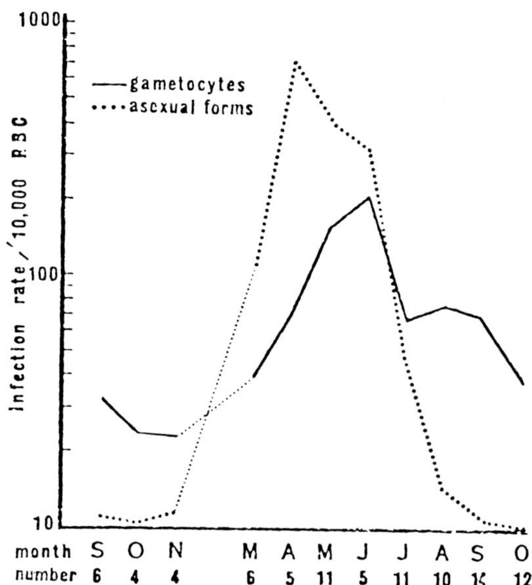

Fig. 3–36. Seasonal variation in parasitemia in adult lizards from Hopland Valley, California, naturally infected with *P. mexicanum*. Monthly rates are averages from several lizards (numbers) examined each month. (From Ayala, S.C.: A new strain of *Plasmodium mexicanum* from California lizards. J. Parasitol. 56:417–425, 1970.)

there is no evidence that malaria is a significant direct cause of mortality in adult lizards. However, malaria causes hemolysis and some anemia. It is probable that *P. mexicanum* is lethal to some yearling fence lizards during the spring and summer transmission season.

Classification and biology of reptilian malaria is discussed further in the text by Garnham[105] and in numerous articles by Telford, some of which are cited in this book.[271,272,273] A classic paper on the life cycle of one species of lizard malaria, *P. mexicanum*, was written by Thompson and Huff,[275] and these two authors have made numerous contributions on the subject of saurian malaria (see the bibliography in the article by Huff[133]).

I am aware of only one report on chemotherapy of saurian malaria. Thompson demonstrated that quinine was active against stages of *P. mexicanum* found in erythrocytes, but was ineffective against exo-erythrocytic forms.[274]

Haemoproteus. This genus is closely related to *Plasmodium* and also causes the deposition of pigment in parasitized cells. It differs from *Plasmodium* in that schizogony does not occur in erythrocytes. Gametocytes are found in the red blood cells and extra-erythrocytic forms are found in the endothelium of blood vessels. Representatives of the genus *Haemoproteus* have been found in lizards, turtles, and snakes.

Babesiosoma and Dactylosoma. These two genera, which collectively can be referred to as **babesioids**, are in the same superfamily (Babesioidea) as *Babesia*, a genus familiar to veterinarians. These relatively small intraerythrocytic parasites have been described in toads, frogs, and salamanders. The biology and taxonomy of the babesioids of cold-blooded vertebrates were reviewed by Jakowska and Nigrelli.[150] These parasites cause little ill effect on the host. Schmittner and McGhee infected leopard frogs *(Rana pipiens)* with *Babesiosoma stableri* and found no deaths attributable to the organism despite the presence of parasitemia up to one year postinoculation.[246] Two of their frogs did show a hematopoietic response to infection.

Several piroplasmid organisms that are closely related to the babesioids have been described in reptiles. Pienaar has reviewed the literature on reptilian piroplasms and on other protozoa inhabiting the blood of reptiles.[225] The piroplasms and babesioids are relatively small (compared to plasmodia and hemogregarines), roughly oval to round, nonpigmented, intraerythrocytic parasites. Because of their small size they cause little or no displacement of the red cell nucleus. (In malaria and hemogregarine infections, the erythrocytic nucleus is commonly displaced to one side.)

Nuttallia guglielmi is a piroplasm found in a European tortoise, *Testudo marginata*.[233] Pienaar discusses in some detail the piroplasms *Tunetella emydis*, found in a Tunisian tortoise, *Emys leprosa*, and *Sauroplasma thomasi*, found in South African lizards in the genus *Cordylus (Zonurus)*. He also describes a new species, *Serpentoplasma najae*, in a black-necked cobra, *Naja nigricollis*.[225] The piroplasms of reptiles may be associated with mild anemic changes in the blood, but have not been associated with overt clinical disease.

Organisms of Uncertain Classification

A number of microorganisms formerly had been classified as *Protozoa*, but are now considered to be more like *Rickettsia*. As a matter of editorial convenience, they are considered here because, like the Haemosporidia, they parasitize red blood cells. Kreier and Ristic list the following members of the genera *Haemobartonella* and *Grahamella* as parasites of herpetofauna (Table 3–2).[173]

Haemobartonella and *Grahamella* spp. appear as pleomorphic coccobacillary forms, staining well with Giemsa stain, and are found in or on red blood cells. Little is known about their pathogenicity in herpetofauna.

Pienaar described two new species in South African lizards which are of questionable classification.[225] *Pirhaemocyton zonurae* was found in the erythrocytes of the girdled lizard, *Cordylus vittifer*, where it appeared as Anaplasma-like bodies 1 to 1.4 μ in diameter as well as larger spherical, stellate, and filamentous forms. The parasite was often associated with the presence of pale albuminoid globules in the cytoplasm of the parasitized red cell. Pirhaemocytonosis causes severe hemolytic anemia with marked anisocytosis and poikilocytosis, pycnosis, and karyorrhexis of erythrocytic nuclei and fragmentation of erythrocytic cytoplasm. The lizard hosts were found to mount an erythropoietic response to the infection, and erythroblastic cells were found in the peripheral circulation. Pienaar thought it likely that severe infections would terminate fatally.

Pirhaemocyton tarenteola was found in a North African gecko, *Tarenteola mauritanica* with progressive anemia. *P. lacertae* was found in a green lizard from Italy, *Lacerta viridis*.[225] *Pirhaemocyton* was first thought to be protozoan, but electron microscopy indicates the intraerythrocytic body is a viral inclusion body.[149b]

Another Anaplasma-like parasite, *Sauromella haemolysus*, was found in a South African gecko, *Pachydactylus c. caponsis*.[149b] The hemoglobin around the coccobacillary parasites was destroyed, and heavy parasitism resulted in a severe hemolytic anemia with hematologic changes similar to those just described in pirhaemocytonosis.

Table 3–2.* *Haemobartonella* and *Grahamella* spp. in Herpetofauna

PARASITE	HOST
Haemobartonella batrachorum	Frog *(Leptodactylus ocellatus)*
H. ranarum	Frog *(Leptodactylus ocellatus)*
H. sp.	Greek tortoise *(Testudo graeca)*
H. sp.	Gecko *(Phylodactylus mauritanicus)*
H. sp.	Lizard *(Lacertilia* sp.)
H. sp.	Lesson's Peruvian lizard *(Tropidurus peruvianus)*
Grahamella sanii	Greek tortoise *(Testudo graeca)*
G. thalassochelys	Loggerhead turtle *(Thalassochelys caretta = Caretta caretta)*

*Adapted from Kreier, J.P., and Ristic, M.: Diseases caused by protista. *In* Infectious Blood Diseases of Man and Animals. Edited by D. Weinman and M. Ristic. Academic Press, New York, 1968.

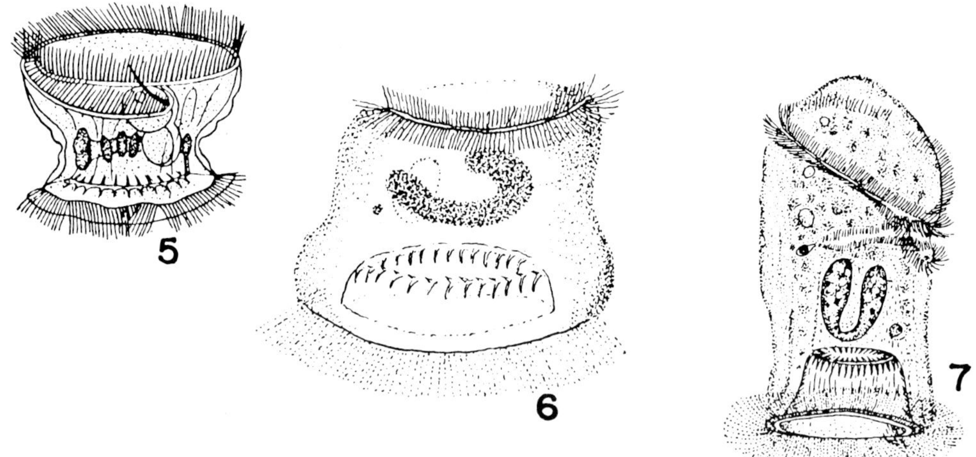

Fig. 3–37. 5, *Trichodina pediculus*, a peritrichous ciliate found on *Hydra* and on the gills of *Necturus* and salamanders. (After James Clark.) **6**, *Trichodina* sp. from the skin and gills of frog and toad tadpoles. (Redrawn after Diller, 1928.) **7**, *Trichodina urinicola*, a peritrichous ciliate from the urinary bladder of *Bufo* sp. and in frogs. (After Fulton, 1923.) (From Cheng, T.C.: The Biology of Animal Parasites. Philadelphia, W.B. Saunders Co., 1964.)

Protozoan Infections of the Skin

*Charchesium polysinum** is a protozoan that grows on the skin of tadpoles. It can cause death by covering the gills. The infection can be treated by placing the tadpoles in distilled water for two to three hours.[226]

Oodinium pillularis is a flagellated protozoan ectoparasite of fish and aquatic amphibians such as tadpoles, axolotls, and aquatic newts. It attaches itself to the skin and gills of these animals, and in heavy infestations the host may appear to be covered by a greyish deposit. The organism swims from one host to another; introduction of one infected animal in a colony can lead to an epizootic in which all are infected. Diagnosis is confirmed by microscopic examination of a skin impression smear for the parasitic stage of the protozoan. Recommended treatment is copper sulphate (2 mg/l of water) or Trypaflavin (10 mg/l of water).[233]

Trichodina spp. are spherical, ciliated protozoa that are ectoparasites of freshwater crustaceans, molluscs, other invertebrates, fish, tadpoles, and salamanders. In addition, certain *Trichodina* spp. reportedly parasitize the urinary bladder of some amphibians (Fig. 3–37). Reichenbach-Klinke and Elkan recommend treating cutaneous trichodinosis with a bath of Trypaflavin (1:1000 to 1:100 concentration).[233]

Dermocystidium and *Dermosporidium* (in the Sporozoan order *Haplosporida*) form cysts in the skin of fish and aquatic amphibians[42] (Figs.

*The spelling *"Charchesium polysinum"* is taken from Pollack.[226] I can find no further reference to this organism, and I assume that he refers to *Carchesium polypinum*, a stalked ciliate often found attached to freshwater animals.

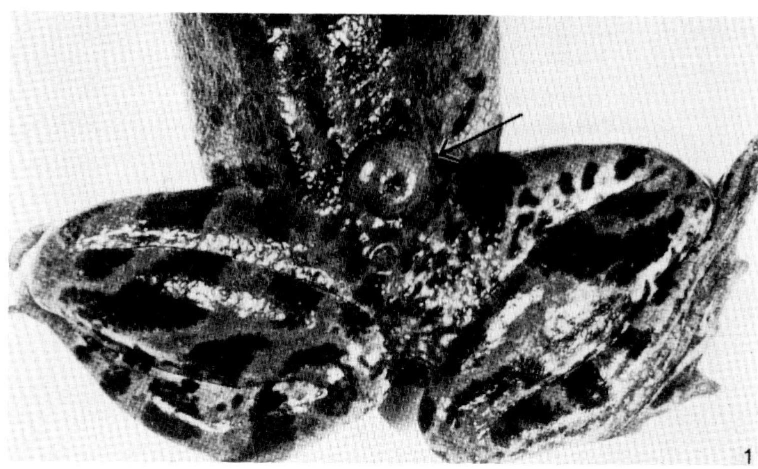

Fig. 3–38. Nodule on the skin of a grass frog *(Rana temporaria)* from Czechoslovakia containing a cyst of *Dermosporidium granulosum*. (From Broz, O. and Privora, M.: Two skin parasites of *Rana temporaria: Dermocystidium ranae* Guyenot and Naville and *Dermosporidium granulosum* n. sp. Parasitology, *42*:65–69, 1952.)

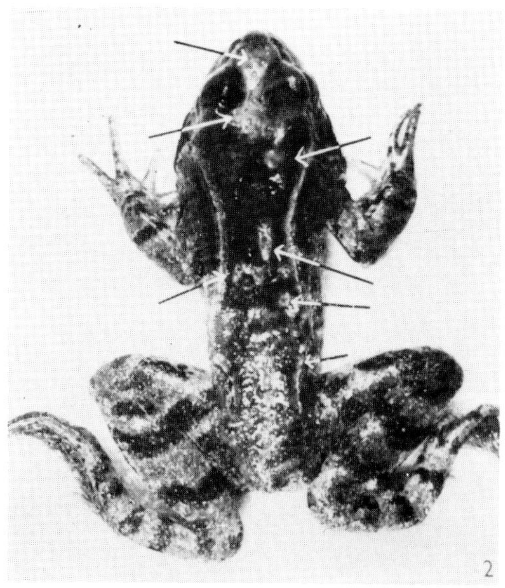

Fig. 3–39. *Dermocystidium ranae*. Cysts (arrows) on the skin of a grass frog *(Rana temporaria)* from Czechoslovakia. (From Broz, O. and Privora, M.: Two skin parasites of *Rana temporaria: Dermocystidium ranae* Guyenot and Naville and *Dermosporidium granulosum* n. sp. Parasitology, *42*:65–69, 1952.)

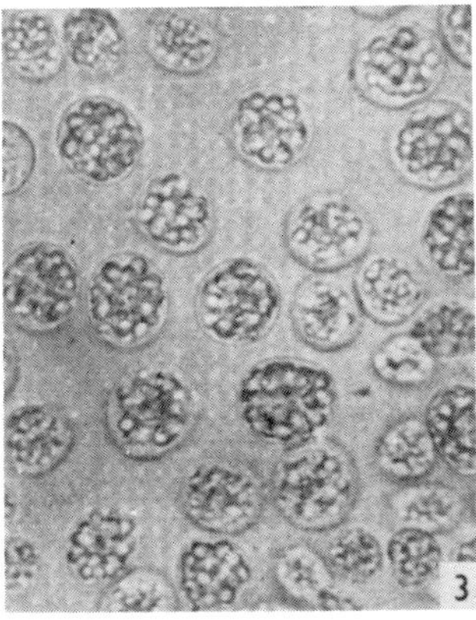

Fig. 3–40. *Dermosporidium granulosum* living spores. (From Broz, O., and Privora, M.: Two skin parasites of *Rana temporaria: Dermocystidium ranae* Guyenot and Naville and *Dermosporidium granulosum* n. sp. Parasitology, *42*:65–69, 1952.)

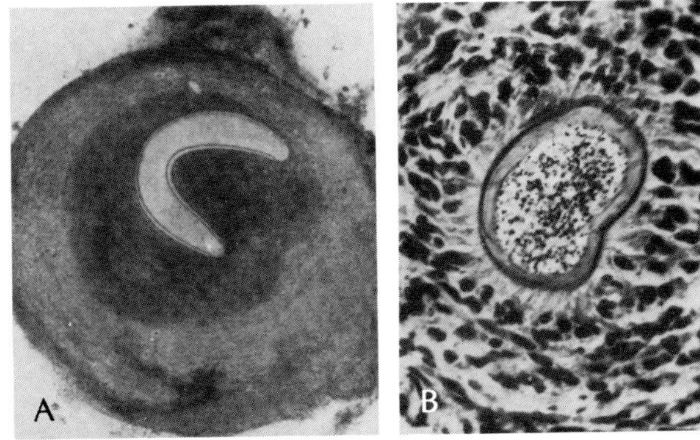

Fig. 3–41. *Dermocystidium ranae.* **A.** Fresh preparation of an immature cyst. **B.** Section through an immature cyst surrounded by fibroblasts and histiocytes. (From Broz, O., and Privora, M.: Two skin parasites of *Rana temporaria: Dermocystidium ranae* Guyenot and Naville and *Dermosporidium granulosum* n. sp. Parasitology, *42*:65–69, 1952.)

3–38 and 3–39). These cysts may be multiple, disfiguring, and debilitating to the host. Diagnosis is made by direct smear or microscopic section of the cyst (Figs. 3–40 and 3–41). No drug treatment is known.

Protozoan Infections of Deep Tissues

Myxosporidea and Microsporidea: These two classes in the subphylum Cnidospora contain only a few species that parasitize reptiles and amphibians.[132] Most of the Myxosporidea are parasites of fish and most Microsporidea parasitize fish or arthropods.

Plistophora myotrophica[53] is a microsporidian parasite of the common toad *(Bufo bufo)* that invades skeletal muscle and causes chronic illness with severe wasting of flesh (Fig. 3–42) and high mortality. In the

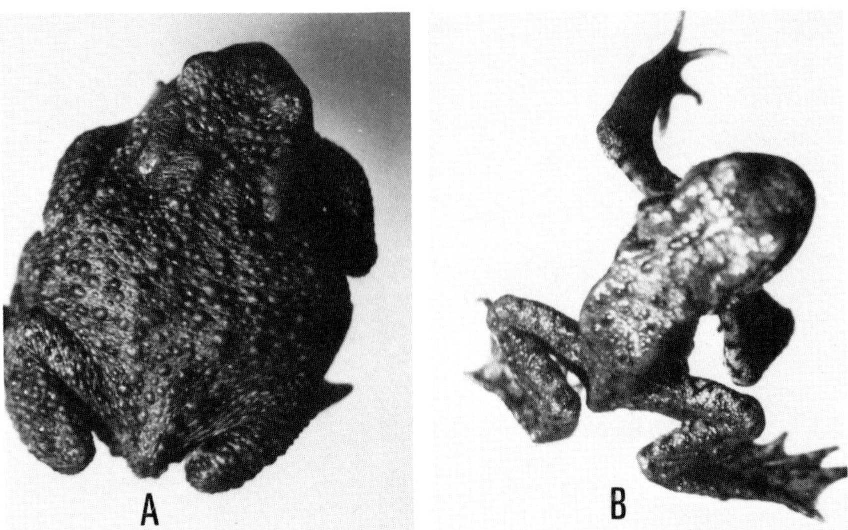

Fig. 3–42. *Plistophora myotrophica* infection in common toads *(Bufo bufo)*, adult males. **A.** In a toad infected for two months there is no deterioration in general condition. **B.** After two years there is severe emaciation. (From Canning, E.U., Elkan, E., and Trigg, P.I.: *Plistophora myotrophica* spec. nov. causing high mortality in the common toad *Bufo bufo*. J. Protozool., *11*: 157–166, 1964.)

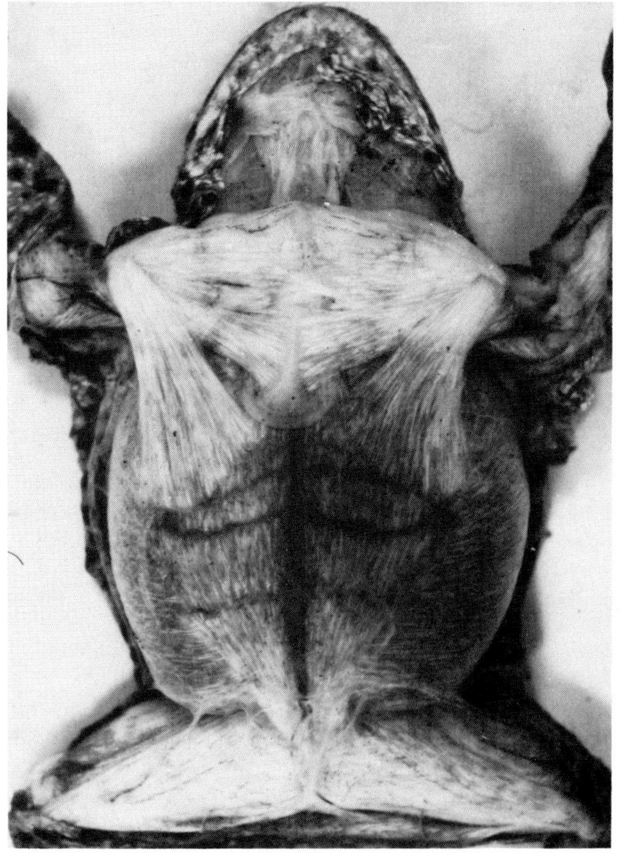

Fig. 3–43. Common toad *(Bufo bufo)*, adult male, skin removed. Heavy infection of pectoral, abdominal, and thigh muscles with *Plistophora myotrophica* (white streaks). (From Canning, E.U., Elkan, E., and Trigg, P.I.: *Plistophora myotrophica* spec. nov. causing high mortality in the common toad *Bufo bufo*. J. Protozool., *11*:157–166, 1964.)

outbreak described by Canning, Elkan, and Trigg, about one third of a large laboratory colony of toads developed anorexia after 3 to 12 months of captivity and then suffered progressive emaciation usually terminating in the death of the host.[53] Postmortem examination revealed white fusiform streaks in all skeletal muscles, the myocardium being spared (Fig. 3–43). Microscopic examination revealed these streaks to be sporoblasts, each containing 60 to 100 spores, in the muscle fiber (Fig. 3–44). The disease could be induced in healthy toads by feeding them meat from infected animals, and the authors postulate that the disease may be spread in nature by ingestion of spores that contaminate the environment when the body of an infected animal decomposes. It is possible that carrion-eating insects, e.g., maggots, could act as a vehicle for transmitting this disease.

Toads die in 3 to 12 months after experimental inoculation. There is no known treatment. South African clawed toads *(Xenopus laevis)* kept in the same laboratory as the infected toads did not become ill.

Sarcosporidiosis: Sarcosporidian cysts commonly infect the heart and skeletal muscle of wild and domestic birds and mammals. Sexual stages are found in the intestinal mucosa of various carnivores. *Sarcocystis* or related genera are occasionally seen in the muscle and intestines of reptiles.[213a,213b]

Renal coccidiosis: *Klossiella boae* was described by Zwart in the kidney of a boa constrictor.[310] Various stages of this coccidian parasite

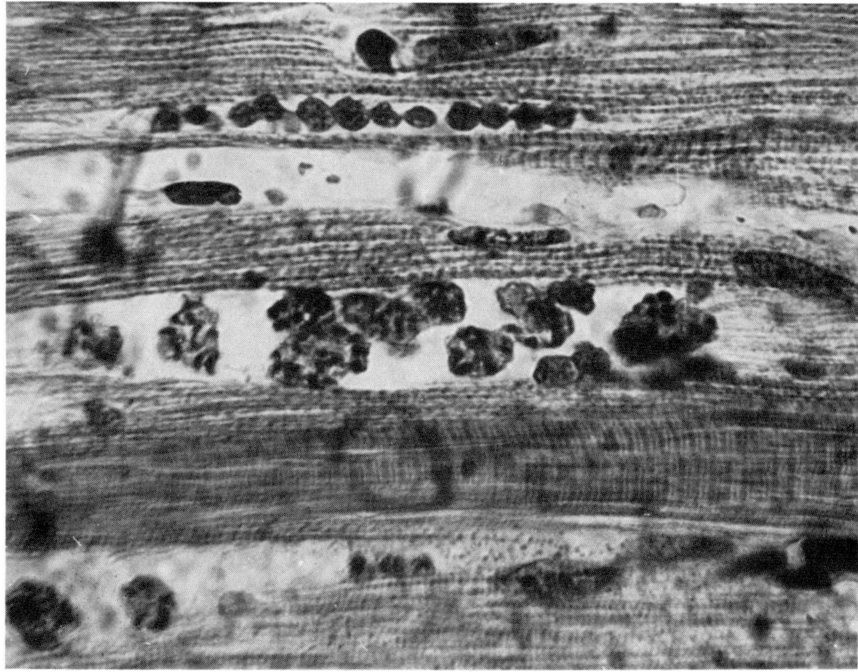

Fig. 3–44. *Plistophora myotrophica* in the skeletal muscle of a common toad *(Bufo bufo)*. The parasites are not encapsulated. (Courtesy of Dr. E. Elkan and Dr. Elizabeth Canning.)

are found in the renal tubular epithelium. As is the case with *K. muris* in the mouse and *K. equi* in zebras, renal coccidiosis in boas seems to be an incidental microscopic finding without apparent ill effects on the host. *Isospora lieberkühni* infects the kidney of European frogs and toads, but it too is not known to be significantly pathogenic.[292]

Toxoplasmosis: There are a few reports of *Toxoplasma*-like organisms occurring in herpetofauna.[185a] To date, these reports are more of academic and biologic interest than of public health or clinical veterinary concern.

Cestodes

Cestodaria is a subclass of primitive flatworms composed of a single segment and having a single set of reproductive organs. Most members of Cestodaria are parasitic in fish, but one species, *Austramphilina elongata*, has been found in the body cavity of the long-necked terrapin from Australia *(Chelodina longicollis)*.

Cestoda is the subclass that contains all the tapeworms of major veterinary and medical importance. These worms, in the adult stage, have segmented bodies and are hermaphroditic. Reichenbach-Klinke and Elkan state that 11 species of tapeworms have been recognized as adults in amphibians,[233] three of which are discussed below.

Nematotaeniid cestodes are unarmed (i.e., lacking a rostellum) and are unique among tapeworms in that their bodies are cylindrical rather than flattened. They have been found in the alimentary tract of amphibians and lizards. *Nematotaenia dispar* is found in the intestine of several species of frogs, toads, and salamanders from Asia, Africa, North America, and Europe. It is 5 to 22 cm long and 0.5 to 0.6 mm in diameter. One case of jejunal obstruction and gangrene caused by a mass of *N. dispar* has been described in the common toad, *B. bufo*.[81] The life cycle of this worm is not known.

The South African clawed toad, *Xenopus laevis*, is commonly parasitized by the cestode, *Cephalochlamys nomaquensis*. It has been reported that parenteral bromphenol is a safe and effective vermifuge for this parasite.[233] (This therapy was fortuitously discovered by Elkan who was using this dye as a reagent in the pregnancy test for which *X. laevis* has commonly been used. Dosage is not discussed in his report.[81])

Ophiotaenia filaroides is a tapeworm of the tiger salamander, *Ambystoma tigrinum*. Eggs passed in the salamander's stool enter the water and are ingested by copepods (e.g., *Cyclops vernalis)* in which they develop into plerocercoids. The salamanders become infected by ingesting this stage in the copepods. Plerocercoids have also been described in the bodies of *A. tigrinum*; these larval stages become adult worms in the salamander's gut either by penetrating the intestinal wall or through cannibalism.[206] Copepods are probably the only intermediate host required in the life cycle of *O. gracilis*, a tapeworm of the bullfrog *(Rana catesbeiana*.[47])

Ophiotaenia is the genus of tapeworm most commonly found in snakes; it is also seen in turtles. As was described above for *O. filaroides*, members of this genus typically use *Cyclops* spp. or other copepods as the first intermediate host. Amphibians commonly act as the second intermediate host. The life cycle of *O. perspicua*, which is a common endoparasite of water snakes *(Natrix rhombifera, N. sipedon)* and of garter snakes *(Thamnophis sirtalis)* is as follows.[55]

The adult worm in the snake's intestine deposits eggs that are passed in the stool. Eggs that enter the water hatch into ciliated onchospheres which actively penetrate the body cavity of copepods where they develop into procercoids in 14 days. Tadpoles ingest these infected copepods, and the worm develops into plerocercoids in the liver and mesentery of the tadpoles. The plerocercoid persists through the amphibian's metamorphosis and may migrate into the body cavity of the adult frog. When the frog is eaten by a snake, the worm develops into an adult in the snake's gut.

Acanthotaenia is a genus of tapeworms commonly found in lizards, especially monitors *(Varanus* spp.). Like *Ophiotaenia, Acanthotaenia* is in the order Proteocephala.

Adult tapeworms have the same potential pathogenicity in herpetofauna as in higher forms, i.e., they compete for nutrients, or cause enteritis, especially at the point of attachment, or intestinal obstruction. Infection with Pseudophyllidean tapeworms *(Bothridium* sp.) in two green tree pythons *(Chondrophython viridis)* was associated with mild, chronic enteritis, characterized by hypertrophy and hyperplasia of intestinal glands and focal discrete nodules containing cholesterol clefts in the lamina propria.[278] Cestodiasis in reptiles usually produces little in the way of clinical signs or demonstrable lesions, however. Diagnosis is made by finding segments or eggs in the stool.

Reptiles have been treated for adult tapeworms with dichlorophene (Dicestal, May and Baker Co.), Diphenthane 70 (Pitman-Moore Co.), using 182 mg/kg body weight,[149] or niclosamide (Yomesan, Chemagro Co.), 300 mg/kg[73] or one 500 mg tablet/7 lb.[27] Bush recommends niclosamide at 165 to 220 mg/kg (75 to 100 mg/lb).[49]

Herpetofauna are often host to larval cestodes, a situation which is of greater veterinary and medical significance than their being host to the adult worms. *Mesocestoides* spp. are tapeworms found as adults in the intestine of carnivorous birds and mammals, including dogs, cats, and raccoons. These carnivores become infected by ingesting tetrathyridea (sparganum-like second-stage larvae) which are found in the tissues of various vertebrates, including snakes, lizards, and amphibians (Fig. 3–45). Tetrathyridea have been found in the kidney, intestinal wall, mesentery, and other organs of North American frogs *(Rana pipens)* and toads *(Bufo americanus, B. cognatus.*[151]*)*

Reptiles and amphibians harbor the spargana or plerocercoids of various Pseudophyllidean tapeworms, including *Diphyllobothrium* spp. and *Spirometra* spp. These spargana may be found in the subcutis, where they cause obvious swellings, and in the liver, where they may cause extensive damage, in the peritoneum, and other tissues (Fig. 3–46). The life cycle is completed when a carnivore that is a suitable final host ingests the spargana-infected animal. If the predator cannot support the adult worm, it may become a paratenic host, i.e., the sparganum will

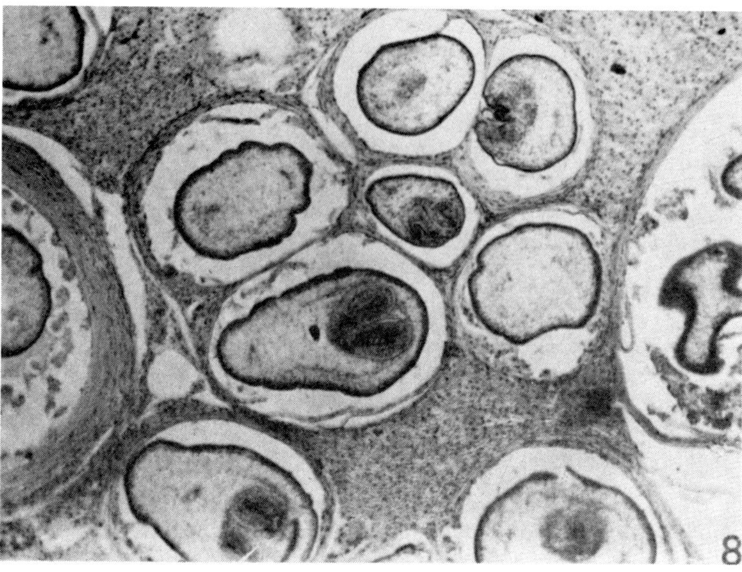

Fig. 3–45. Tetrathyridea of *Mesocestoides corti* in the liver of a lizard, *Uta stansburiana*. (From Telford, S., Jr.: Parasitic diseases of reptiles. J. Am. Vet. Med. Assoc., *159*:1644–1652, 1971.)

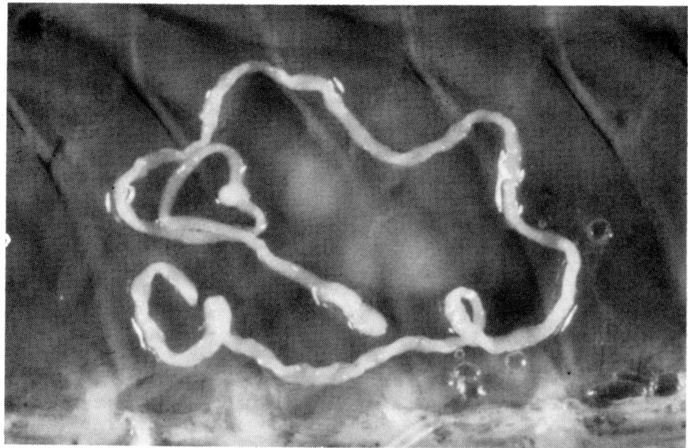

Fig. 3–46. Sparganum larva in an eastern indigo snake *(Drymarchon corais cooperi)*. Larva was encapsulated in a nodule in the body wall, similar to the nodules (light spots) behind the worm. (Courtesy of Dr. Marilyn Anderson and the Ohio State University, Department of Veterinary Pathobiology.)

invade its tissues and persist in the sparganum stage. Several cases of human sparganosis ascribed to the eating of raw snake (especially snake liver) have been described. This is not an unusual dietary custom in the Far East where it is thought to have some medicinal value.[298] Another Far Eastern custom that may result in human sparganosis is the application of fresh-cut frogs to wounds and ocular lesions; spargana in the frog can migrate directly into the human tissue.

Sparganosis is unlikely to be diagnosed ante mortem in herpetofauna unless the parasite is producing a subcutaneous swelling or is accidentally discovered during laparotomy. Once observed, the parasite can be surgically removed.

The text by Wardle and McLeod offers a broad review of tapeworms, and has data on morphology and taxonomy of those infecting herpetofauna.[296]

Trematodiasis

Reptiles and amphibians commonly harbor flukes. Adult worms are usually found in the host's respiratory, urinary, or alimentary tracts, and larval trematodes occur in various tissues. The majority of these flatworms are in the order Digenea, which includes all the trematodes of man and domestic animals. Adult digenetic flukes have one or more ventral suckers for adhesion and are internal parasites of vertebrates in which they reproduce sexually. In most digenetic life cycles fluke eggs are passed in stool or urine. An infective stage enters a suitable mollusc (usually a snail) and, as a larva, reproduces asexually. An infective larval stage eventually enters the definitive host either by direct penetration (e.g., the schistosomes) or by ingestion of the larvae that are encysted either in the mollusc, on vegetation, or within another intermediate host.

Some of the common digenetic trematodes of herpetofauna and the way in which the definitive host is infected are listed in Table 3–3. Some of the host-parasite relationships listed in Table 3–3 are extremely common [e.g., *Ochetosoma (Neorenifer) aniarum*, *Pneumoneces (Haematoloechus)* spp. (Fig. 3–47), and *Dasymetra* spp.] and may be expected to occur in the majority of reptiles or amphibians coming from enzootic areas. The vast majority of digenetic trematodes listed in Table 3–3 cause little if any damage in their natural hosts and are likely to be significant pathogens only in aberrant hosts, or in aberrant sites in the usual hosts, or when they are present in unusually large numbers.

Renifers are a group of flukes including the genera *Renifer*, *Dasymetra*, *Ochetosoma*, *Stomatrema*, *Pneumatophilus*, and *Lechriorchis*. They are commonly found in the mouth, pharynx, esophagus, trachea, or lung of certain snakes, e.g., indigo snakes *(Drymarchon corais cooperi)* (Fig. 3–48A), kingsnakes *(Lampropeltis* spp.), water snakes *(Natrix* spp.), hognose snakes *(Heterodon contortrix)*, and garter snakes *(Thamnophis* spp.*)*.[116] These trematodes usually crawl away with exposure to light when the snake's mouth is opened. They are thought to be nonpathogenic, but they may be associated with gaping of the mouth.

Table 3–3. Some Common Digenetic Trematodes of North American Herpetofauna

SITE IN WHICH ADULT FLUKE IS FOUND	FLUKE SPECIES	DEFINITIVE HOST	MEANS OF INFECTION
Mouth	*Ochetosoma (= Neorenifer) aniarum*	Water snakes (*Natrix* spp.)	Ingestion of tadpoles
	Halipegus spp.	Frogs (*Rana* spp.)	Ingestion of dragonflies
Lungs	*Pneumoneces (Hematoloechus)* spp.	Frogs (*Rana* spp.)	Ingestion of dragonflies
Trachea	*Pneumatophilus* spp.	Water snakes (*Natrix* spp.)	Ingestion of tadpoles
Esophagus	*Dasymetra* spp.	Water snakes (*Natrix* spp.)	Ingestion of tadpoles
Small intestine	*Brachycoelium* spp.	Salamanders of various genera	Ingestion of snail slimeballs or snails
	Crepidostomum serpentinum	Queen snake (*Natrix septemvitata)*	Probably ingestion of crayfish
	Plagitura parva	Newts (*Notophthalmus viridescens)*	Ingestion of snails or insect larvae containing metacercariae
	Glypthelmins spp.	Frogs (*Rana* spp.)	Metacercariae encyst in skin of adult frog which ingests its sloughed skin during molting
Large intestine, rectum	*Megalodiscus temperatus*	Frogs (*Rana* spp.)	Metacercariae encyst in skin; sloughed skin is ingested by the host.
	Diplodiscus spp.	Frogs (*Rana* spp.)	Metacercariae encyst in skin which is ingested after sloughing; also, ingestion of tadpoles
Biliary system	*Loxogenoides bicolor*	Frogs (*Rana* spp.)	Probably ingestion of dragonfly adults or nymphs
Urinary bladder	*Gorgoderina* spp.	Frogs (*Rana* spp.)	Ingestion of crayfish
Blood	*Spirorchis* spp.	Turtles (various genera)	Direct percutaneous penetration by cercariae

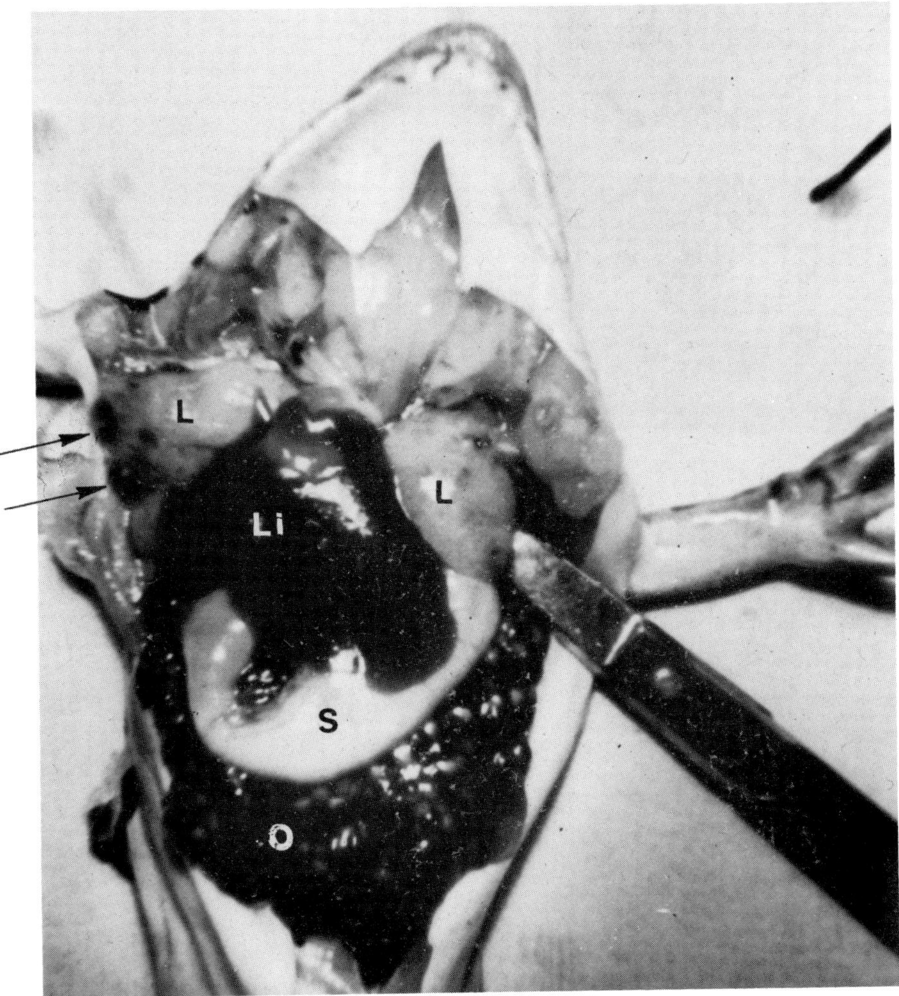

Fig. 3–47. Pulmonary trematodiasis in a female leopard frog *(Rana pipiens). Pneumoneces (Haematoloechus)* sp. are the dark spots in the lungs (over the tips of the scissors, right; arrows, left). **L**, lungs; **Li**, liver; **O**, ovary; **S**, stomach.

Snakes get infected by ingesting the metacercariae which encyst subcutaneously in amphibians, e.g., *Rana, Bufo,* and *Amphiuma* spp.

Cooper found large numbers of renifers *(Ochetosoma* and *Mesocoelium* spp.) in the mouth of newly caught bush vipers *(Atheris* spp.) (Fig. 3–48B) and was able to remove them with a moist swab.[64] Nelson recommends treating oral trematodiasis *(Lechriorchis tygarti)* in water snakes *(Natrix s. sipedon)* with 0.2 ml tetrachlorethylene per kg of body weight, given in capsule form, p.o., at least four days after the last feeding, with a second dose given no sooner than three weeks after the first.[216] Because of possible toxicity of the drug (liver damage) and the low pathogenicity of the flukes, such treatment is indicated only if the infection is unusually heavy and manual removal of the flukes impossible or impractical.

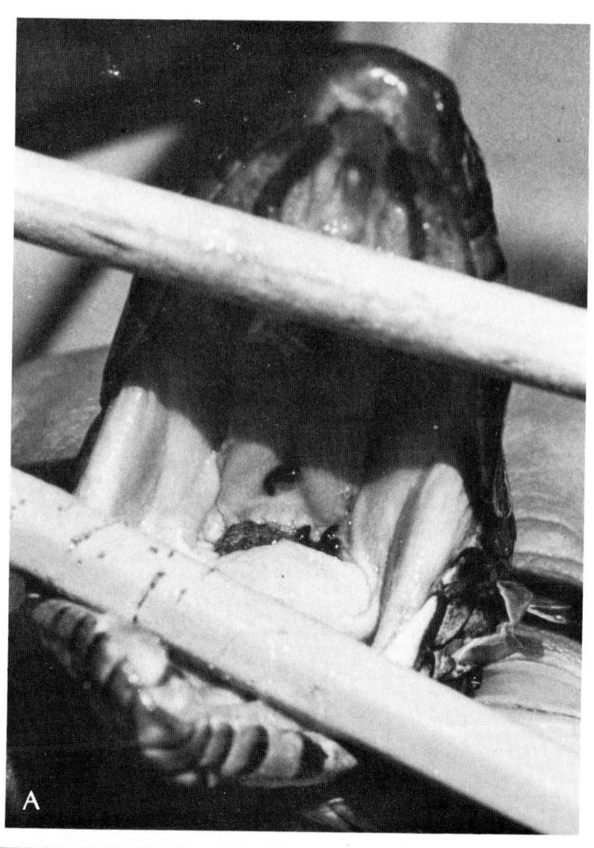
A

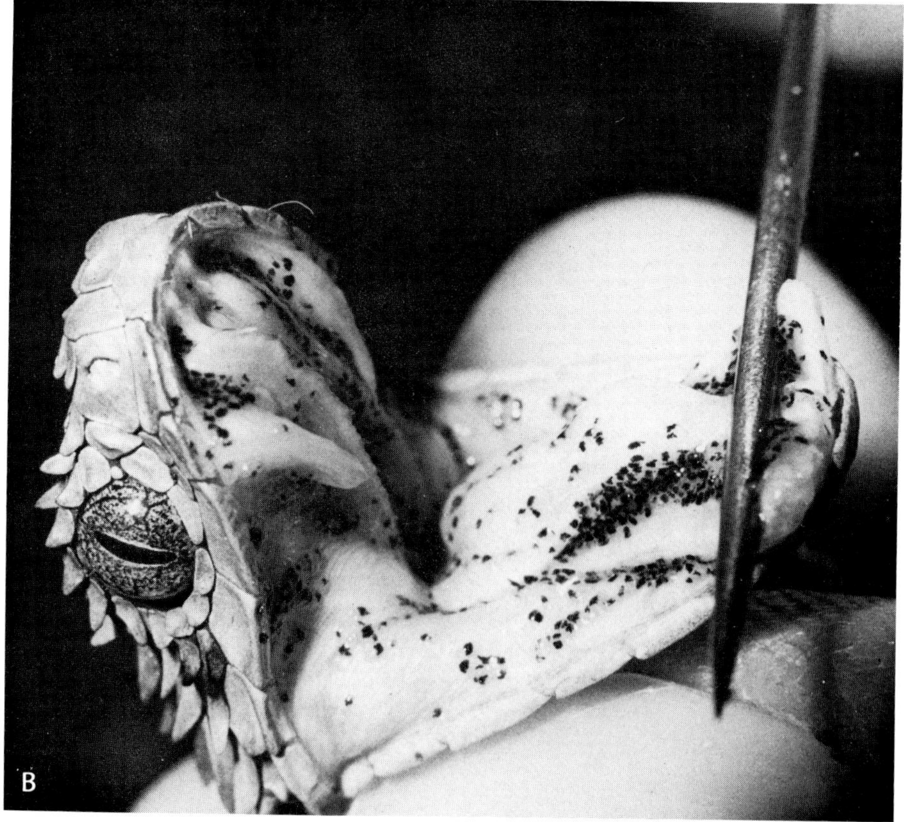
B

Adult flukes in the genus *Styphlodora* have been found in the renal tubules, ureters, or cloaca of kingsnakes (*Lampropeltis* sp.), cottonmouth moccasins (*Agkistrodon piscivorus*), indigo snakes (*Drymarchon corais*), tropical rat snakes (*Spilotes pullatus*), black-striped snakes (*Coniophanes sp.*), bushmasters (*Lachesis muta*), and boa constrictors (*Constrictor constrictor*). These flukes can cause renal tubular damage, including mineralization.[170a]

Herpetofauna act as secondary intermediate or carrier hosts for some digenetic flukes. For example, frogs and tadpoles harbor mesocercariae of *Alaria* spp. (strigeid flukes). When these amphibians are eaten by mice, rats, or raccoons, the next stage (mesocercaria) develops. The cycle is completed when a wild or domestic cat or dog eats the mesocercaria-bearing host, the adult fluke developing in the canine or feline gut. Mesocercaria of other strigeid flukes develop in frogs, tadpoles, salamanders, and water snakes, the definitive host being various aquatic birds that eat these animals. Strigeid larvae may be found in large numbers, causing severe necrosis and inflammation in their migratory path and probably causing some debility. Mesocercariae of the strigeid fluke, *Diplostomulum* sp., in the brain of *Triturus* newts is associated with "tumor" formation in the meninges;[182] the lesions were not adequately described, however, to determine if they were inflammatory or truly neoplastic. The mesocercaria of the strigeid, *Tylodelphis excarata*, may be found swimming in the cerebrospinal fluid of aquatic frogs, the definitive host being a stork. The mesocercaria of another strigeid, *Diplostomulum xenopi*, is commonly found encysted in the pericardium of the South African clawed toad, *Xenopus laevis*; heavy infections can cause epicardial hemorrhage and fatal pericardial effusion.[218]

A fatal *Alaria* infection occurred in a young man who may have eaten raw or undercooked frogs' legs.[93a] The hind legs of one bullfrog can harbor more than 3,000 mesocercariae, each larva barely visible (~300 μ long).[93a] Careful handwashing after handling tissue of frogs and other possible hosts of *Alaria* larvae seems prudent.

Larval strigeid flukes in Michigan were found to cause a "bloat disease" of tadpoles. Eight to 10 days following heavy infections, tadpoles developed abdominal distention, became sluggish, lost their equilibrium, floated on their backs, and died within a few days after onset of signs. Lighter infections result in a more prolonged illness.[66]

A remarkable infection by strigeid mesocercariae encysted within the lateral line system (see p. 46) of African clawed toads (*Xenopus laevis*) was described by Elkan.[81] All of the neural patches in the system were

←

Fig. 3–48. **A.** Flukes, family Ochetosomatidae, in the mouth of an indigo snake (*Drymarchon corais*). (From Soifer, F.: Parasitic diseases of reptiles. *In* Zoo and Wild Animal Medicine. Edited by M.E. Fowler. Philadelphia, W.B. Saunders Co., 1978. Photograph courtesy of Dr. Murray E. Fowler.) **B.** Oral trematodiasis in a bush viper (*Atheris* sp.). (From Cooper, J.E.: Veterinary aspects of recently captured snakes. Br. J. Herpetol., 5:368–374, 1973. Photograph courtesy of Dr. J.E. Cooper.)

infected and became hyperpigmented, while the rest of the toad's skin became pale, resulting in a neat, symmetrical design, as if the skin had been stitched (Fig. 3–49). Infected toads lost their equilibrium, stopped feeding, and died within two weeks after clinical onset.

The presence of metacercariae of various trematode species in the skin of amphibians is often marked by the deposition of melanocytes around the larval flukes. With the exception of the lateral line infection mentioned previously, cutaneous infection with larval flukes usually does not cause serious disease, so treatment is not indicated. But it is possible to pick out the encysted worms with a needle and the aid of a magnifying glass.

Spirorchidae is a family of flukes in which the adults are found in the blood of reptiles, especially turtles. Infection occurs by cercariae, shed by snails, penetrating directly through the host's skin or mucous membranes as in mammalian or avian schistosomiasis. The penetration apparently causes local irritation, manifested by clawing at the site, gaping, and snapping the jaws.[115,131] The flukes mature in the chambers of the heart and within the lumens of blood vessels. They deposit eggs that penetrate the vessel wall and often lodge in various organs where

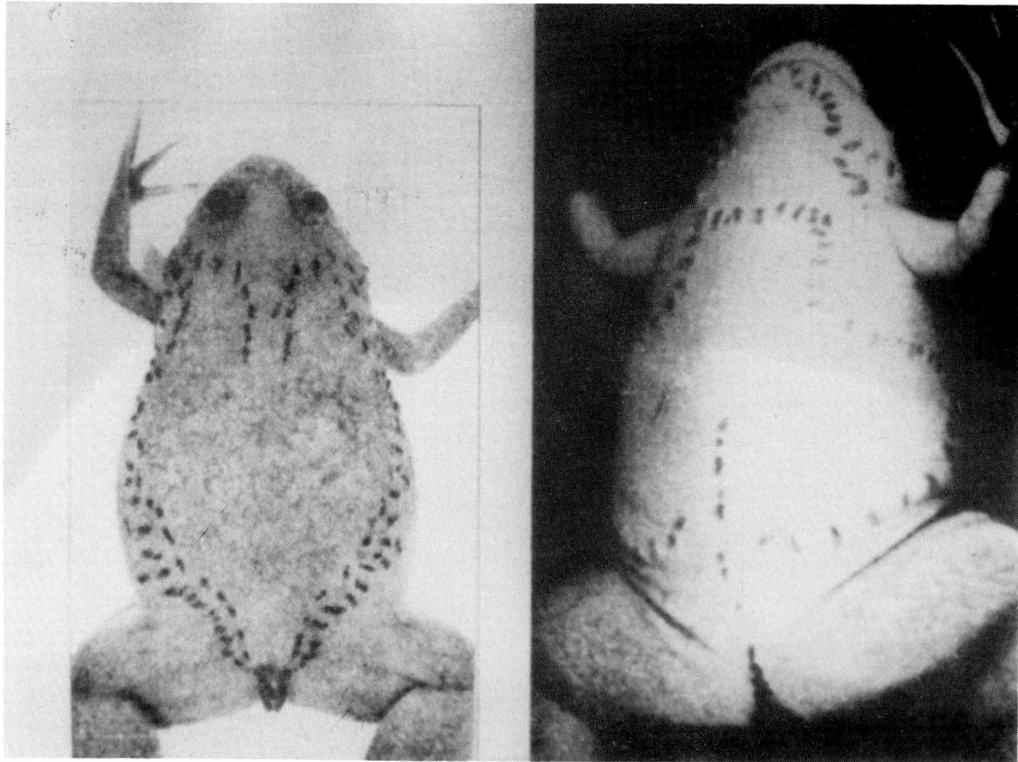

Fig. 3–49. *Xenopus laevis*. Adult female with cercarial infection of the lateral line system. Cercarial cysts below each neuromast with intense melanosis. Left, dorsal; right, ventral view. (From Reichenbach-Klinke, H. and Elkan, E.: The Principal Diseases of Cold Blooded Vertebrates. New York, Academic Press, 1965. Photograph courtesy of Dr. E. Elkan and the Zoological Society of London.)

they excite a granulomatous response. Only those eggs that enter the lumen of the gut and are passed via the feces into water can develop further. A miracidium hatches from the egg and burrows into a suitable snail where the larva multiplies asexually, finally producing cercariae which bore out of the snail and actively seek a new turtle host.

Spirorchid flukes, which often infect the arteries and veins of the painted turtle, *Chrysemys picta*, include *Spirorchis elegans*, which has a prepatent period of six to 10 weeks, and *S. parvus, S. elephantis,* and *S. artericola,* which have prepatent periods of three and a half to four months.[115] *Proparorchis artericola* is a blood fluke found in the arteries of freshwater turtles, including *Chrysemys (Pseudemys)* spp., and *Malaclemys (Malacoclemmys) leseierrii.*[295,302] The eggs of *P. artericola* incite granuloma formation in the lung and abdominal viscera.

A painted turtle with a five-centimeter (two-inch) shell length was presented with marked hydropic swelling of all four feet (Fig. 3–50). Paracentesis of the abdomen yielded a sterile, clear, colorless fluid with specific gravity 1.005 and a protein content of 1.4 g/dl. The animal died within two weeks and postmortem examination revealed multiple granulomata of heart, liver, kidneys, thyroid,

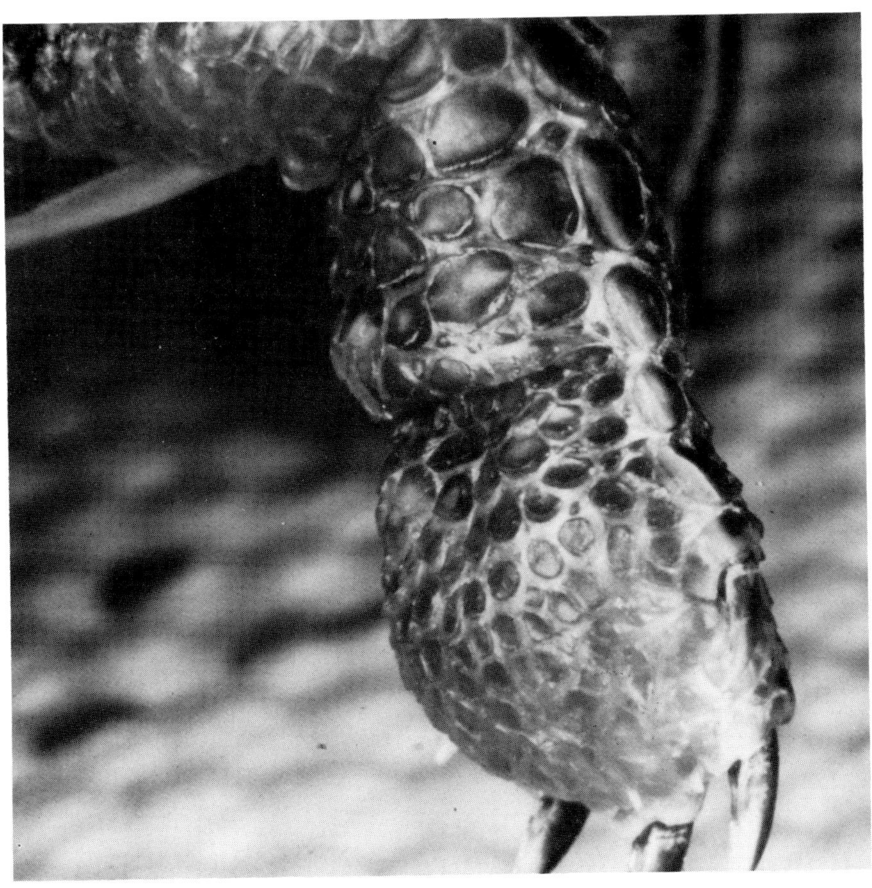

Fig. 3–50. Pedal edema in a western painted turtle *(Chrysemys picta belli)* with severe spirorchiasis.

intestine, spleen, pancreas, and lung containing eggs of a spirorchid fluke (Fig. 3–51). Adult flukes could not be found, which is usually the situation, apparently because they live a relatively short time while producing many eggs.

Spirorchids can cause severe lesions, including fluid accumulation, in turtles. Infected turtles become listless and may die if heavily parasitized or suffering from concurrent illness. Light infections may be subclinical.[131]

Diagnosis of spirorchiasis can be made by demonstrating the eggs in feces or tissue. Eggs are expelled in the stool in greater numbers if the turtle is kept on a soft diet for several days followed by roughage, e.g., lettuce.[131] Treatment for spirorchid infection has not been described.

Besides being host to digenetic trematodes, herpetofauna may harbor species of the other two trematode orders, Aspidobothrea and Monogenea.

The Aspidobothrea have been found as external and internal parasites of molluscs, fish, frogs, and turtles, but most of the Aspidobothrean parasites of herpetofauna are in the alimentary tract of turtles. Reproduction is sexual, and some species have alternate hosts in their life cycle. The adherent organ is an oval sucker (the opisthaptor) that

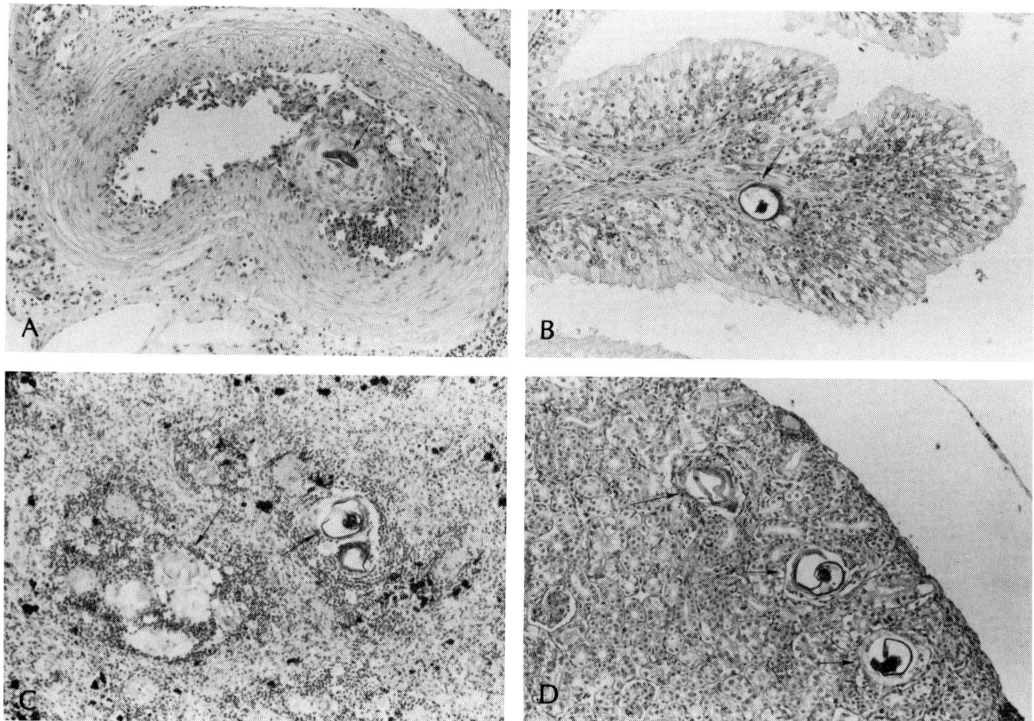

Fig. 3–51. Spirorchid eggs (arrows) in a western painted turtle *(Chrysemys picta belli)*. 125×. **A.** In a thrombus, with a giant cell formation, mesenteric artery. **B.** Intestine. **C.** Spleen. **D.** Kidney. Similar lesions were seen in the heart, thyroid, pancreas, liver, and lung of this animal.

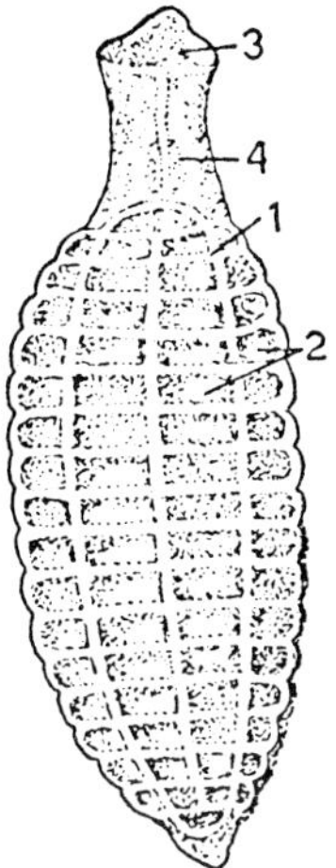

Fig. 3–52. Adult *Aspidogaster conchicola*, an internal parasite of clams which can also infect turtles eating parasitized clams. **1**, sucker; **2**, alveoli; **3**, mouth funnel; **4**, pharynx. (From Cheng, T.C.: The Biology of Animal Parasites. Philadelphia, W.B. Saunders Co., 1964.)

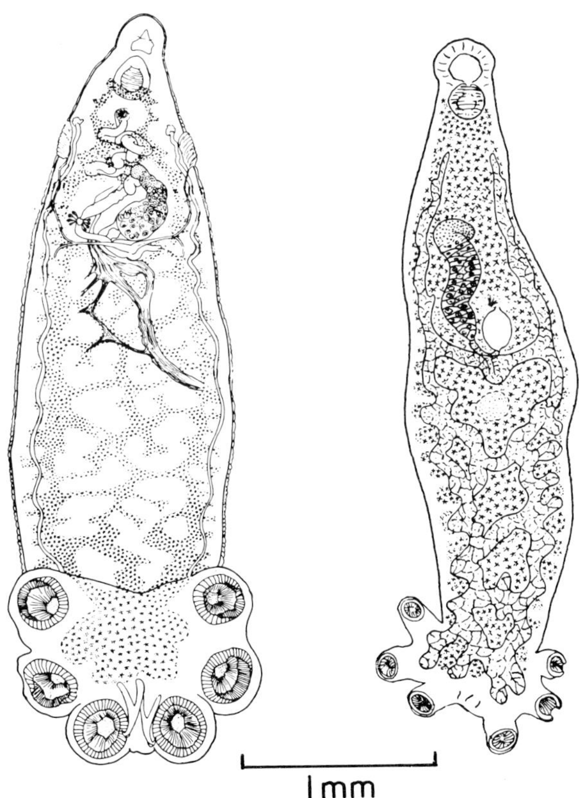

Fig. 3–53. *Polystoma integerrimum (nearcticum)* from the urinary bladder of the tree frog *Hyla versicolor*. Bladder generation (left); gill generation (right). (Reprinted with permission from Parasites of Laboratory Animals by Robert J. Flynn © 1973 by the Iowa State University Press, Ames, Iowa.)

covers the ventral surface of the body and is usually divided by septae into multiple alveoli (Fig. 3–52).

Monogenetic trematodes, like the Aspidobothrea, have no asexual reproduction. Their life cycle is direct and is limited to one host. Their adherent organ is a posteroventral sucker that has multiple smaller suckers and which may also have hooklets (Fig. 3–53). The majority of monogenetic flukes are ectoparasites of fish, but about two dozen species have been described in herpetofauna, the great majority of these being found in the urinary bladder of turtles. Others are found in the urinary bladder of frogs and toads, in the nose, mouth, and esophagus of turtles, and as ectoparasites of turtles and the mudpuppy *(Necturus maculosus)*.

The life cycle of *Polystoma integerrimum (nearcticum)* (Fig. 3–53), the most common monogenetic trematode of amphibians, is representative of the Monogenea infecting herpetofauna.[55,233] The monoecious adults live in the urinary bladder of various frogs and toads. The worms copulate in the spring, and the female worms lay eggs for one week, during the spawning season of their hosts. Anurans mate in water, so most of the eggs laid by the worms reach an aqueous environment. Maturation of the trematode larva is temperature-dependent; above 10°C (50°F) a ciliated larva, the onchomiracidium, emerges from the egg in about three weeks. The onchomiracidium attaches itself to the gills of tadpoles, which are at an appropriate stage of development to be parasitized. Most of the tadpoles have internalized their gill structure by this time, and if the larva finds such a host, it enters the tadpole's gill chamber and attaches to the gill filaments, where, for the next two months, the larval fluke subsists on mucous and sloughed cells from the host. When the gills are lost, as the tadpole metamorphoses into a frog, the worm migrates down the alimentary tract and eventually reaches the frog's urinary bladder where the trematodes subsist on blood derived from mucosal vessels. Sexual maturity is reached in three years, and the parasite can live for another three years after this. If the onchomiracidium attaches itself to the external gills of a younger tadpole it becomes a neotenic ectoparasite, i.e., it reaches sexual maturity while maintaining the larval form.

The most remarkable aspect of the life cycle of *P. integerrinum* is that the maturation of the worm is closely linked to the maturation and seasonal changes in the host, this synchronization apparently being controlled by the amphibian's endocrine balance.

Sphyranoura oligorchis, S. polyorchis, and *S. osleri* are monogenetic flukes found on the gills of mudpuppies *(Necturus maculosus)* in North America. They suck blood, fray the gills, and may cause asphyxiation.[159] Otherwise, little is known about the pathogenicity, and nothing has been published on the treatment of aspidobothrean and monogenetic trematodes of herpetofauna. Reichenbach-Klinke and Elkan list the members of these orders which parasitize reptiles and amphibians.[233] Further information on the biology of these parasites can be derived from the text by Cheng and from the references listed by him.[55]

Acanthocephalan Infections

The larvae of thorny-headed worms are occasionally found in the abdomen or subcutis of amphibians and terrestrial reptiles. No specific signs have been associated with such infections, they are not likely to be diagnosed clinically, and no drug treatment is known. The larvae are acquired by ingestion of arthropod intermediate hosts.

Adult thorny-headed worms are frequently found in the small intestine of certain aquatic turtles, these animals becoming infected by eating specific snail intermediate hosts. Frogs, toads, and newts acquire adult Acanthocephalids by ingestion of infected arthropods. These adult worms can cause nodular granulomas of the intestinal wall at the site of attachment and can also cause intestinal perforation. Diagnosis of infection can be made by finding the characteristic thick-shelled oval eggs containing rostellar hooklets. (These eggs must be differentiated from Cyclophyllidean tapeworm eggs which also contain hooklets, but are rounder.) Chemotherapy of acanthocephaliasis in amphibians and turtles has not been studied, but therapeutic agents used for the analogous condition in swine could be tried.

Nematode Infections

Among the great variety of nematodes found in the alimentary tract of herpetofauna a relatively few deserve specific mention because of their pathogenicity or frequency. Anthelminthics found effective against various intestinal nematodes in reptiles include piperazine citrate (40 to 60 mg/kg), dichlorvos (Task, Shell Chemical Co.) (12.5 to 25 mg/kg daily for two days), mebendazole (Telmin, Pitman-Moore Laboratories) (20 mg/kg daily for two days), and thiabendazole (Thibenzole, Merck) (50 mg/kg), all given p.o., and levamisole (Tramisole, Cyanamide) (5 mg/kg, subcutaneously). Where known, drugs of choice for specific nematode infections are given later in this section. Doses given for reptiles in general should be halved for turtles.

Ascarids are found in many reptiles, the best known being *Polydelphis* and *Ophidascaris* spp. which snakes acquire by eating infected intermediate hosts such as frogs, marsupials, or rodents.[260,261] The adult worms, which superficially resemble the ascarids of dogs and cats, live in the snake's esophagus, stomach, or small intestine (Fig. 3–54). Eggs are passed in the stool (Fig. 3–55), and the embryo develops in the soil into a second-stage larva, which is infective via the oral route for the appropriate intermediate host within whose tissues it develops, awaiting ingestion by a suitable ophidian definitive host. Sprent has demonstrated that *Ophidascaris moreliae* larvae survive decomposition of the intermediate host (mouse).[260] Such larvae can be infective for pythons if they are released into water.

The extent of somatic migration by ophidascarid larvae within the snake varies among the nematode species. For example, third-stage *O. moreliae* larvae migrate to the lung of their python host, probably after direct penetration of the esophagus.[260] Third- and fourth-stage larvae migrate from the lung, up the trachea, and into the esophagus.

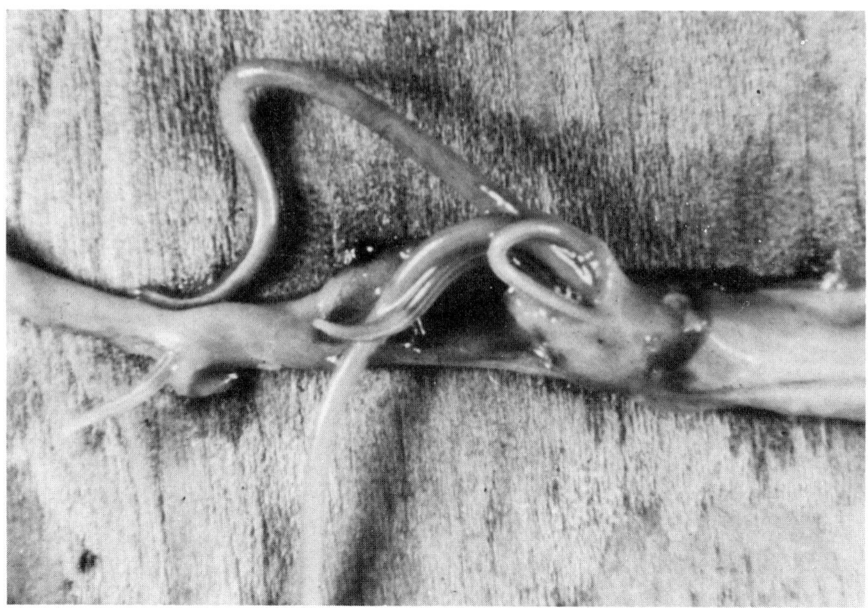

Fig. 3–54. *Ophidascaris* sp. adults emerging from an incision in the small intestine of a green palm viper *(Trimeresurus gramineus)* (Armed Forces Institute of Pathology Accession No. 1058159.)

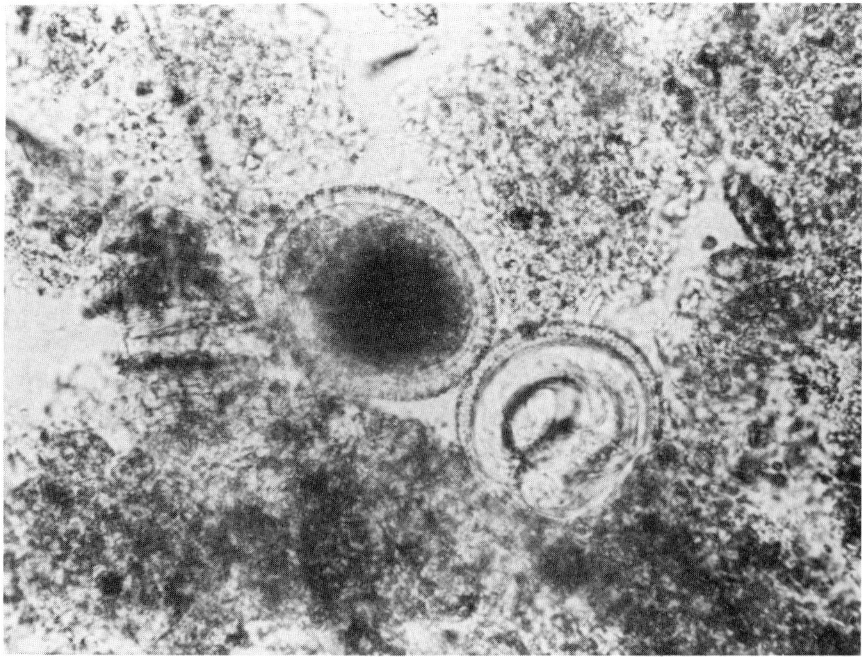

Fig. 3–55. Ophidascarid eggs in the stool of a reticulated python *(Python reticulatus)*. The egg, lower right, contains an infective (first-stage) larva. Embryonation occurred in 10% formalin.

Polydelphis anoura, another ascarid of Australian pythons, develops to an infective third stage in the tissues of intermediate hosts. After these are ingested by the snake, the worms develop to maturity within the esophagus and stomach of the reptile without further somatic migration.[261]

A green palm viper *(Trimeresurus gramineus)* which had been well and was killed for investigative purposes had several adult ascarids in the small intestine (Fig. 3–54) and three larvae encapsulated on the surface of the liver (Fig. 3–56). The worms were in the genus *Ophidascaris*, species undetermined. The larvae were so well encapsulated that they could have matured to adulthood only if the host were eaten by another snake.

A peculiar characteristic of many ophidascarids is that the fourth-stage larvae and adults develop partially buried in the wall of the esophagus or stomach of the snake, clumped tightly together. Their heads are imbedded in the gastric mucosa while their bodies protrude into the lumen giving a "Medusa-head" effect (Fig. 3–57). *Ophidascaris labiatopapillosa* actually threads its way into and back through the stomach wall so that the middle of the worm's body is imbedded in the stomach wall and may even extend up to one centimeter into the mesentery while the head and tail ends of the worm protrude into the lumen of the stomach. *O. labiatopapillosa* is a parasite of North American snakes, e.g., water snakes *(Natrix s. sipedon, N. c. cyclopion)*, black

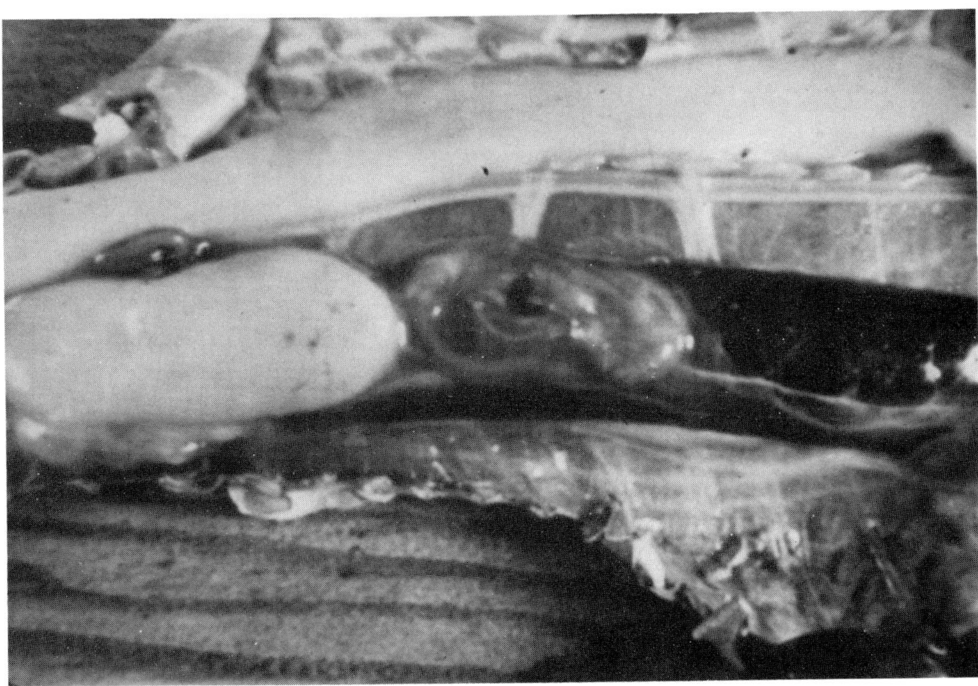

Fig. 3–56. *Ophidascaris* larvae encapsulated on the surface of the liver of a green palm viper *(Trimeresurus gramineus)*. The capsule on the left has been incised (upper edge), permitting the worm to emerge. (Armed Forces Institute of Pathology Accession No. 1058159.)

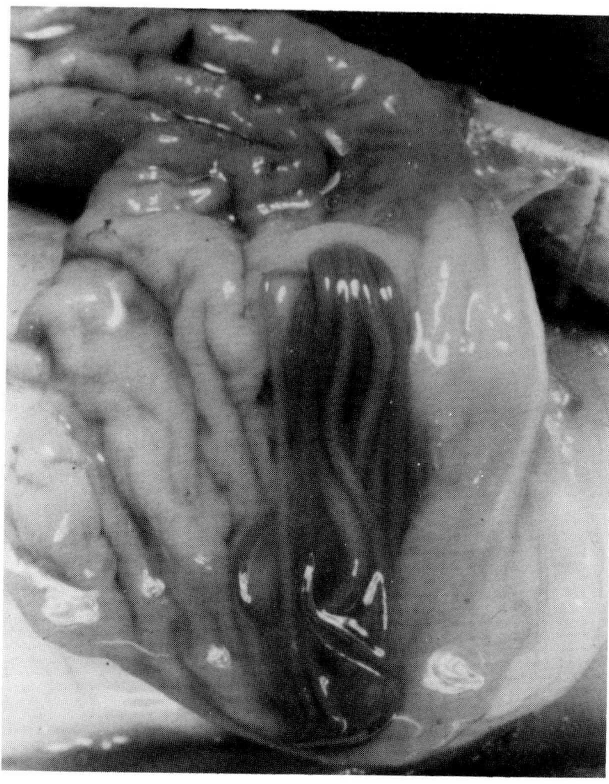

Fig. 3–57. Fourth-stage *Ophidascaris* larvae attached in a tight clump to one focal area in the gastric mucosa of a lesser Indian rat snake *(Elaphe carinata)*. (Armed Forces Institute of Pathology Accession No. 1058270.)

racer *(Coluber constrictor)*, hognose snake *(Heterodon platyrhinos)*, and the kingsnake *(Lampropeltis getulus)*, which utilizes frogs and other amphibians as intermediate hosts.[13]

Snakes can tolerate moderate ascarid loads without apparent ill effects. However, abscesses can form at the site of larval penetration of the stomach, resulting in separation of the muscular and submucosal layers.[87] In the presence of heavy infection or accompanying stress, e.g., intercurrent disease, these worms may compete significantly with their host for nutrients and can cause gastrointestinal perforation and intestinal, biliary, or pancreatic duct obstruction.[175] Developing and migrating larvae cause purulent and ulcerative lesions in the lung, trachea, and other sites which can prove fatal.

The presence of ascarids is apparent if the snake vomits or defecates the worms, but diagnosis is usually made by stool examination. Ophidascarid eggs resemble the eggs of ascarids of domestic animals in size and shape, being subglobular with thick shells (Fig. 3–56). The eggs of *Polydelphis anoura* measure 81 to 90 × 60 to 71 μ,[261] those of *Ophidascaris moreliae* average 81 × 78 μ,[260] and the eggs of *O. labiatopapillosa* measure 90 to 100 μ in diameter.[13] Reptilian ascariasis can be treated with 2,2 dichlorvinyl dimethyl phosphate (Atgard V, Shell Chemical Co.) using one oral dose of 24 mg per kg of body weight.[77a] Treatment can be repeated in a week if necessary. Alternative treatments are thiabendazole (Mintezol, Merck, Sharpe & Dohme), 50 mg per kg p.o., or 4 chlorophenol/methylbenzene (Vermiplex, Pitman-Moore, Inc.), 0.25 ml per lb. of body weight. The latter drug is given in capsule form; the number 2 capsule contains 2.5 ml of liquid. Care must be taken to avoid breaking the capsule in the snake's mouth because Vermiplex is caustic; flushing the capsule down the esophagus with water is advised. The therapeutic ratio of Vermiplex is low, and doses as low as 1.5 times the indicated level can cause convulsions in snakes.[111]

Kalicephalus is a genus of strongyloid nematodes parasitic in snakes which shows little host specificity. Depending on the species, these worms can be found anywhere in the alimentary tract from the esophagus to the rectum. Their presence has been associated with hemorrhagic ulcers (Fig. 3–58), accumulation of inflammatory debris, and obstruction of the GI tract.[63,85] Heavy infections may result in anorexia, debility, and death. Differential diagnosis includes bacterial, amebic, other parasitic, and toxic gastroenteritis.

Kalicephalus infections can be diagnosed by demonstrating the thin-walled, transparent oval eggs in the stool or in swabs of the esophagus. The eggs are in the morula stage when laid, but may contain the first-stage larva (Fig. 3–59) by the time they pass in the stool. The eggs of *K. parvus* measure 80 to 100 μ in length by 40 to 50 μ in width. The eggs of *K. agkistrodontis* and *K. rectiphilus* are the same width as

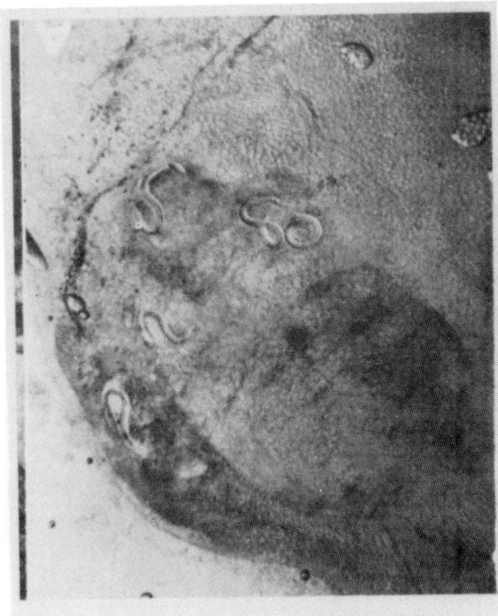

Fig. 3–58. Gastritis in a gopher snake (*Pituophis* sp.), two weeks post-infection, showing encysted third-stage larvae of *Kalicephalus parvus*. (Reproduced by permission of the National Research Council of Canada from the Canadian Journal of Zoology, *34*:425–452, 1956.)

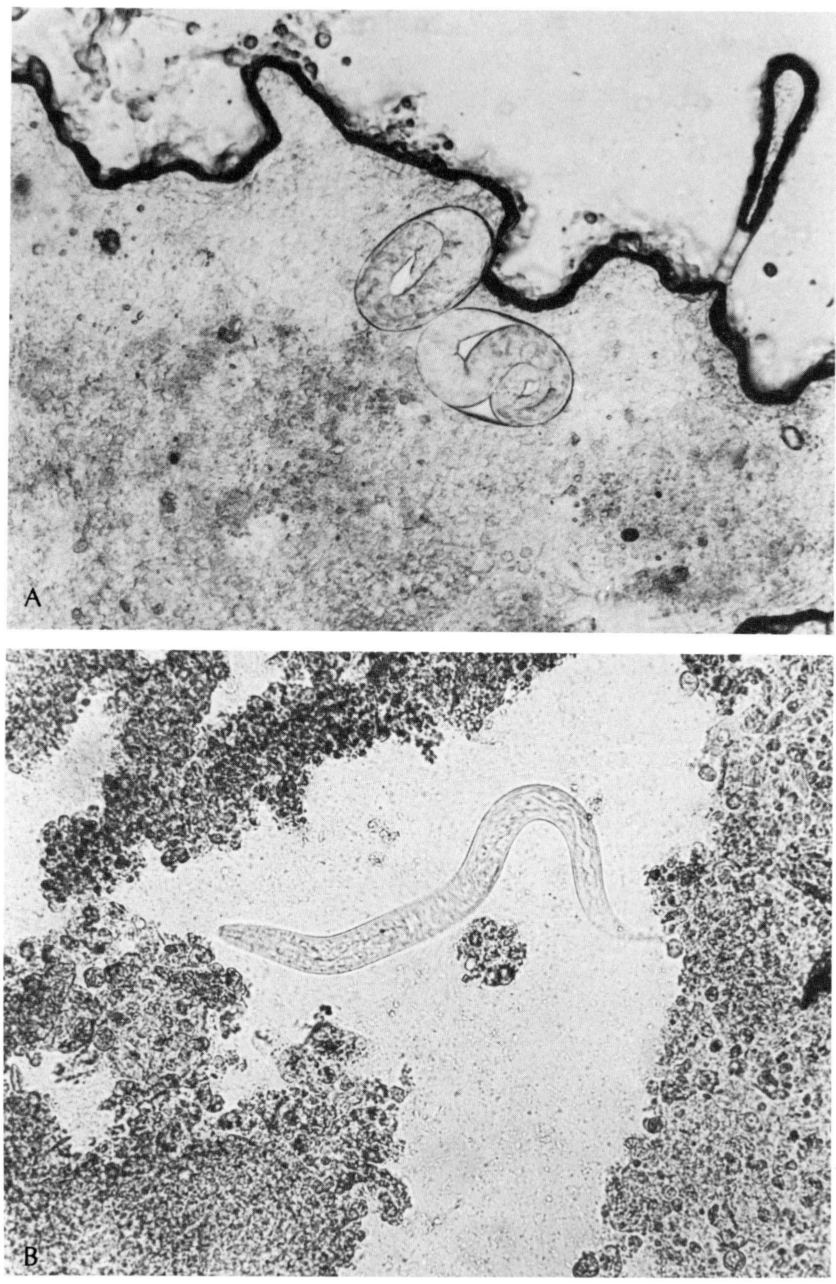

Fig. 3–59. **A.** Two eggs of *Kalicephalus* both containing developing larvae. **B.** A young larva of *Kalicephalus* among oesophageal debris. (From Cooper, J.E.: Disease in East African snakes associated with *Kalicephalus* worms (Nematoda: Diaphanocephalidae). Vet. Rec., *89*:385, 1971. Photographs courtesy of Dr. J.E. Cooper.)

those of *K. parvus*, but 10 μ shorter. The first-stage (rhabditiform) larvae of these three species average ⅓ mm long by 0.02 mm wide.[243]

The life cycle of *Kalicephalus* is direct. Infection can occur by ingestion of infective larvae and by percutaneous penetration.[243] This parasite can increase in numbers in captive reptiles. Prevention depends on keeping the cage dry and adequately removing stools from the cage. Treatment of *Kalicephalus* is with thiabendazole, 50 mg per kg, given as a drench that can be repeated in two weeks. If infection has become established in a snake colony, redosing should be done every six weeks after the first two doses.[63] This repeated treatment and adequate sanitation should eliminate kalicephaliasis.

Camallanus microcephalus, C. trispinosus, and *Spiroxys contortus* are nematodes commonly found in the stomach and duodenum of North American freshwater turtles. The first intermediate host is a copepod. Amphibians or fish that ingest the copepod become carrier hosts. Turtles become infected by ingesting the copepod or the carrier hosts. The worms imbed deeply in the gastric or duodenal wall and may cause abscesses.[159] Specific treatment has not been described, but broad spectrum anthelminthics (p. 151) could be tried.

Oxyurids are among the most common and numerous intestinal helminths of lizards and turtles. Unlike *Kalicephalus* spp., oxyurids show relatively high host specificity. Like their counterparts in man *(Enterobius vermicularis)*, rabbits *(Passaleuris ambiguus)*, and horses *(Oxyuris equi)*, these pinworms usually live in the lower GI tract and cause little overt or significant disease. There is one case report of a Fiji Island iguana *(Brachylophus fasciatus)* that suffered a fatal impaction of the colon owing to an intertwined mass of oxyurids *(Alaeuris brachylophi)*.[155]

Oxyuriasis is diagnosed by finding eggs or intact adults in the stool. In many species the eggs are oval with one flattened side. Some reptilian oxyurid eggs are embryonated at the time of deposition. Oxyurid life cycles are direct. Usually, no treatment is indicated for reptilian pinworms, but thiabendazole can be used, 50 mg per kg of body weight, giving two doses two weeks apart.

Nematodes in the superfamily Spiruroidea are often found in the stomach of herpetofauna. Infection is acquired by ingesting larvae encysted in intermediate hosts (copepods or insects). For example, *Skrjabinoptera phrynosoma* is often present in massive numbers in horned lizards *(Phrynosoma cornutum)*, the intermediate host being ants, which are the main dietary item of the lizard.[184] The life cycle of *S. phrynosoma* is remarkable because the adult female worm, containing encapsulated eggs in her uterus, is passed, intact, in the stool and is then picked up by certain ants that carry the worm to their nest. The worm is then eaten by larval ants that become infected with larval worms. When these ants become adults and are eaten by horned toads, the life cycle is completed.

Herpetofauna also act as intermediate hosts for spirurid larvae, the definitive host being a carnivore, such as a dog, cat, or man, which ingests the infected reptile or amphibian. For example, cats became infected with adult *Physaloptera rara* after being fed third-stage larvae removed from the stomach of rattlesnakes.[301] *Gnathostoma spinigerum* is the most important of the zoonotic spirurid larvae. The usual definitive hosts are wild and domestic canids and felids in Asia. The eggs, passed in their stool, get into water where a larva is released which is ingested by a minute crustacean *(Cyclops* spp.) which, in turn, is ingested by a fish, amphibian, or aquatic reptile. The worm remains in the larval stage if these cold-blooded animals are eaten by an inappropriate vertebrate, e.g., another reptile or man, but the life cycle is completed if the secondary intermediate host is eaten by a canid or felid. In man, *G. spinigerum* larvae produce an inflammatory reaction as they migrate in the subcutis, eye, or wall of the digestive tract.

Frogs *(Rana pipiens, R. clamitans, R. septentrionalis, R. catesbeiana)* and certain fish, e.g., pike or bullheads, are paratenic hosts for the giant kidney worm, *Dioctophyma renale*. The eggs of this nematode are passed in the urine of definitive carnivore hosts, e.g., mustelids and dogs. The eggs are ingested by freshwater oligochaetes *(Lumbricus variegatus)*, in which they develop to the infective (third) stage. If suitable frogs or fish eat the infected oligochaetes, the larvae encyst in their stomach, abdominal wall, or mesentery. The cycle is completed when definitive hosts eat infected oligochaetes, fish, or frogs.[190a]

Lungworms, mostly in the genus *Rhabdias*, are found in many species of frogs, toads, snakes, chameleons, and the slowworm, *Anguis fragilis*. In some areas, infection with lungworms is almost universal in some of these species, and individual worm burdens may be very high. Many of these cases show few, if any, clinical signs and may show minimal

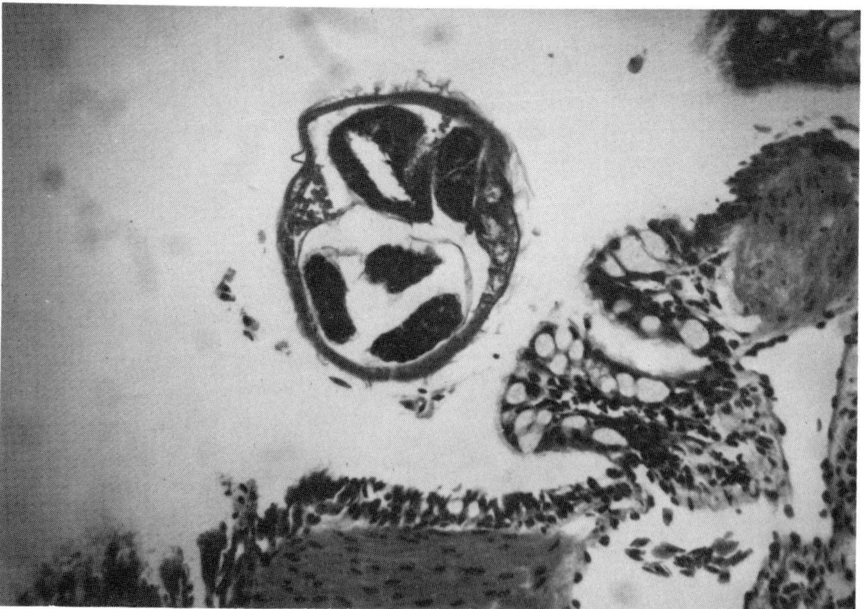

Fig. 3–60. Lungworm seen in cross section in the lung of a leopard frog *(Rana pipiens)*. As is usually seen in frogs, there is no accompanying necrosis and minimal inflammation.

inflammatory response (Fig. 3–60). Lungworms have been described, however, as a cause of severe respiratory distress in snakes which can terminate fatally. In such cases there is exudative pneumonia[312] (Fig. 3–61), and the major differential diagnosis is bacterial pneumonia, which was discussed at the beginning of this chapter (p. 89).

The life cycle of *Rhabdias* spp. is similar to that of *Strongyloides* spp. except that the adults of the former reside in the lung, whereas the latter live in the small intestine of their respective hosts. The adult female lungworm produces embryonated eggs or rhabditiform larvae in the lung. These eggs or larvae pass up the trachea to the mouth, are swallowed, and are passed in the stool, which can be examined to establish the diagnosis. Rhabditiform larvae mature in the soil, mate, and produce infective filariform larvae that enter a suitable amphibian or reptilian host either orally or percutaneously. The larvae then migrate via the bloodstream to the lungs, where they mature.[304] Heavy larval invasion can prove fatal, as demonstrated in *R. sphaerocephala* infection in the giant toad, *Bufo marinus.*[304] Under unsanitary conditions this life cycle can be perpetuated in captivity, so prevention depends on keeping cages clean and dry.

Zwart and Jansen treated lungworm infections in water snakes *(Natrix tessellata, N. natrix)* and garter snakes *(Thamnophis sirtalis)* with apparent success, using tetramisole (Ripenol), 10 mg per kg intrapleuroperitoneally, and oral oxytetracycline.[316] Fiennes has reported some success treating lungworm infections in snakes with piperazine.[87]

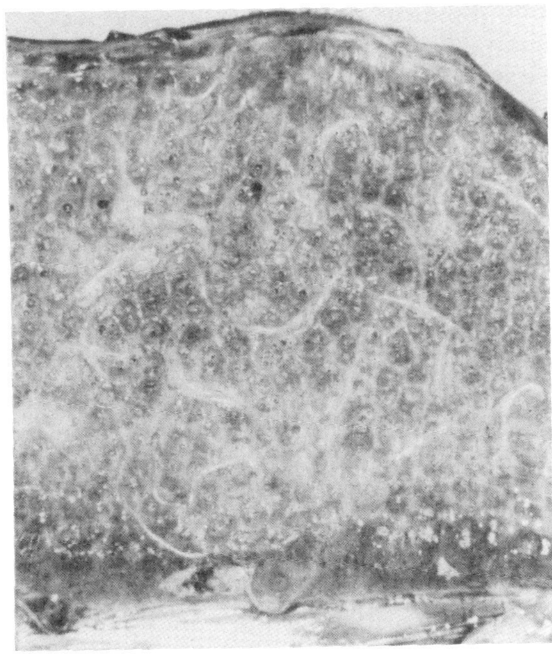

Fig. 3–61. Aesculapian snake *(Elaphe longissima)* with severe verminous pneumonia caused by lungworms *(Rhabdias fuscovenosa)*. (From Zwart, P.: Ziekten van reptielen II: Aandoeningen van de ogen, de oren, de mondholte en de longen. Lacerta, *30*:72–79, 1972.)

Filarial worms are found in various amphibians and reptiles.[69,305] Depending on the species, adult worms may be in major vessels or connective tissue, e.g., the subcutis or mesentery. Filariasis may be subclinical, but in massive infections, especially in abnormal hosts, blood or lymphatic vessels may be occluded, resulting in edema and/or necrosis of the area supplied by the thrombosed vessel.

Cutaneous swellings and severe, necrotic dermal lesions caused by *Macdonaldius oschei*, a filaria of New World snakes, have been described in captive Asiatic pythons[233] (Fig. 3–62). In the aberrant (Asiatic python) hosts, the adult worms are found primarily in the mesenteric arteries (Fig. 3–63). In the natural (New World) hosts, the adult worms are usually found in the posterior vena cava and renal portal vein where they sometimes cause aneurysms and thrombosis[273] (Fig. 3–64). Despite the severity of these venous lesions, *M. oschei* infections in boa constrictors and other Mexican snakes are usually subclinical, and no associated dermal lesions are found.[269]

As in mammalian filariasis, diagnosis is made by finding the microfilariae in the blood (Fig. 3–65) or finding adult filariae or microfilariae in lesions. Prevention of filariasis depends on elimination of the vectors that are blood-sucking arthropods, e.g., ticks and mosquitoes. Chemotherapy for reptilian filariasis has not been reported, to my knowledge, but agents used for analogous veterinary and medical conditions could be tried, e.g., diethylcarbamazine. It has been reported that adult *M. oschei* in boa constrictors *(Constrictor constrictor mexicanus)* can be killed by keeping the snakes at a constant ambient temperature of 35 to 37°C for 24 to 48 hours, although the microfilariae may persist for more than a week.[268]

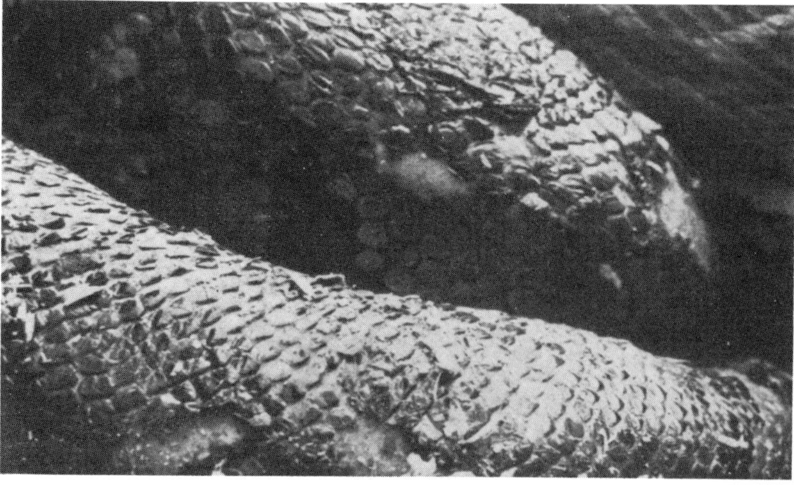

Fig. 3–62. Necrosis of the skin with loss of scales in a reticulated python *(Python reticulatus)* caused by filariasis. (From Reichenbach-Klinke, H. and Elkan, E.: The Principal Diseases of Lower Vertebrates. New York, Academic Press, 1965.)

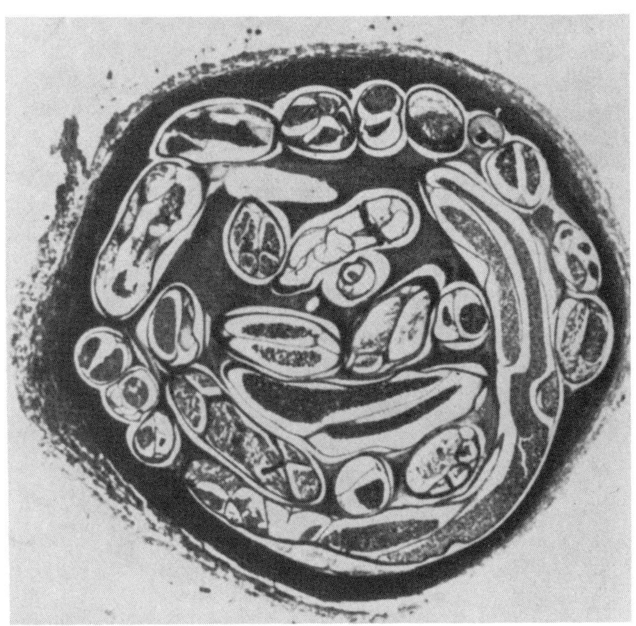

Fig. 3–63. Section through the mesenteric artery of *Python molurus bivittatus* Kühl filled with adult filarial worms of *Macdonaldius oschei* Chabaud and Frank. (Photo by W. Frank. From Reichenbach-Klinke, H. and Elkan, E.: The Principal Diseases of Lower Vertebrates. New York, Academic Press, 1965.)

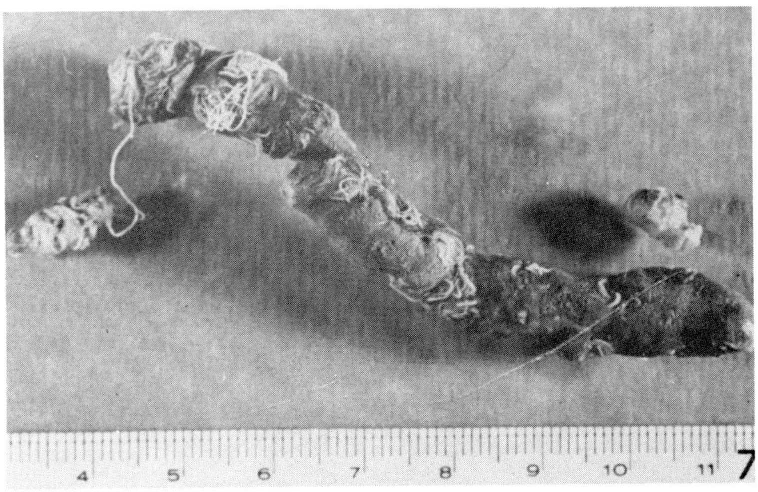

Fig. 3–64. A mass of filarial worms, *Macdonaldius oschei*, which occluded the posterior vena cava of a *Boa constrictor*. (From Telford, S.R., Jr.: Parasitic diseases of reptiles. J. Am. Vet. Med. Assoc., *159*:1644–1652, 1971.)

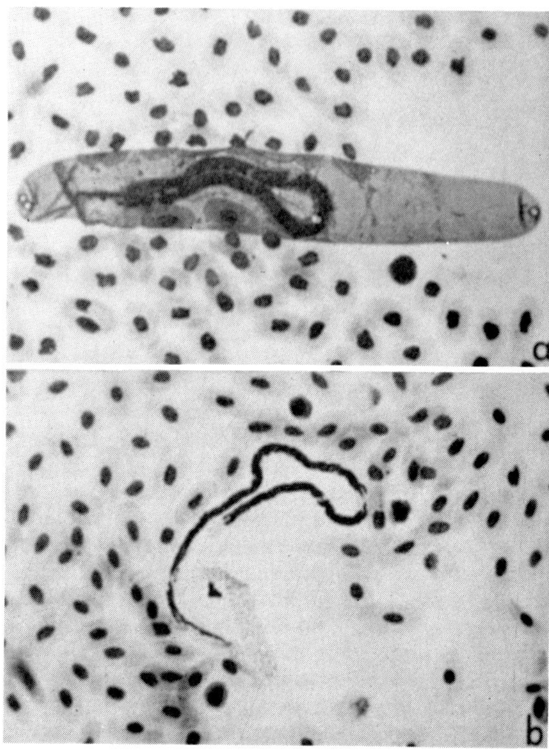

Fig. 3–65. Microfilariae of a Mexican boa constrictor *(Constrictor constrictor)*. **A**, *Macdonaldius oschei*. **B**, *M. colimensis*. (From Telford, S.R., Jr.: Parasitic diseases of reptiles. J. Am. Vet. Med. Assoc., *159*:1644–1652, 1971.)

Leeches

Leeches are common ectoparasites on aquatic reptiles and amphibians, especially turtles. After these blood-sucking annelids feed to repletion they drop off the host, so they are not commonly seen in captive herpetofauna. Adequate quarantine procedures before introducing new specimens in a collection should effectively prevent these worms from becoming established in such potentially suitable environments as a turtle pond in a zoo.

Leeches should not simply be pulled off as this may traumatize the host's skin or may leave the mouthparts imbedded in the host. Topical application of concentrated salt solutions, alcohol, or vinegar can encourage the leech to release its hold. Some of the leeches that attack reptiles are not very host-specific and may attack man and other animals. The same treatment to remove the leeches can be used on these hosts.

A very remarkable and unique situation has been reported by Mann and Tyler, in which a leech, *Philaemon* sp. (probably *Ph. grandidieri*), was found as an internal parasite of five species of frogs in New Guinea.[193] Most of the leeches were found singly and located subcutaneously in the dorsal lymph sac (Fig. 3–66), and some of them were

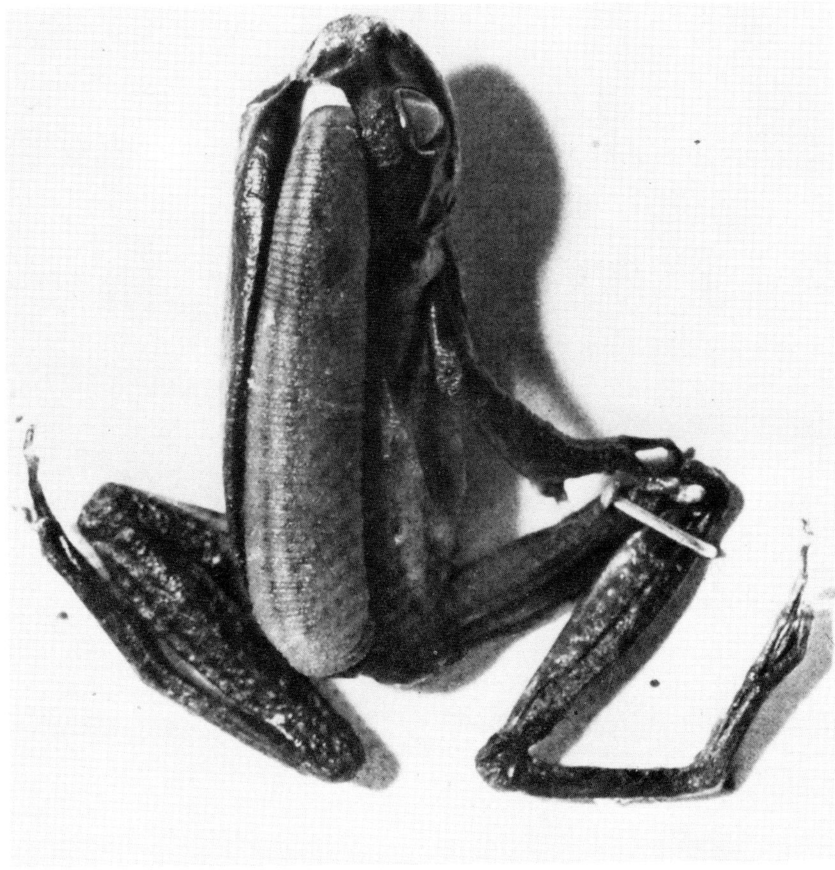

Fig. 3–66. A leech *(Philaemon)* in the dorsal lymph sac of a small frog of New Guinea. (From Reichenbach-Klinke, H. and Elkan, E.: The Principal Diseases of Lower Vertebrates. New York, Academic Press, 1965. Courtesy of B.N. Dovetil, Esher, Surrey.)

even in the body wall and body cavity. The only possible treatment for this unusual endoparasitism would be surgical removal of the leech.

In addition to their role as bloodsuckers, leeches are also intermediate hosts for hemogregarines and for trypanosomes in aquatic herpetofouna. Leeches *(Ozobranchus branchiatus)* have been found in association with cutaneous fibroepitheliomas in green sea turtles *(Chelonia mydas)*, but a causal relationship has not been proven (see p. 207).

Pentastomiasis

Pentastomes are a phylum of parasites which show some of the characteristics of arthropods and annelid worms. The great majority of pentastomes are found as adults in reptiles.

For the pentastomes considered here, the life cycle pattern is as follows: The adult worm resides in the respiratory tract (usually the lungs) of snakes, lizards, or crocodilians (a few species are found in turtles). Eggs are deposited (Fig. 3–67) containing the primary larva

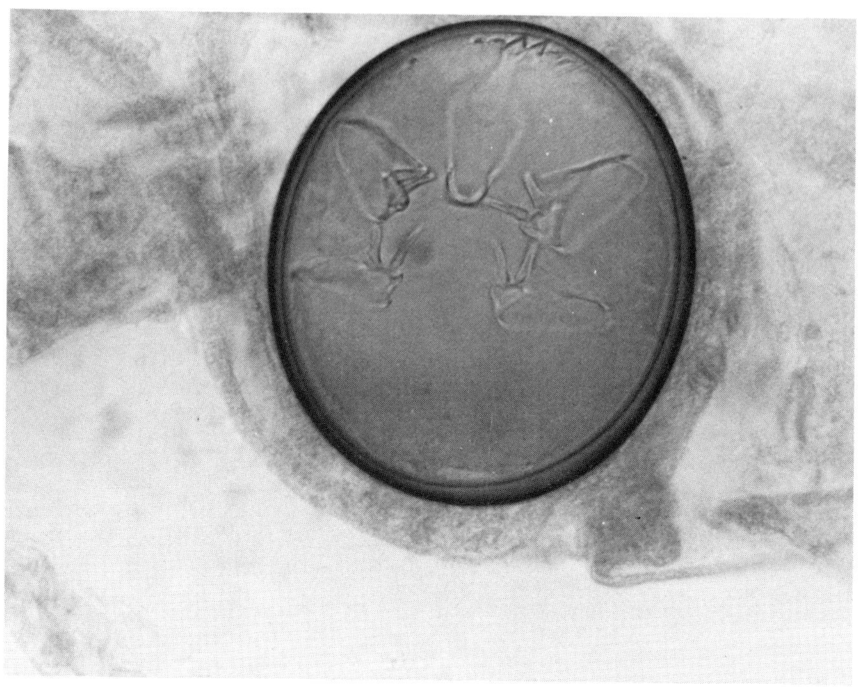

Fig. 3–67. Egg (125 μ diameter) containing primary larva of *Raillietiella orientalis* from a cobra *(Naja naja philippinensis)*. 320×. (Courtesy of Dr. D.E. Deakins. From Deakins, D.E.: *Raillietiella orientalis* (Pentastomida) hyperinfection in *Naja naja philippinensis* (Reptilia: Serpentes). M.S. thesis, University of Oklahoma, 1969.)

which may have four nonjointed leg-like appendages (Fig. 3–68), giving it superficial resemblance to a mite. The eggs are brought up in the sputum, passed in the stool, and then develop to an infective stage and are swallowed by a suitable intermediate host such as a rodent, primate, or ungulate. It is likely that insects act as intermediate hosts for certain *Raillietiella* spp. in lizards. Man may also enter the pentastome life cycle as an intermediate host (see p. 167). The larvae develop into infective nymphs in the mesentery, liver, and other tissues of the intermediate host and develop into adults in the reptilian respiratory tract after the intermediate host is swallowed by the definitive reptilian host. The body of the adult worm is pseudosegmented by a series of thickened cuticular annulations which, in some species, look like a series of rings (Fig. 3–69).

Pentastomes have a great capacity to bore through tissue and, on occasion, adult worms may bore through the lung and body wall and protrude from the skin (Fig. 3–70). They have also been seen to emerge from the mouth or nares (Fig. 3–71), especially when the hosts are stressed or anoxic. Pentastomes often occur in great numbers, both as adults in the definitive host and as larvae and nymphs in intermediate hosts. Despite their numbers and their capacity to migrate through tissue, most larval and adult pentastome infections in natural hosts are

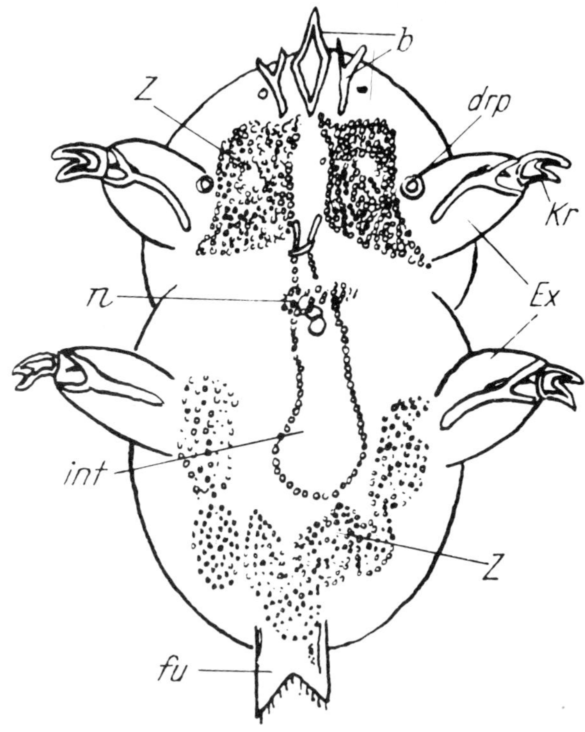

Fig. 3–68. Primary larva of *Porocephalus clavatus*. From Osche (1963). **b**, penetrating apparatus; **drp**, gland pore; **ex**, appendage; **fu**, forked terminal appendage; **int**, intestine; **Kr**, claws (appendage hooks); **n**, rudiments of nervous system; **z**, large gland cells. (From Self, J.T.: Biological relationships of the Pentastomida; a bibliography on the Pentastomida. Exp. Parasitol., *24*:63–119, 1969. Photograph courtesy of J. Teague Self.)

asymptomatic and may cause little inflammatory reaction.[252] In some cases, however, there may be significant damage to the reptilian host, e.g., by direct destruction of tissue or by occlusion of the trachea.

Reptiles can suffer autoinfection with some pentastomes, e.g., *Raillietiella, Sambonia,* and *Kiricephalus* spp., resulting in tissue invasion by larvae, nymphs, and adults, with hemorrhagic, acute inflammatory, or chronic granulomatous reaction in various organs, especially the colon, liver, and lungs.[74] Deakins has described massive granulomatous colitis with severe fibrosis of the gut wall and severe granulomatous inflammation of portal areas in the liver in such cases.[74] The larvae of *Sebekia oxycephala* caused hemorrhagic necrosis in the liver and the adults caused hemorrhagic necrosis in the lungs of American alligators *(Alligator mississippiensis)*.[123a] The severity and nature of the response to pentastomes is influenced by the immunologic status of the host, prior sensitization, intercurrent disease, and number and stages of the invading worms. Nymphs and adult pentastomes feed on parenchymal cells and blood, and massive infections can cause significant hemorrhage and destruction of tissue.

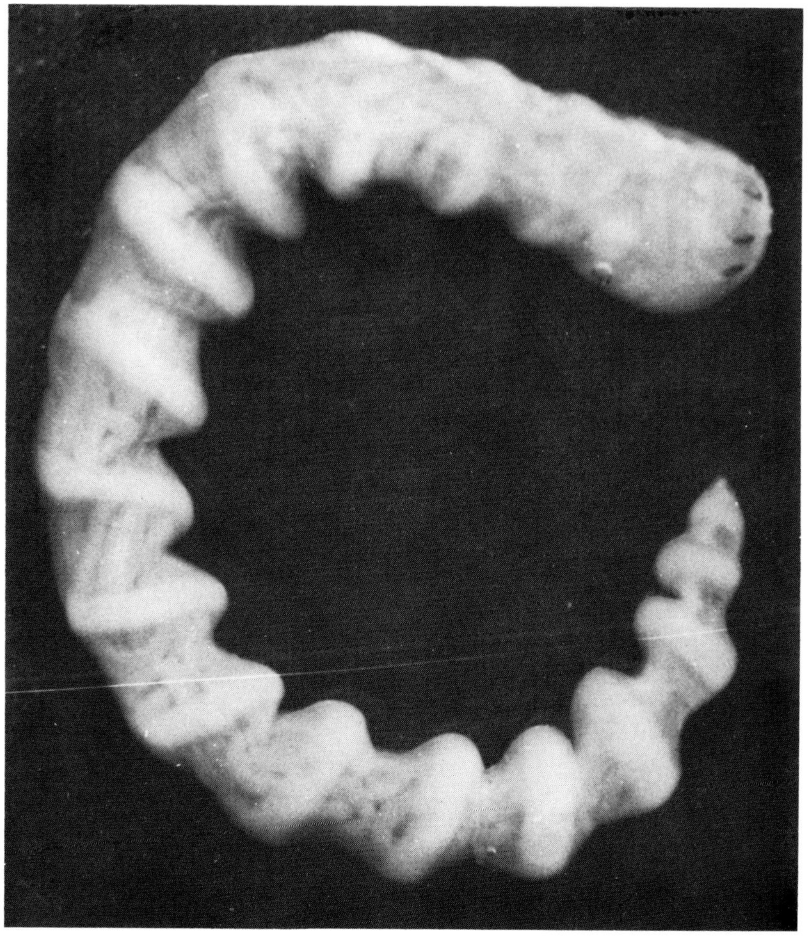

Fig. 3–69. Adult *Armillifer armillatus*, a common pentastome of African pythons and vipers. (Courtesy of George L. Graham, Ph.D.)

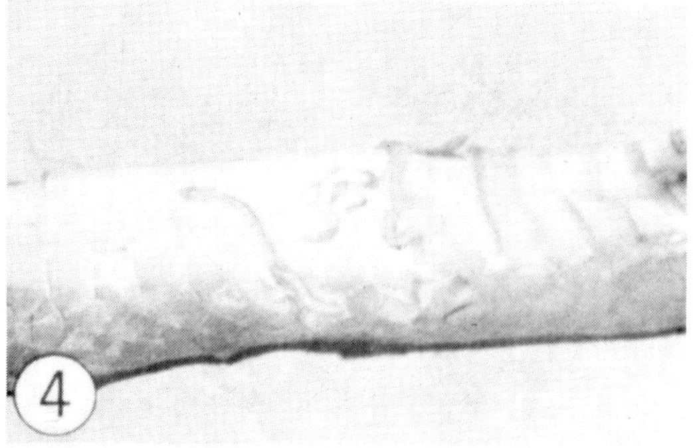

Fig. 3–70. Pentastomes, *Kiricephalus pattoni*, emerging through the skin of a green snake (*Opheodrys* [*Liopeltis*] *major*). (From Self, J.T. and Kuntz, R.E.: Host-parasite relations in some Pentastomida. J. Parasitol., *53*:202–206, 1967.)

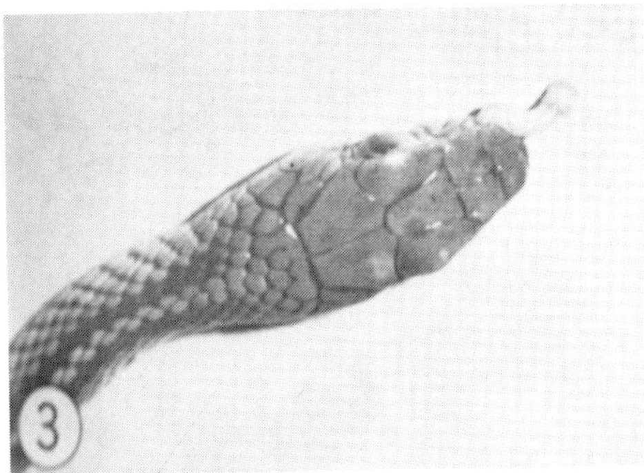

Fig. 3–71. A pentastome, *Kiricephalus pattoni*, emerging from the nostril of a green snake *(Opheodrys [Liopeltis] major)*. (From Self, J. T. and Kurtz, R. E.: Host-parasitic relations in some Pentastomida. J Parasitol., *53*:202–206, 1967.)

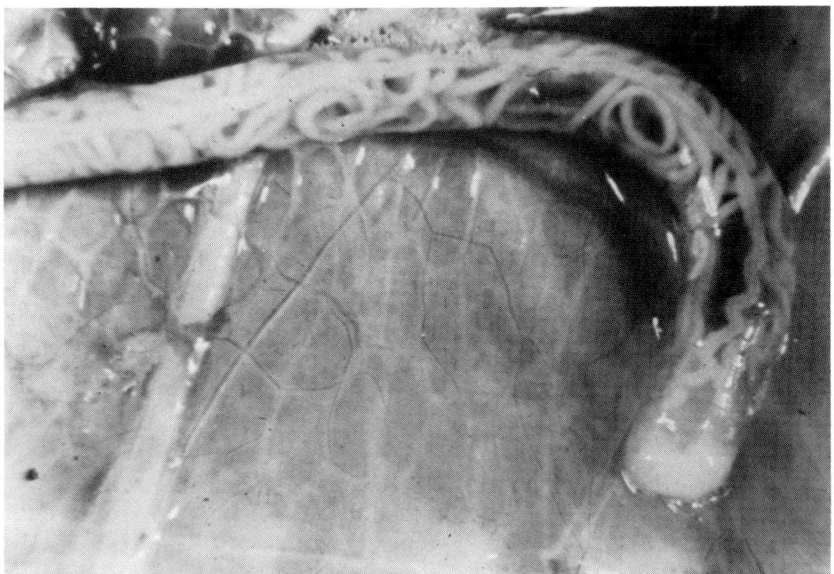

Fig. 3–72. Cranial half of an adult female pentastome, *Porocephalus crotali*, in the lung of a cottonmouth moccasin *(Agkistrodon piscivorus)*. The head of the worm is attached to the lung (lower right). The coiled genital tract can be seen through the transparent cuticle. (Armed Forces Institute of Pathology Accession No. 1058160.)

Examples of common adult pentastomes in reptiles include *Armillifer armillatus* (see Fig. 3–69) in African pythons and vipers, *Porocephalus crotali* (Fig. 3–72) in the cottonmouth moccasin *(Agkistrodon piscivorus)* and North American rattlesnakes *(Crotalus* spp.*)*, *Kiricephalus* spp. in colubrid snakes (including many of the nonpoisonous snakes of the United States), *Raillietiella* spp. in lizards and snakes, and *Sebekia* spp. in crocodilians.

Armillifer armillatus commonly uses primates, rodents, and small antelopes as intermediate hosts; man is commonly an accidental host in

Africa. Despite the fact that the great majority of human infections are asymptomatic, appropriate sanitary precautions should be taken to prevent ingestion of eggs in the event someone has an infected snake.

There is no known effective treatment for pentastomiasis in reptiles. An extensive review and bibliography of the Pentastomida has been published.[251]

ACARIASIS

According to Reichenbach-Klinke and Elkan, 250 species of mites have been described as reptilian parasites.[233] The most common and best known among these is the snake mite, *Ophionyssus natricis (serpentium)* (Fig. 3–73), a major pathogen in captive reptiles. This mite is red, grey, or black and approximately one mm long. It is found between and under the scales of snakes (and, less commonly, lizards), especially in the areas of the chin, eye, and cloaca.

Infested snakes often rub and twist their body and may remain immersed in water for an unusually long time. Mites drowned by this immersion can be seen in the water dish.[166] Under unsanitary conditions in captivity the mite population can increase enormously; heavily infested reptiles become debilitated through blood loss. These mites

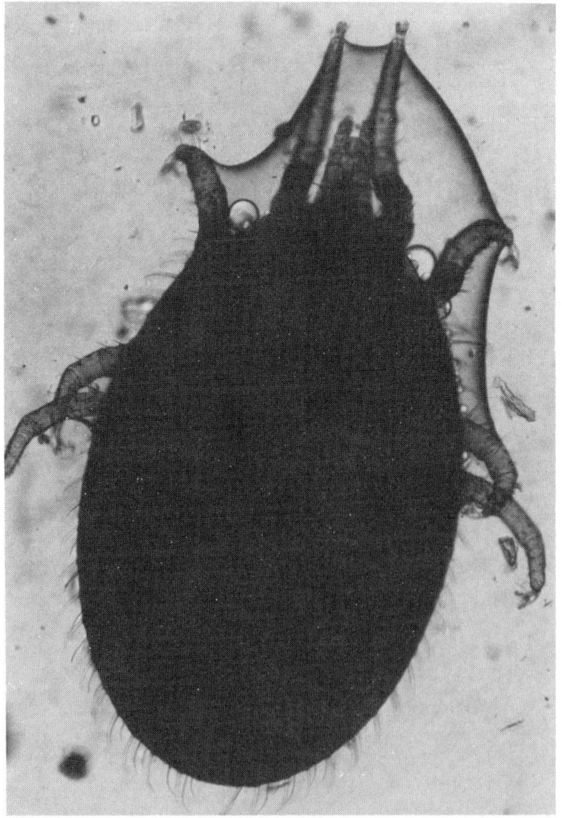

Fig. 3–73. *Ophionyssus natricis (serpentium)*, adult, 60×.

also transmit *Aeromonas hydrophila*,[51] a gram-negative rod that causes pneumonia and hemorrhagic septicemia in reptiles (see p. 89). *O. natricis* can cause dermatitis in humans.[248]

Some lizards reduce their ectoparasite load by eating the mites.[48] By doing this, they may infect themselves with certain hematozoa. Inspection for mites should always be included in the physical examination of snakes.

Infestation with mites can be treated topically with a silica gel powder (Dri-Die 67, Neil A. Maclean Co.), which dehydrates the mites. This powder should be used with caution on very small reptiles because it can also have a dehydrating effect on them. Another undesirable side effect is aerosolization and inhalation by the patient and the person applying the dust. Hanging DDVP-impregnated fly strips (Vapona, Shell Chemical Corp.) reportedly eliminates the mites, but in my experience such compounds can be toxic to small reptiles such as anole

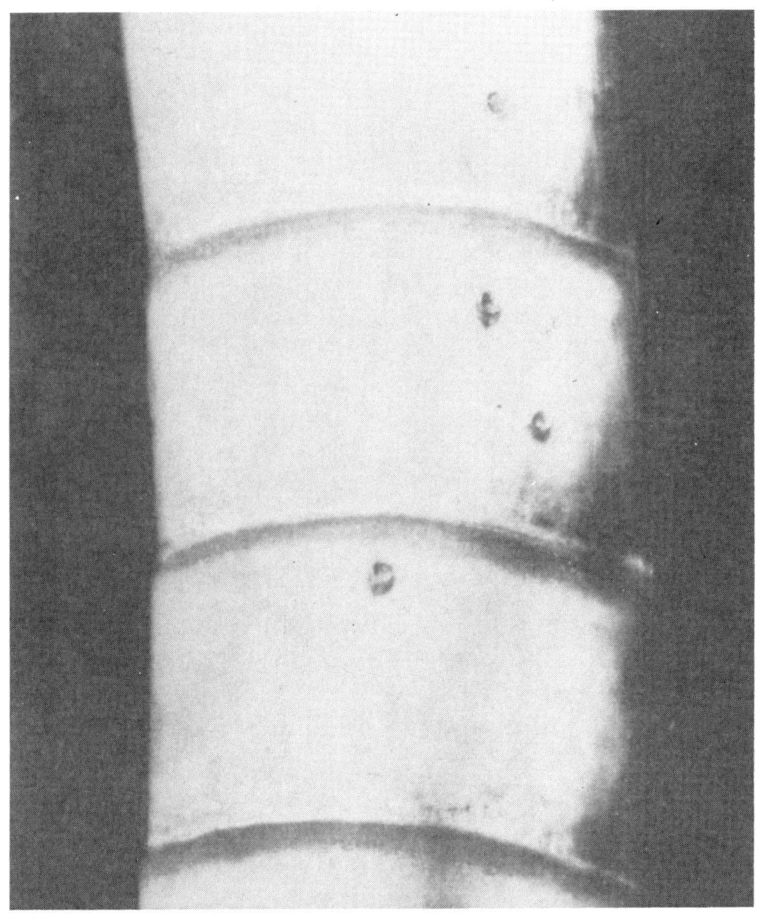

Fig. 3–74. Pits caused by the mite *Ophioptes tropicalis* in the ventral scales of a marsh snake, *Erpetodryas carinatus*. 6×. (From Ewing, H.E.: A new pit-producing mite from the scales of a South American snake. J. Parasitol. *20*:53–56, 1934.)

lizards *(Anolis carolinensis)*. (See the section on toxicology on pages 196 to 197.) Acariasis has been controlled at the Nairobi Snake Park by spraying all new arrivals with 1% trichlorophon (Neguvon, Bayer Laboratories) and repeating this every four to six weeks.[64]

Two agents that reportedly are highly effective miticides are Ortho Dibrom 8–E (California Chemical Co.), 2 to 4 ml per gallon of water, and Diazinon 25E (Geigy), diluted 1:240 to 1:480 in water. Both agents are used as sprays and can be reapplied, if needed, in 2 to 4 weeks.[52] The safety of these products has not been fully established. Diazinon 25E diluted 1:240 was apparently tolerated well by anole lizards, but 5 ml of this dilution killed two out of five ring-necked snakes *(Diadophis punctatus arnyi)* within a week.[52] Two adult Paraguayan false water cobras *(Cyclagras gigas)* died within two hours after brief immersion in a 1:360 dilution of Diazinon 25E even though they were rinsed with water immediately after treatment.[120a] Diazinon 25E diluted 1:480 was safely tolerated by ring-necked snakes,[52] so the therapeutic ratio of this product for reptiles is apparently low.

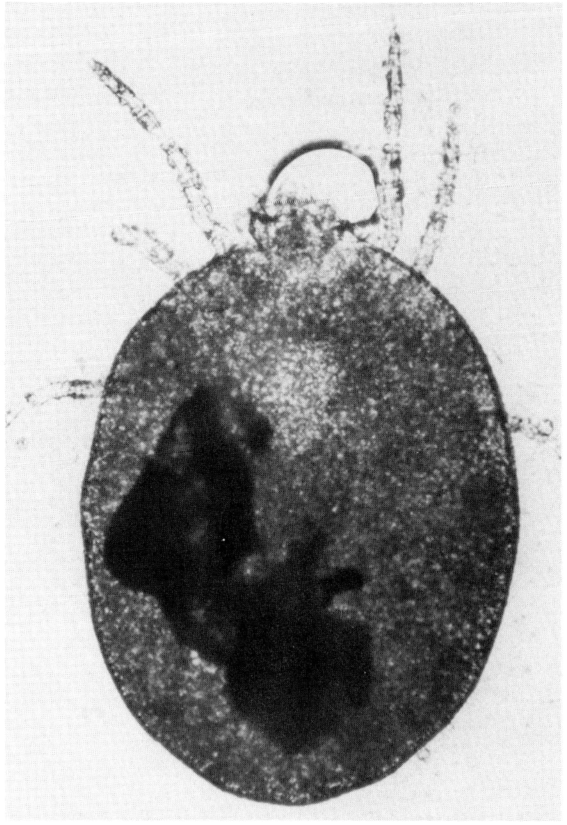

Fig. 3–75. A chigger, removed from an anole lizard *(Anolis carolinensis)*. The larval Trombiculid mite has six legs. 125× (Photograph courtesy of Dr. Steven Engler.)

Reptiles can be routinely treated for mites before they are introduced into a collection to prevent infestation of other specimens. Sanitary measures that help reduce mite populations include removing from the cage shed skins, pieces of bark, and other items where the mites can hide.

Ophioptes tropicalis is a mite found on South American snakes, producing characteristic pitted lesions on the scales in which they live[83] (Fig. 3–74). Treatment recommended for *Ophionyssus natricis* would probably also be effective for *Ophioptes tropicalis*.

Two genera of lung mites are found in snakes: *Entonyssus* and *Ophiopneumicola*.[245] Little has been written about their pathogenicity or clinical significance. Treatment has not been reported.

Chiggers are six-legged larvae of Trombiculid mites which parasitize the skin of reptiles, birds, and mammals, including man (Fig. 3–75). The eight-legged Trombiculid nymphs and adults are free-living, feeding on other small arthropods and their eggs. Chiggers have been

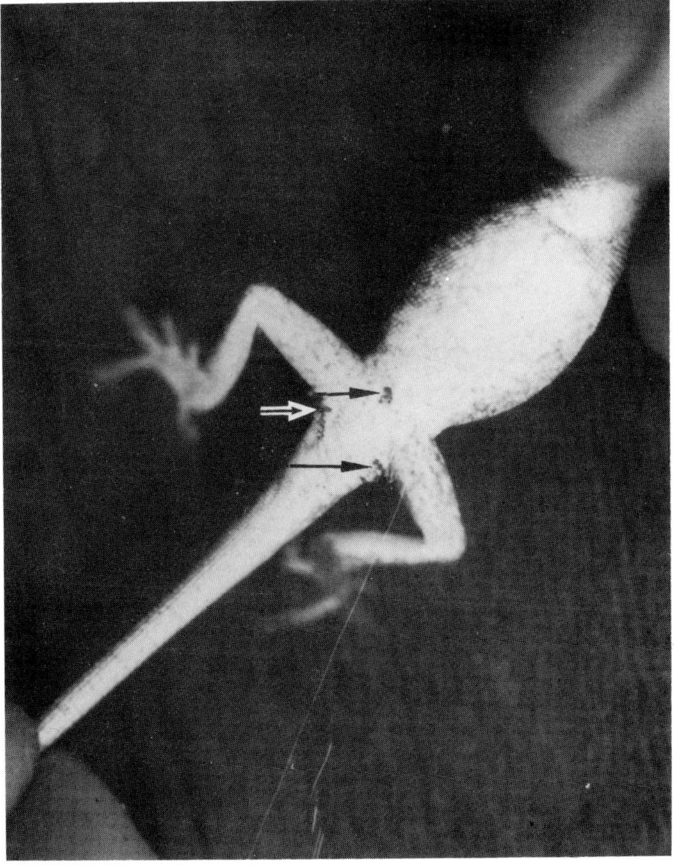

Fig. 3–76. Chiggers (arrows) on the caudal aspect of the thigh and base of the tail on an anole lizard (*Anolis carolinensis*).

given the colloquial name "red bugs," and in heavy infestations, which can be debilitating, clumps of these larval mites are grossly apparent as red spots on the host's skin. They often prefer to attach at skin folds, e.g., axilla and hip (Fig. 3–76). Because the free-living nymphs and adults do not readily survive indoors, infestation with chiggers is usually limited to newly arrived specimens. In light infestations, chiggers can be individually picked off with very fine forceps, taking care to remove the imbedded mouthparts and swabbing the site of attachment with an antiseptic. In heavy infestations one of the treatments for mites, described previously, can be used.

One genus of chiggers, *Hannemania*, is parasitic in the larval stage in amphibians.[138,139] *H. dunni* in pickerel frogs *(Rana palustris)* and various salamanders in eastern United States and *H. penetrans* in other frogs in eastern United States cause orange-red vesicles (Fig. 3–77) less than one mm in diameter on the thighs and perineum. Diagnosis is made by teasing the mite from the vesicle or demonstrating it histologically (Fig. 3–78).

Ticks are commonly found on terrestrial reptiles. Like chiggers, these ectoparasites most often attach to body folds (Fig. 3–79A). In one instance I saw a tick with its mouthparts imbedded in the carapace of an African tortoise (Fig. 3–79B).

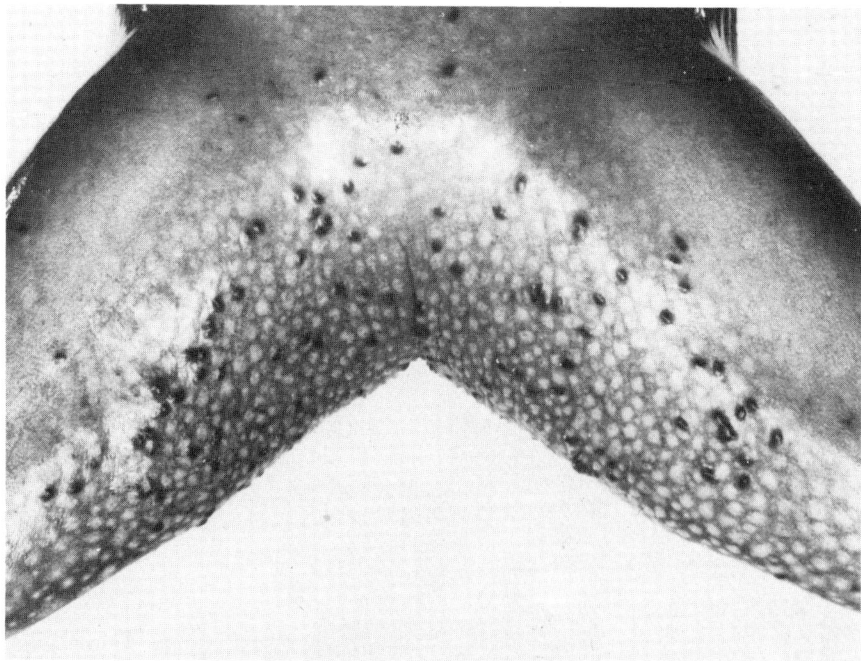

Fig. 3–77. *Hannemania* infection in a frog. Note vesicles produced by mites embedded in skin. (From Worms 1967. Courtesy J. Institute of Animal Technicians. Reprinted with permission from Parasites of Laboratory Animals by Robert J. Flynn © 1973 by the Iowa State University Press, Ames, Iowa.)

Ticks are bloodsuckers, but are rarely present in sufficient numbers to cause significant blood loss. They should be removed with forceps, taking care not to leave the mouthparts imbedded in the skin.

Ticks may be vectors of certain blood parasites. Some ticks that parasitize reptiles will also feed on mammals. Therefore, all exotic reptiles should be examined and treated for ticks because of the potential hazard of importing foreign diseases of man or domestic animals with these vectors. For example, nymphs of the sheep tick, *Ixodes ricinus*, a vector of tularemia, louping ill, and Russian spring and summer encephalitis, were found on lizards *(Lacerta vivipara)* in England.[223]

An outbreak of Q fever *(Coxiella burnetii* infection) occurred among workers who handled a shipment of tick-infested ball pythons *(Python*

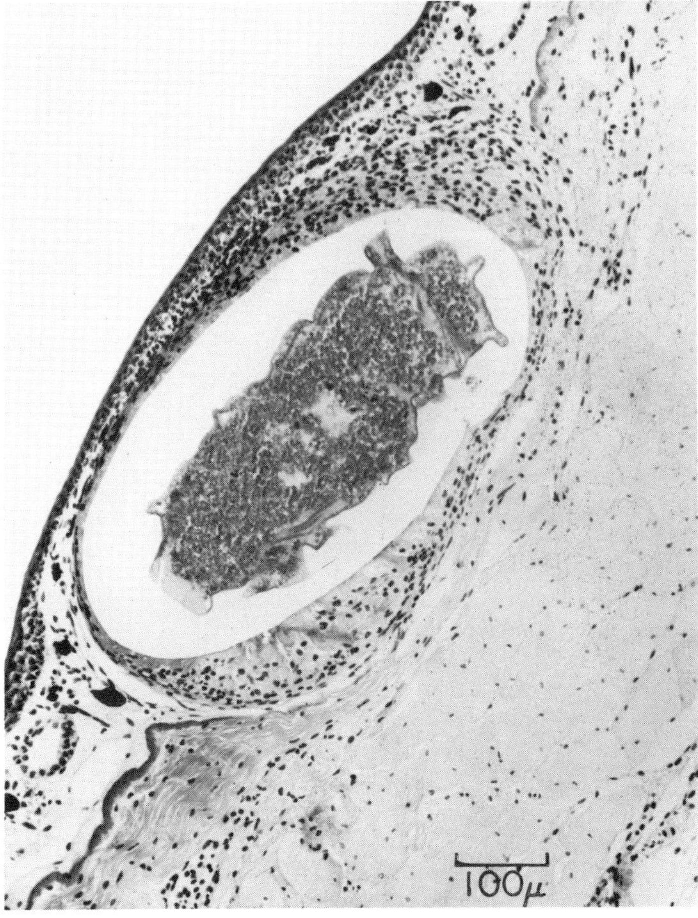

Fig. 3–78. *Hannemania* infection in a frog. Note mite in section of vesicle. (From Worms 1967. Courtesy J. Institute of Animal Technicians. Reprinted with permission from Parasites of Laboratory Animals by Robert J. Flynn © 1973 by the Iowa State University Press, Ames, Iowa.)

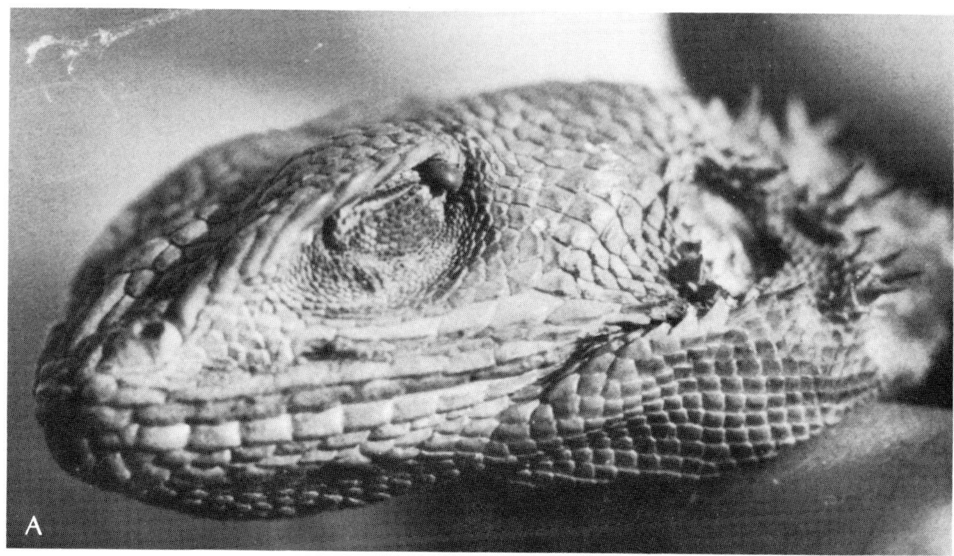

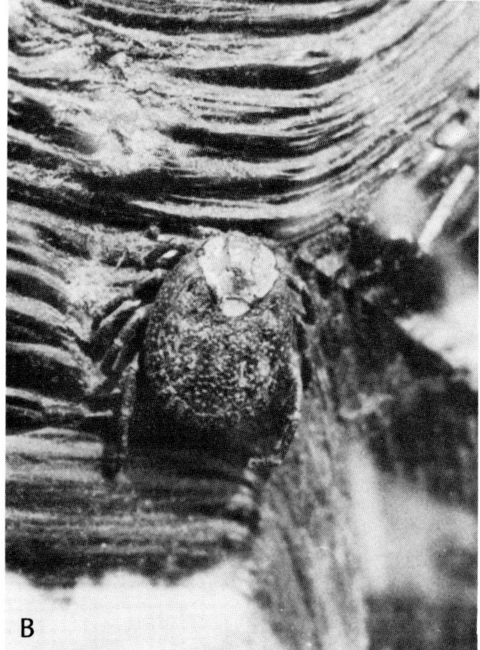

Fig. 3–79. **A.** Tick with mouthparts imbedded in the lateral canthus of the eye in an Agamid lizard. **B.** Adult female ixodid tick feeding on the carapace of an East African tortoise.

regius). Rickettsiae were seen, but not identified, in some ticks. Attempts to isolate the pathogen from python blood and tissue were unsuccessful.[8a] *C. burnetii* was cultured from the liver and spleen of a python, a monitor lizard, and a tortoise, and antibodies to the organism were found in rat snakes and water snakes caught in India.[308a]

PARASITIC COPEPODS

Certain copepods that parasitize fish and are commonly known as "fish lice" are occasionally found as ectoparasites of tadpoles and salamanders.[17,114] Little is known about their pathogenicity in amphibians.

DIPTERA

In the wild, reptiles are commonly attacked by mosquitoes and biting flies. This may have agricultural and public health significance since reptiles might be a reservoir for such arthropod-borne diseases as eastern and western encephalitis and Japanese B encephalitis. Some of the flies and mosquitoes that attack reptiles will also bite birds and mammals, including man.

Myiasis occurs in toads and tortoises in the wild. Recently caught animals are occasionally presented with this condition. The toad fly *(Bufolucilia buforivora)* and some related species deposit their eggs on toads and other amphibians. The larvae migrate in the nostrils, destroying the nasal mucosa, and boring through tissue to devour orbital contents. They may even penetrate the cranial cavity and destroy the brain. The condition is mutilating and is usually fatal.[159,233]

Various species of flesh flies can produce myiasis in land tortoises, preexisting wounds being a favored entry site for the maggots.[146] Treatment consists of removal of the maggots, surgical debridement, and antiseptic treatment of the wound. Vigorous flushing of the fistulous tract with 3% hydrogen peroxide may help drive out the invading larvae.

NONINFECTIOUS AND NEOPLASTIC DISEASES

NUTRITIONAL, METABOLIC, AND IDIOPATHIC DISEASES

The normal feeding habits, diet, and digestive processes of herpetofauna have been described in the first two chapters. One of the major contributing causes of death in captive wild animals is failure to provide an adequate, balanced diet. Rarely can the owner duplicate natural feeding patterns, especially for species that have unique dietary requirements. Specific nutritional requirements have not been determined for most wild animals, including herpetofauna. It should be presumed, until proven otherwise, that reptiles and amphibians require the same vitamins, minerals, and other nutrients required by mammals, and that carnivorous species require a high-protein diet with all the amino acids considered essential for mice and men.

Reptiles may refuse to eat because of disease or failure to adapt to captivity, a situation described by Cowan as the "maladaptation syndrome."[68] Progressive weight loss becomes clinically obvious because of increasing prominence of bony structures and loose folds of skin. Any underlying disease should be treated and the animal should be maintained by parenteral or forced oral nutrition (see p. 65). There may be better absorption and response to vitamins given parenterally than orally.[92] Reluctant feeders reportedly can be induced to feed by using a wide spectrum light source (see p. 62).

Female boa constrictors often refuse to eat during pregnancy and may lose considerable weight.[93] Male boas feed irregularly during the mating period.[93]

Among herpetofauna, nutritional disorders have been most clearly defined for young aquatic turtles partly because they have been so popular as pets, partly because certain nutritional problems are patently reflected in defective growth of the shell, and partly because their dietary needs have been so grossly and widely abused. Commercial turtle food, consisting of dried insects, is totally inadequate to sustain life, let alone growth, in young chelonians. The most obvious results of giving such food are swollen orbital contents (squamous metaplasia of the ophthalmic glands) owing to vitamin A deficiency and a soft or deformed shell owing to vitamin D deficiency and/or an imbalanced Ca:P ratio.

Hypovitaminosis A. When young turtles are fed a diet deficient in vitamin A, they develop squamous metaplasia and keratinization of the harderian and lacrimal glands (see p. 44), resulting in enlargement of these glands which, in turn, causes protrusion and eversion of the eyelids (Fig. 3–80). Turtles affected bilaterally are blind, do not feed, and die of starvation or intercurrent disease.[82] The condition has been described in aquatic turtles in the genera *Clemmys, Emys, Chinemys, Chrysemys (Pseudemys),* and *Graptemys.*

In addition to the ocular adnexal lesions, there often is squamous metaplasia and keratinization in pancreatic ducts, renal collecting tubules, ureters, and the urinary bladder. Inflammation marked by an exudate of eosinophilic granulocytes usually accompanies the epithelial changes in the ocular glands and other organs. Proliferative glomerulonephritis, renal interstitial fibrosis, degenerative and inflammatory lesions of the thyroid, and fatty degeneration of the liver are also found in vitamin A deficient turtles.[82]

Hypovitaminosis A can be prevented by using appropriate vitamin supplements or by feeding the turtle bits of raw liver. If cases are far advanced or complicated by other deficiencies and concurrent infections at the time of presentation, cure is unlikely. Early cases may respond to oral or parenteral vitamin A. One half to one ml (25,000 to 50,000 units) of a commercial vitamin A preparation (Aquasol) can be given IPP, one dose usually being sufficient if cure is still possible.[27a] Hime recommends giving two doses of 5,000 IU vitamin A seven days apart.[125a]

Thiamine Deficiency. Thiamine (B_1) deficiency occurs in reptiles, especially those fed diets containing the thiamine destroying enzyme,

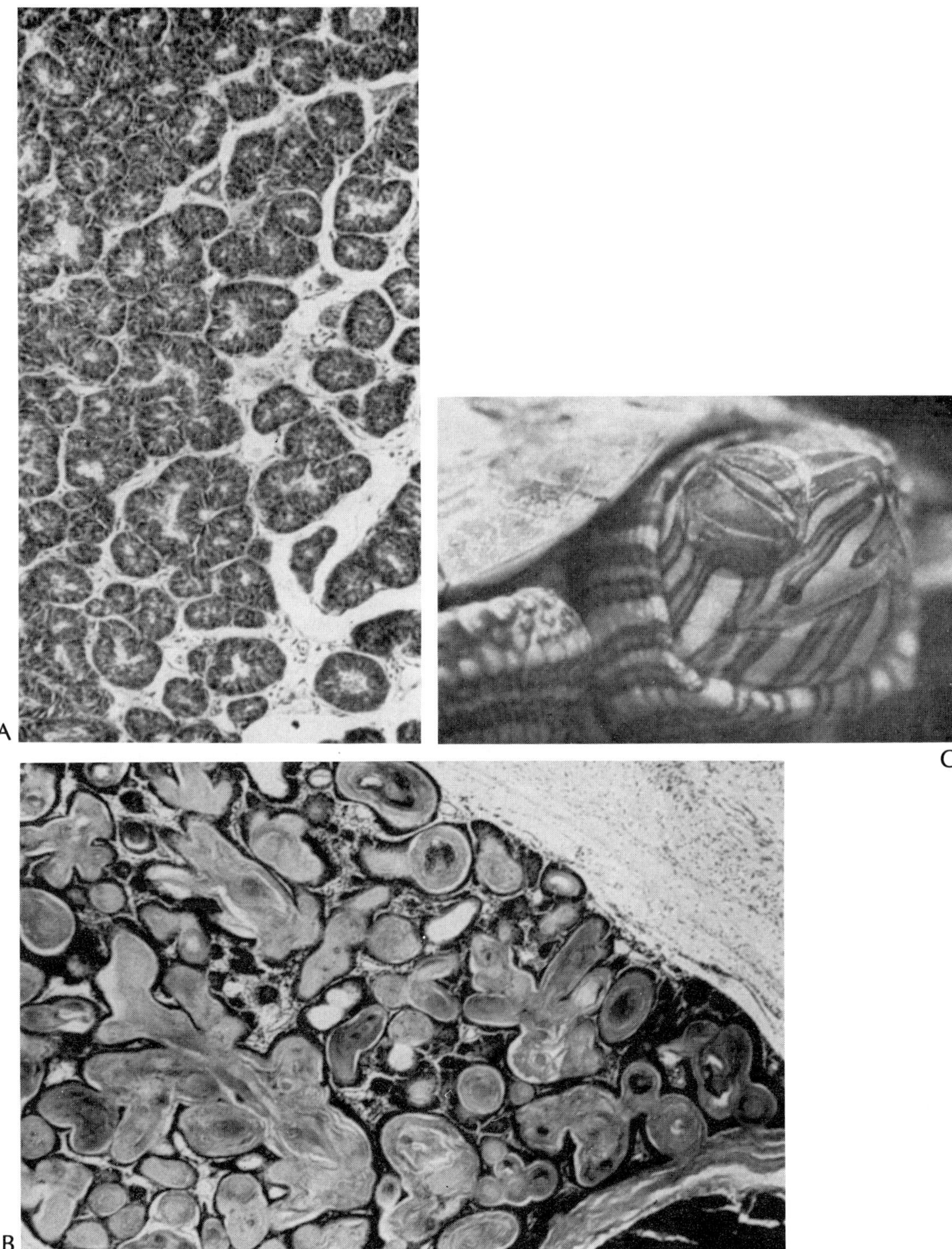

Fig. 3–80. **A.** Normal lateral lachrymal gland of *Clemmys leprosa*. Masson's trichrome stain. 137×. **B.** Almost complete squamous metaplasia of the glandular portion of the lateral lachrymal gland of *Chrysemys scripta elegans*. H and E stain; 55×. **C.** Painted turtle *(Chrysemys scripta elegans)*, with swollen orbit caused by hypovitaminosis A induced squamous metaplasia of ophthalmic glands. (From Elkan, E. and Zwart, P.: Ocular disease of young terrapins. Pathol. Vet., 4:201–222, 1967.)

thiaminase. Fish-eating snakes and turtles are the most frequently affected.

Early clinical signs include progressive emaciation, enteritis, and pulmonary edema. Incoordination and paralysis precede death.

Diagnosis of thiamine deficiency may be made by evaluating the diet and clinical signs. A history of being fed fish containing thiaminase (e.g., smelt, minnows, goldfish) will add support to the diagnosis.

Treatment should include the parenteral administration of 15 to 50 mg of thiamine IM and a correction of the diet. A supplementation of 15 mg of dietary thiamine is required to offset the thiaminase activity of each pound of smelt fed.

Hypovitaminosis E. This condition results in steatitis and has been described most frequently in crocodilians,[103,289] but it occurs in other reptiles also. This disease, which resembles pansteatitis in cats, mink, and swine, occurs on diets low in vitamin E and relatively rich in polyunsaturated fatty acids (PUFA), such as are found in rancid fish oils. Steatitis is also said to occur in snakes fed obese laboratory rats.[96,287] The antioxidant properties of vitamin E are destroyed by the oxidizing properties of the PUFA.

Crocodilians fed all-fish diets (especially smelt and mackerel) are likely to be affected. They often show progressive anorexia and listlessness, but in some cases they may continue to eat until the time of death. Clinically, they appear to be in good flesh. A Marcy garter snake *(Thamnophis marcianus),* which was fed a diet composed principally of smelt, developed steatitis and suffered incoordination, anorexia, and paralysis.[181]

Gross lesions consist of multiple foci of induration of subcutaneous, intermuscular, perivisceral, and abdominal fat depots (Fig. 3–81). The foci are yellow to brown, greasy, and soaplike. Adhesions may occur between abdominal viscera.[96] The liver may be fatty and contain foci of necrosis. Histologically, there is dense, diffuse infiltration of adipose tissue by fibroblasts and inflammatory cells, including macrophages and giant cells. Much of the fat is replaced by a globular, acid-fast pigment, ceroid, which may be engulfed by the phagocytic cells. Ceroid is also found in the liver and spleen.

Prevention of steatitis depends on providing an adequate vitamin E level in the diet and reducing the PUFA level. This can be accomplished by feeding entire rodents, chicks, or other birds to crocodilians and reducing their fish intake. Crocodilians should never be fed rancid fish. Vitamin E supplements may be added to the food. Feeding obese rodents to crocodilians should be avoided, especially those rodents fed a diet high in polyunsaturated oils.

Early cases may be treated by the prophylactic dietary measures outlined previously. Vitamin E can also be given parenterally.

Hypovitaminosis K. This condition is said to occur in crocodilians and is associated with gingival bleeding.[96] Treatment is intramuscular injection of vitamin K; Frye suggests giving 0.5 mg/kg body weight.[96]

Disorders of Bone and Calcium Metabolism. Commonly seen in captive herpetofauna, most of these diseases are caused by feeding the

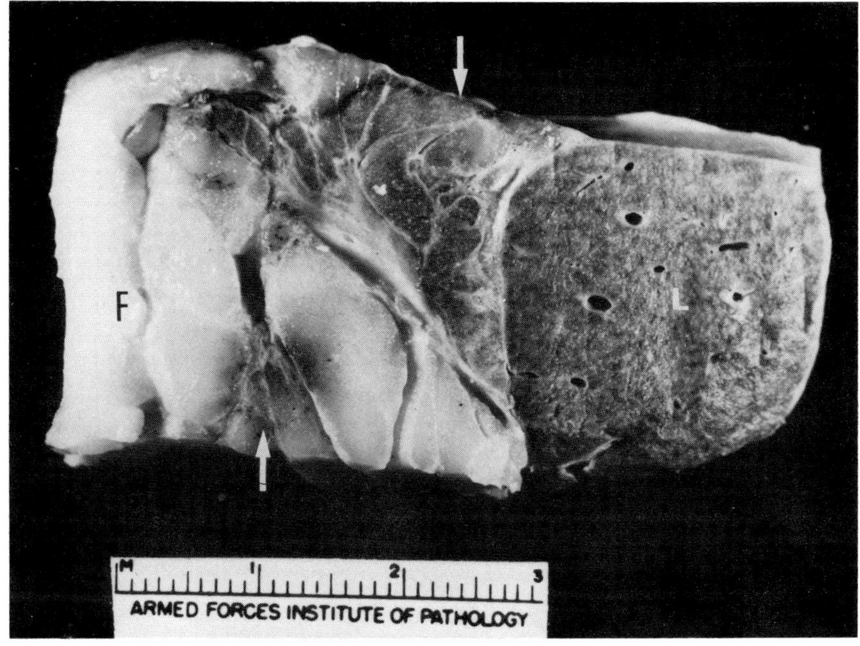

Fig. 3–81. Steatitis in a caiman. Normal abdominal fat **(F)** is white. Areas of steatitis (arrows) are reddish brown. The liver **(L)** is dark brown. (Courtesy of the National Zoological Park, Washington, D.C. and the Armed Forces Institute of Pathology.)

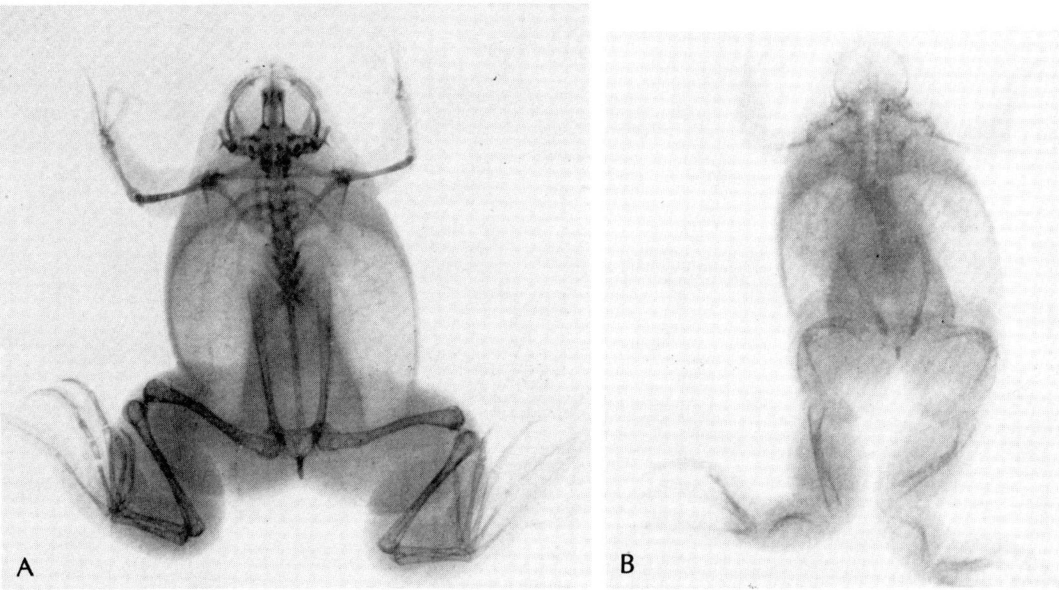

Fig. 3–82. **A.** Radiograph, normal adult male African clawed toad *(Xenopus laevis)*. **B.** Radiograph, 14-month-old African clawed toad *(Xenopus laevis)* fed horse liver exclusively. There is generalized deficient skeletal calcification with deformities of the pelvis, urostyle, spinal column, femora, and tibiofibulae. (From Bruce, H.M. and Parkes, A.S.: Rickets and osteoporosis in *Xenopus laevis*. J. Endocrinol., *7*:64–81, 1950.)

animals diets too low in calcium or in the ratio of calcium to phosphorus, or by providing inadequate vitamin D.[43,287,317] As a result of these nutritional deficiencies or imbalances, the bones become decalcified, soft, thickened, and bent. Demineralization, deformities, and spontaneous fractures of the ribs, mandibles, long appendicular bones, and, to a lesser extent, of the cranium, vertebrae, pelvis, and digits can be seen radiographically (Figs. 3–82, 3–83, 3–84). In advanced cases, the thickening and deformities of bones and loss of teeth may be evident on physical examination. In the turtle, disorders of calcification also result in deformities of the shell.

Terms such as rickets, osteomalacia, osteoporosis, and fibrous osteodystrophy have been used to describe the nutritional bone disorders of reptiles and amphibians.[43,68,287,290,317] Until more is known about the physiology of bone in herpetofauna, including the exact roles of vitamin D, parathormone, thyrocalcitonin, growth hormone, osteoblasts, and osteoclasts, and until controlled experimental studies are done on individual deficiencies in these animals, analogy with the mammalian bone diseases is imperfect. However, the most reasonable supposition, based on available clinical data, is that most nutritional bone disorders in adult reptiles are owing to diets low in calcium or in Ca:P ratio, which result in secondary hyperparathyroidism and fibrous osteodystrophy.[287] Chondroid hyperplasia, not seen in mammalian fibrous osteodystrophy, may be prominent in reptiles.[317] Wallach states

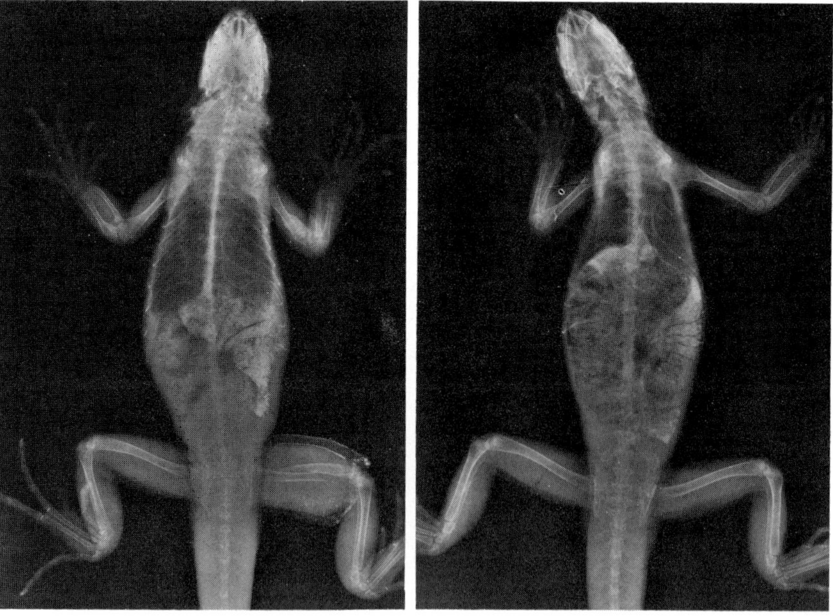

Fig. 3–83. Green iguana *(Iguana iguana)* (left) fed diet deficient in calcium and vitamin D. There are fractures of the femur, humerus, radius, and ulna. Animal on the right, on adequately supplemented diet, is normal. (From Zwart, P. and Van de Watering, C.C.: Disturbance of bone formation in the common iguana *(Iguana iguana L.)* Acta Zool. Pathol. Antverpiensia *48*:333–356, 1969. Photographs courtesy of Dr. P. Zwart.)

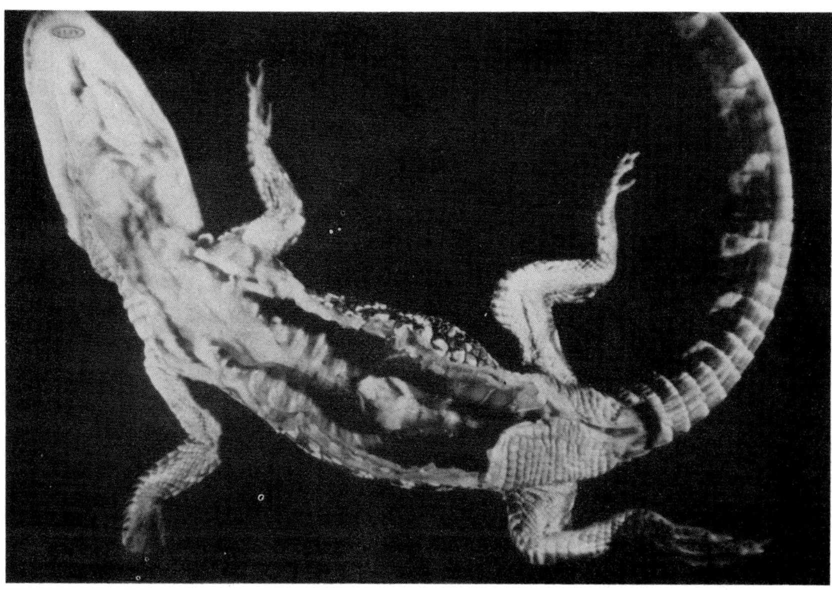

Fig. 3–84. Fractured vertebra with callus formation in a baby American alligator *(Alligator mississippiensis).* The animal had been fed an all-meat diet, resulting in secondary hyperparathyroidism, fibrous osteodystrophy, and pathologic fracture. It probably also suffered from hypovitaminosis D, as a result of being kept indoors, under incandescent light. (Armed Forces Institute of Pathology Negative No. 63-3000-2.)

that bone resorption may be exacerbated in diets relatively or absolutely deficient in calcium if vitamin D is adequate because this may help mobilize available skeletal stores of calcium.[287]

Zwart suggests that hyperparathyroidism in geckos *(Phelsuma* spp.*)* causes mobilization of calcium from the bones to the chalk sacs (see p. 12), causing distention of the latter organs[315] (Fig. 3–85). Herpetofauna fed exclusively on fish, meat, liver, mealworms, or calcium-deficient fruits and vegetables such as lettuce and bananas are most susceptible to nutritional bone disorders. Adequate calcium intake can be assured by feeding herpetofauna nutritionally balanced dog food or whole rodents, or by sprinkling bone meal, ground limestone, or other

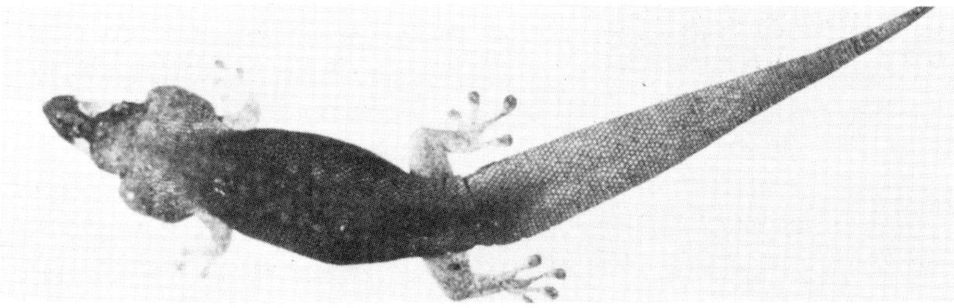

Fig. 3–85. Gecko *(Phelsuma dubia dubia)* with abnormally distended chalk sacs. Eyes were removed by dissection. (From Reichenbach-Klinke, H., and Elkan, E.: The Principal Diseases of Lower Vertebrates. New York, Academic Press, 1965.)

mineral supplement on food, or by adding appropriate mineral supplements to the drinking water. Mineral blocks that can be put in a turtle's tank water are available in pet stores, but they are not adequate, per se, in overcoming a grossly calcium-deficient or imbalanced diet. Progression of disease may be halted by correcting the diet, but it is not likely that deformities secondary to nutritional deficiencies will be reversed.

Adequate vitamin D intake can be assured by vitamin supplementation or by appropriate exposure of the animals to sunlight or ultraviolet light, remembering that such exposure can be deleterious or fatal if excessive.

Hypervitaminosis D is associated with calcification of the media of the aorta, pulmonary, renal, and iliac arteries in green iguanas *(Iguana iguana)*. These vessels may become grossly distorted and brittle. Mineralized casts and degenerative changes in the tubular epithelium of the kidneys may also be found.[284]

Various idiopathic bone disorders in reptiles have been reported. Frye and Dutra described osteocartilaginous exostoses on the legs and ribs of an immature male long-necked monitor lizard *(Varanus bengalensis nebulosus)*.[101] Lesions that were apparently similar to these, but which were designated osteochondromas, were found in three other lizards *(Cyclura macleayi, Iguana iguana,* and *Uromastix hartwickei)*.[142]

A proliferative, ankylosing disease of the spinal column in a four-year-old male boa constrictor *(Constrictor constrictor)* was designated as a case of osteitis deformans (Paget's disease of bone).[98] The density of bone was not described, but published radiographs suggest there was a sclerotic process. If the designation as Paget's disease was correct, the case described was more like the late stage than the acute phase of the human disease.[234] The disease in the boa also bore some resemblance to a case of ankylosing disease of the vertebrae in a female Chinese stripetailed snake *(Elaphe taenura)* diagnosed as "osteoperiostitis" (Fig. 3–86),[68] but descriptions of the two cases were not detailed enough for complete comparison.

Achondroplastic dwarfism was diagnosed in a three-year-old female red-eared turtle Chrysemys *(Pseudemys) scripta elegans*.[99] There was demineralization of the skeleton and marked cartilaginous hyperplasia of the epiphyses, which are not the usual findings in mammalian achondroplasia. In addition, the irregular disarray of chondrocytes, which is the hallmark of the disease in mammals,[154,234] was not described in this turtle, so the case may not have been completely analogous to the hereditary condition in man and domestic animals.

Overgrowth of the horny tissue of the jaw sometimes occurs in turtles, resulting in difficulties in prehension and chewing of food (Fig. 3–87). The cause is unknown. Treatment consists of trimming away the excess tissue with clippers, scissors, or saw.[57]

Developmental Anomalies. A great variety of spontaneous and experimentally produced **developmental anomalies** have been described in amphibians and reptiles. The ones attracting the greatest attention have been two-headed monsters and animals with excess limbs or various degrees of Siamese twinning. Cases of melanism, albinism, and other variants from normal pigmentation have been described in many species. Other congenital defects include brachygnathia, micro-

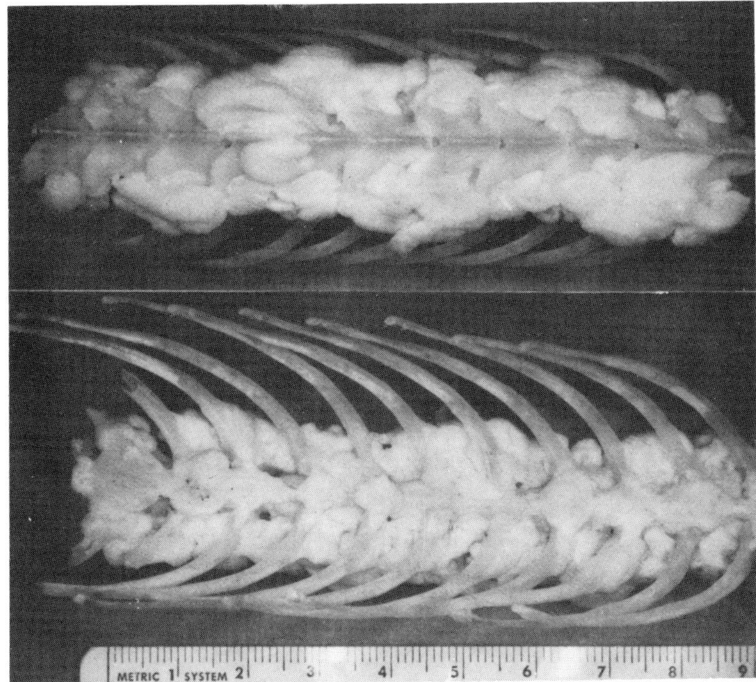

Fig. 3–86. Chinese stripetail snake *(Elaphe taenura,* female). Spine shows osteoperiostitis. Dorsal (top) and ventral (bottom) views show exostosis and fusion. (From Cowan, D.F.: Diseases of captive reptiles. J. Am. Vet. Med. Assoc., *153*:848–859, 1968. Photograph courtesy of Dr. D.F. Cowan.)

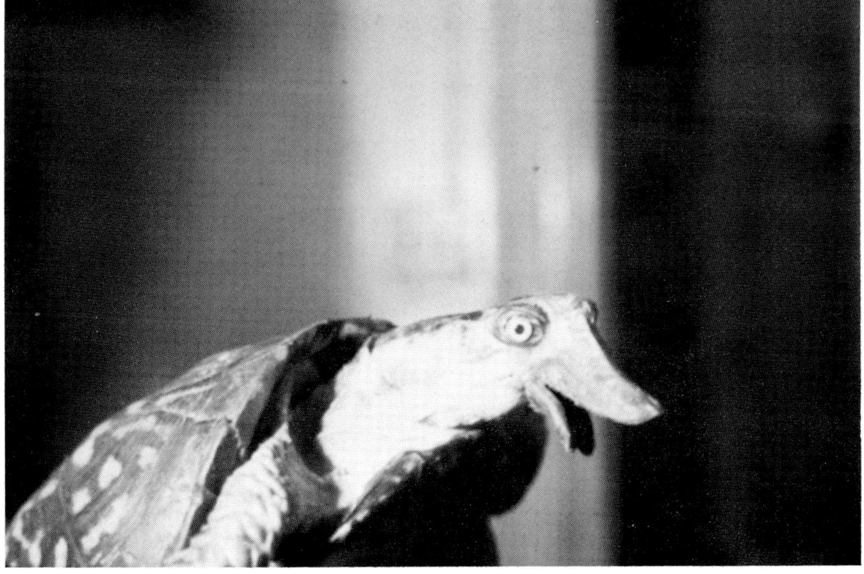

Fig. 3–87. Box turtle *(Terrapene carolina)* with idiopathic overgrowth of the horny tissue of the mouth. (Courtesy of Dr. Robert Altman.)

phthalmia, cleft palate, and hermaphroditism. An introduction to the literature on teratology in herpetofauna can be found in the text by Reichenbach-Klinke and Elkan[233] and in an article by Bellairs.[26]

Hypoglycemic Shock. This condition has been described in crocodilians, especially American alligators *(Alligator mississippiensis).*[291] It is most likely to occur in the winter and spring when the blood glucose level of the alligator is at its lowest level (Fig. 3–88). The alligator has a seasonal physiologic variation in blood glucose, ranging from 50 mg/dl in the late fall to 100 mg/dl in the summer.

Signs of hypoglycemic shock in crocodilians include mydriasis, upward gaze, swimming in circles, opisthotonos, torticollis, and seizures. Untreated, it is likely to terminate fatally. The clinical state may be brought on by stress, such as handling and excess crowding.

Differential diagnosis of hypoglycemia includes poisoning by neurotoxic agents, hypocalcemia, thiamine deficiency, septicemia, and encephalitis. Specific diagnosis can be made by appropriate laboratory tests and response to therapy.

Hypoglycemia should be treated with glucose solutions given parenterally or by stomach tube. The dose should be monitored by clinical response and blood glucose level. Wallach has recommended a dose of 3.3 g glucose/kg (1.5 g/lb) of body weight.[286]

Gout. Gout occurs in snakes, lizards, turtles, and crocodilians.[10,288] It is characterized by deposition of uric acid crystals in joints and thoracic and abdominal viscera. There may be sluggishness and decreased appetite, or no clinical signs may be apparent, and the reptile may be found dead in the cage.

Clinically, gout should be suspected in reptiles with swollen joints and diagnosed by demonstrating elevated uric acid levels in the blood. Normal uric acid levels in American alligators range from 1.0 to 4.1

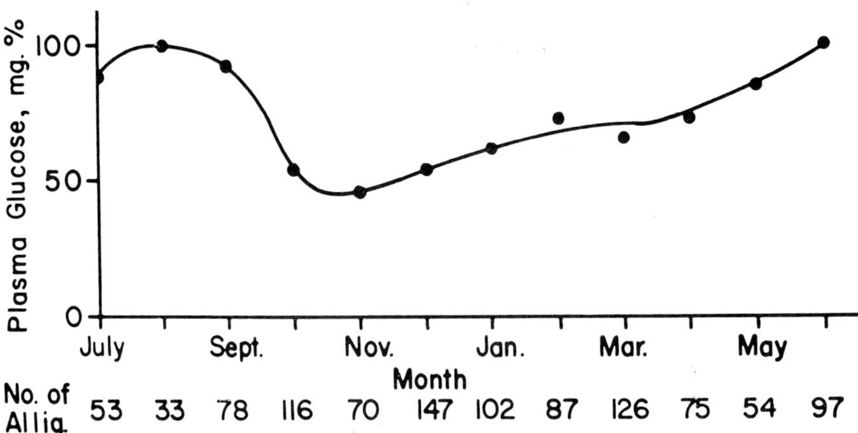

Fig. 3–88. Seasonal changes in blood glucose. The alligators varied in weight from about 300 g to 4 kg. Figures represent "true glucose" values as measured by glucose oxidase. (From Coulson, R.A., and Hernandez, T.: Biochemistry of the Alligator. Baton Rouge, Louisiana State University Press, 1964.)

mg/dl plasma. Levels of 70 mg/dl have been found in alligators with gout.[67]

Chalky or yellowish-white to pink deposits from pinpoint size up to several centimeters in diameter are found in the joints, kidney, liver, and pericardial sac (Figs. 3–89, 3–90, 3–91, and 3–92); joint and visceral involvement may occur concurrently or independently. Lesions may be multifocal or confluent. Tophi, seen histologically, are pathognomonic of gout. Tophi are collections of urate crystals surrounded by an inflammatory response that usually includes multinucleated giant cells (Fig. 3–93). The urates, per se, can be preserved and histologically demonstrated in tissue fixed in absolute alcohol, using special stains (Figs. 3–94 and 3–95) or polarized light (Fig. 3–96). Tissue fixed in aqueous formalin can be used for diagnosis, even though the water-soluble urates are dissolved, because the histopathology of gout is so characteristic.

It has been suggested empirically that gout is brought on by dehydration and either a high-protein diet (unlikely, in my opinion), or endogenous protein breakdown resulting from failure to feed.[68] Overdosage with gentamicin causes gout in snakes because of damage to proximal renal tubules resulting in impaired excretion of uric acid.[212a] Theoretically, gout could be treated by withdrawing nephrotoxic agents, rehydrating with electrolyte and glucose solutions, and nutritionally restoring nitrogen balance.

Articular Pseudogout. This condition was diagnosed postmortem in a two-year-old female red-eared turtle *(Chrysemys [Pseudemys] scripta*

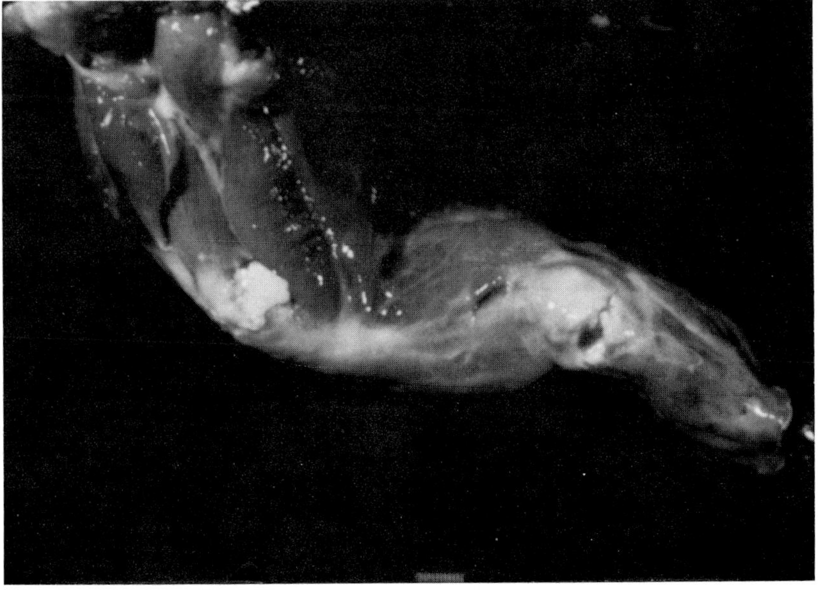

Fig. 3–89. Articular gout, hind leg of a dwarf crocodile *(Osteolaemus tetraspis)*. Chalky white urate deposits are in the knee and tarsal joints. (Courtesy of Dr. Marilyn Anderson and the Ohio State University, Dept. of Veterinary Pathology.)

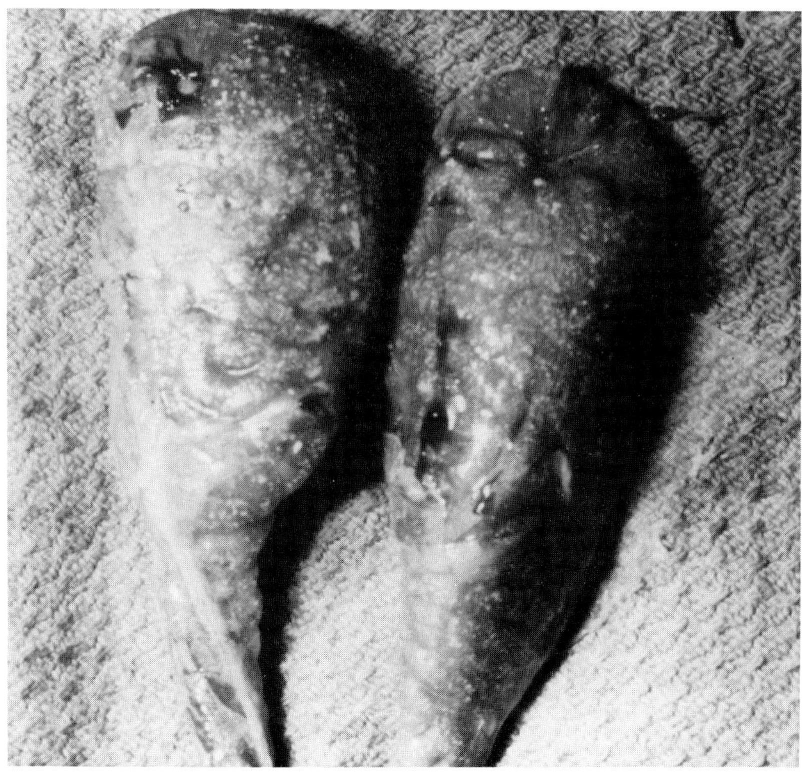

Fig. 3–90. Visceral gout in an Indian monitor lizard *(Varanus bengalensis)*. Urate deposits appeared as yellow-white flecks, 0.5 to 1 mm in diameter. (Armed Forces Institute of Pathology Accession No. 1095008.)

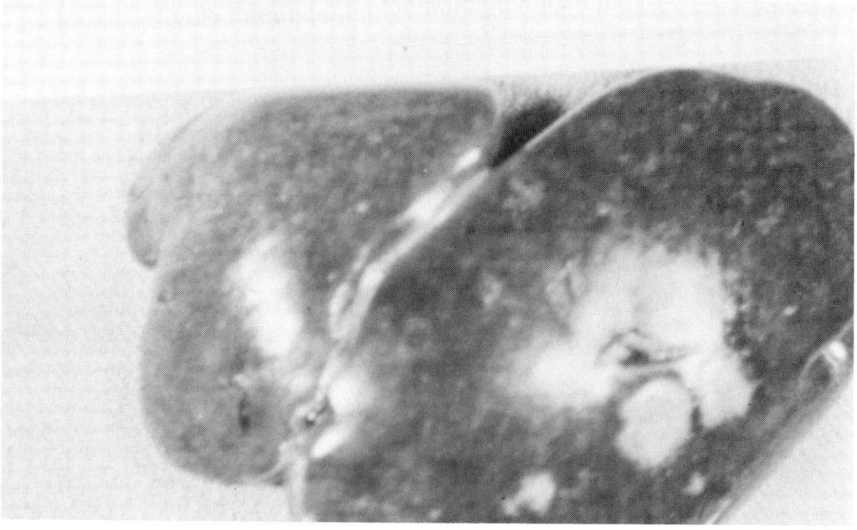

Fig. 3–91. Visceral gout in an Indian monitor lizard *(Varanus bengalensis)*. Chalky white deposits of uric acid are in the liver (cut surface). (Armed Forces Institute of Pathology Accession No. 1095008).

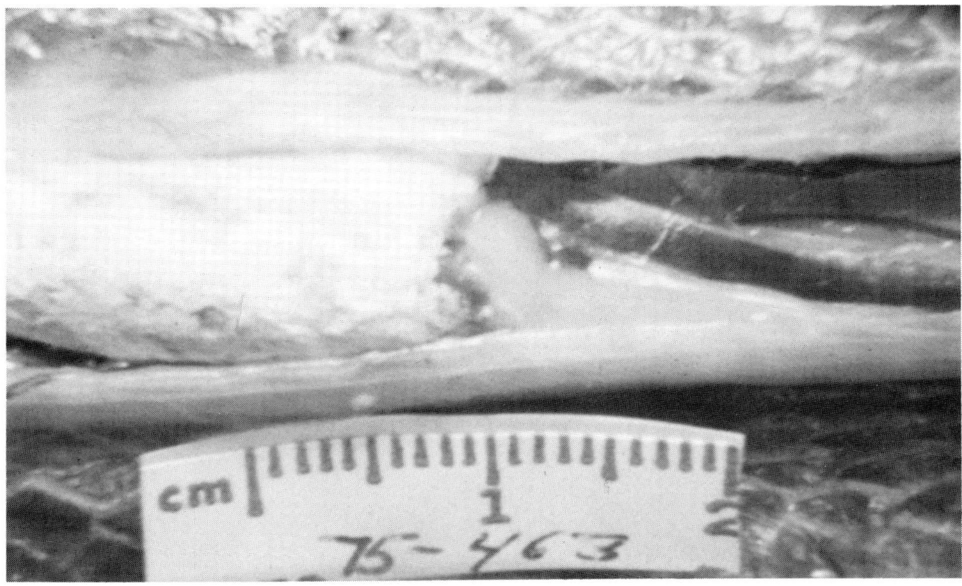

Fig. 3–92. Visceral gout in a green vine snake *(Oxybelis fulgidus)*. Urate-encrusted pericardium (at left) is chalky white. (Courtesy of Dr. Richard Montali, National Zoological Park, Washington, D.C.)

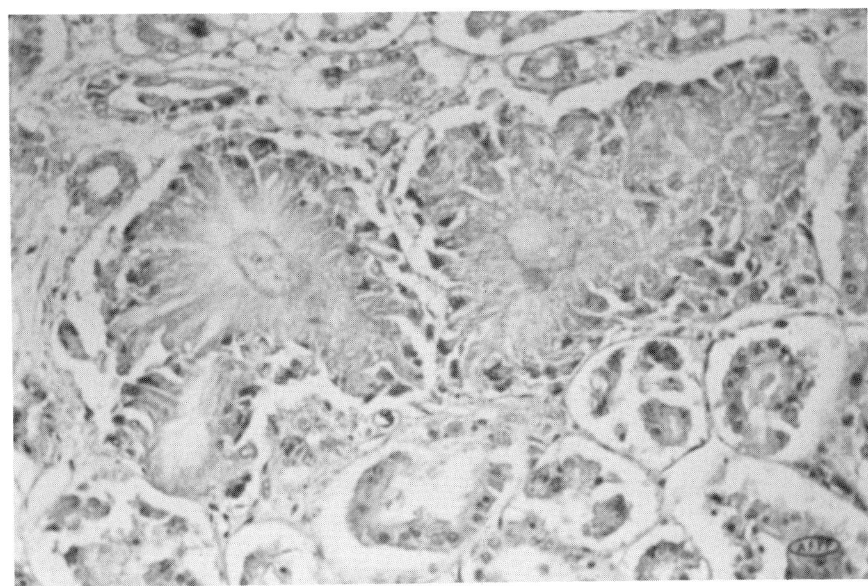

Fig. 3–93. Tophi in the kidney of a Sudan plated lizard *(Gerrhosaurus major)* with visceral gout. The inflammatory cells palisade on the periphery of uric acid deposits. Uric acid crystals, per se, have been removed by dissolving them in the aqueous formalin fixative. Tubular epithelium is artifactually detached from the basement membranes. H and E stain; 135×.

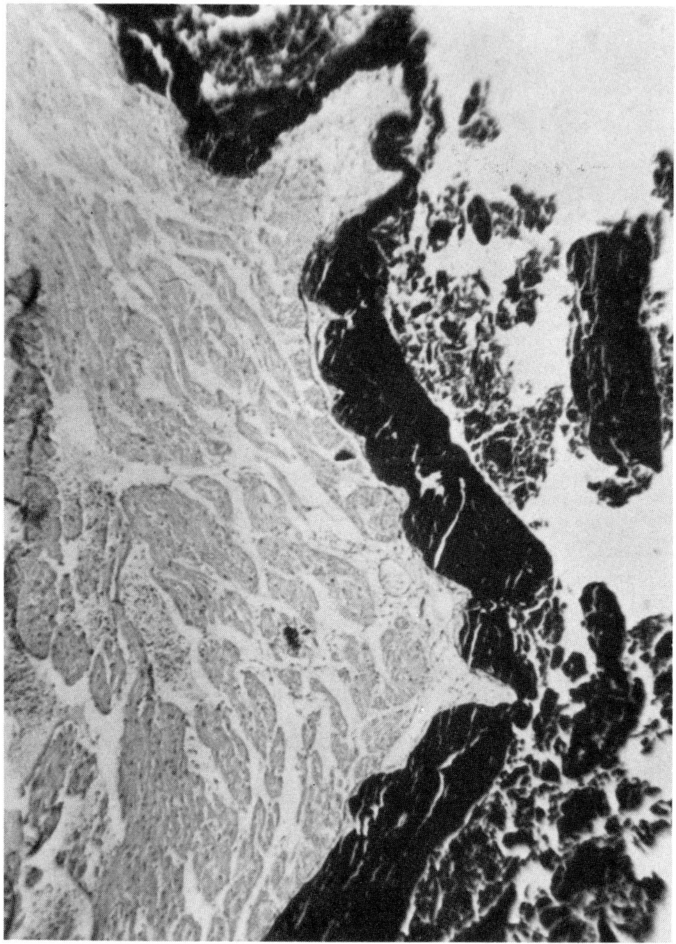

Fig. 3–94. Pericardial urate deposits (black) in an Indian monitor lizard *(Varanus bengalensis)* with visceral gout. Tissue fixed in absolute alcohol. De Galantha stain; 35×. (Armed Forces Institute of Pathology Accession No. 1095008.)

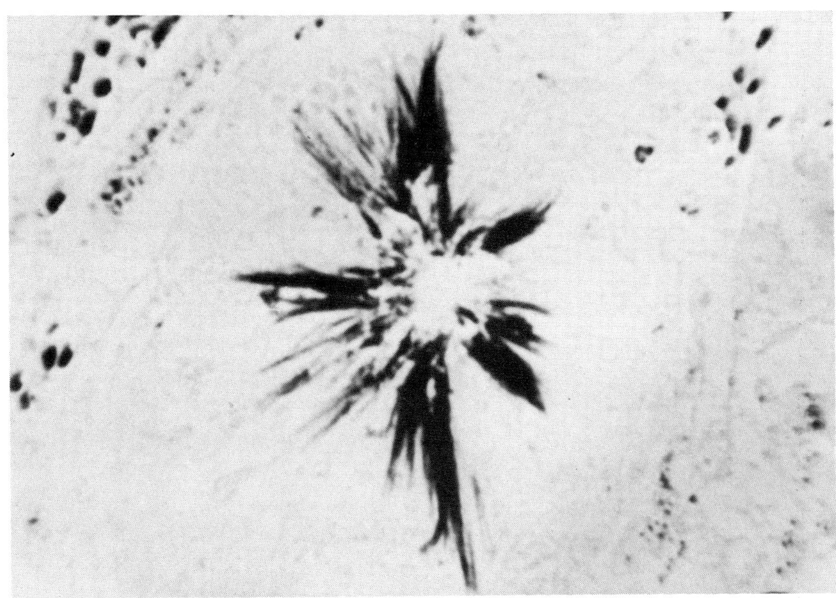

Fig. 3–95. Urate crystals in a tophus in an Indian monitor lizard *(Varanus bengalensis)*. Absolute alcohol fixation. De Galantha stain; 350×. (Armed Forces Institute of Pathology Accession No. 1095008.)

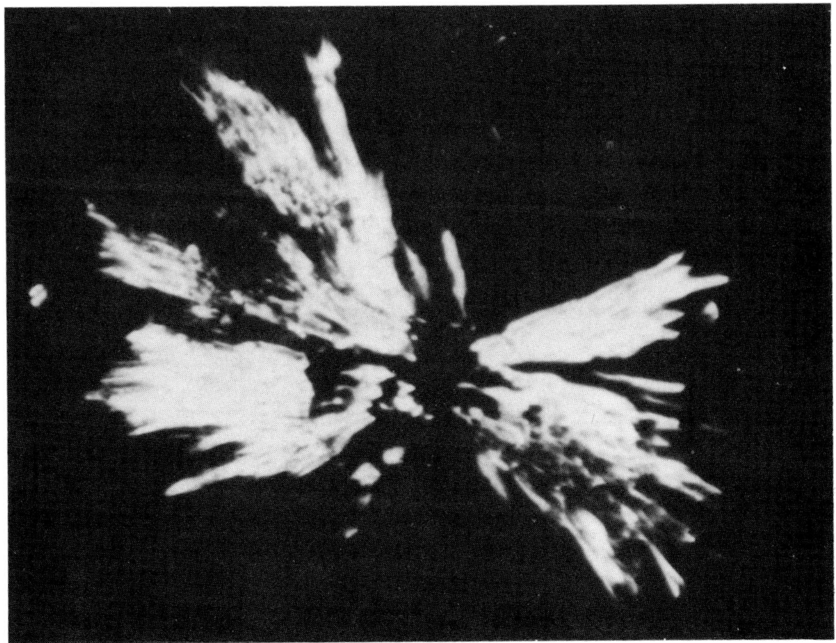

Fig. 3–96. Birefringent urate crystals in a tophus, Indian monitor lizard *(Varanus bengalensis)*. Absolute alcohol fixation. Unstained, polarized light; 350×. (Armed Forces Institute of Pathology Accession No. 1095008.)

elegans).[102a] The turtle, which had been fed a diet of shrimp, had a soft shell and swollen joints and had difficulty moving. Its blood uric acid was 7.8 mg/dl, approximately six times the normal level. On postmortem, it had no visceral lesions, but there was a cream-colored, gritty, nonbirefringent material around major joint capsules, identified by crystallography as hydroxyl apatite, $Ca_{10}(PO_4)_6(OH)_2$.

Arteriosclerosis. Although uncommon in reptiles, arteriosclerosis has been the subject of some interest from the standpoint of comparative pathology.

Atheromas (Fig. 3–97), with fatty deposits in the aortic intima, have been described in a few reptiles,[90,91,282] but they apparently were not associated with clinical illness. Ardlie and Schwartz looked for cardiovascular lesions in 148 Australian reptiles (39 snakes, 109 lizards) and did not find any atheromas, although serum cholesterol values ranged from 21 to 759 mg/dl.[11] They did find that 30.8% of their snakes had saccular aneurysms of the aorta, apparently caused by pentastome larvae (see p. 163).

The most common and the only clinically significant form of arteriosclerosis in reptiles is calcification of arterial walls.[90] Medial calcification in major arteries has been described in a fatal disease of green iguanas (*Iguana iguana*).[247,284] Wallach reported that his cases were caused by hypervitaminosis D[284] (see p. 182).

There are very few reports of noninfectious vascular diseases in amphibians. Intimal thickening and chondroid metaplasia were found in two adult female bullfrogs that also had enlarged, cystic kidneys.[90]

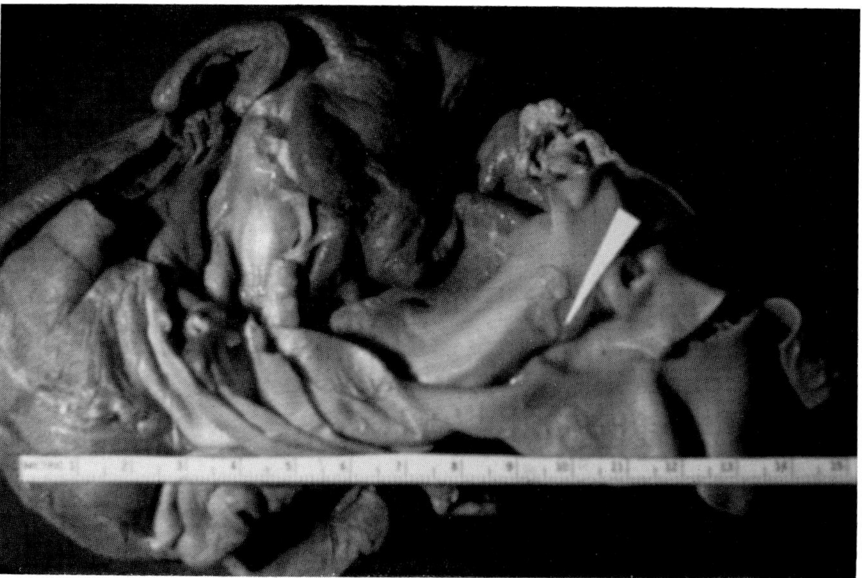

Fig. 3–97. Atheromatous plaques (pointer and above the 10- to 11-cm marks on the ruler) in the right aortic arch of an adult male Komodo dragon (*Varanus komodoensis*). The animal died with congestive heart failure and adenocarcinoma of the colon. (Specimen courtesy of Dr. Richard Montali: National Zoological Park, Washington, D.C.)

Amyloidosis. Amyloidosis was found in the renal glomeruli of a Central American boa *(C. constrictor imperator)* and the spleen of a brown tree snake *(Boa enydris enydris)*. No specific disease was associated with the appearance of amyloid in these two snakes.[68]

Pancreatic Disease. A peculiar form of pancreatic disease occurs in captive snakes. The disease is characterized by multifocal necrosis of pancreatic acini followed by hyperplasia of ductile elements (Fig. 3–98). The regenerative process was originally described as a malignant neoplastic disease,[228] but is now classified as an idiopathic hyperplasia. For unknown reasons the condition has occurred frequently at the Philadelphia Zoo, particularly in snakes dying after prolonged captivity.[68,229]

Diabetes Mellitus. Diabetes mellitus was diagnosed postmortem in a 12-year-old male red-eared turtle *(Chrysemys [Pseudemys] scripta elegans)*.[102b] The turtle was small for its age and sex. It suffered a terminal illness characterized by anorexia and progressive weakness and lethargy. The liver was enlarged, pale, grey, and friable, with decreased

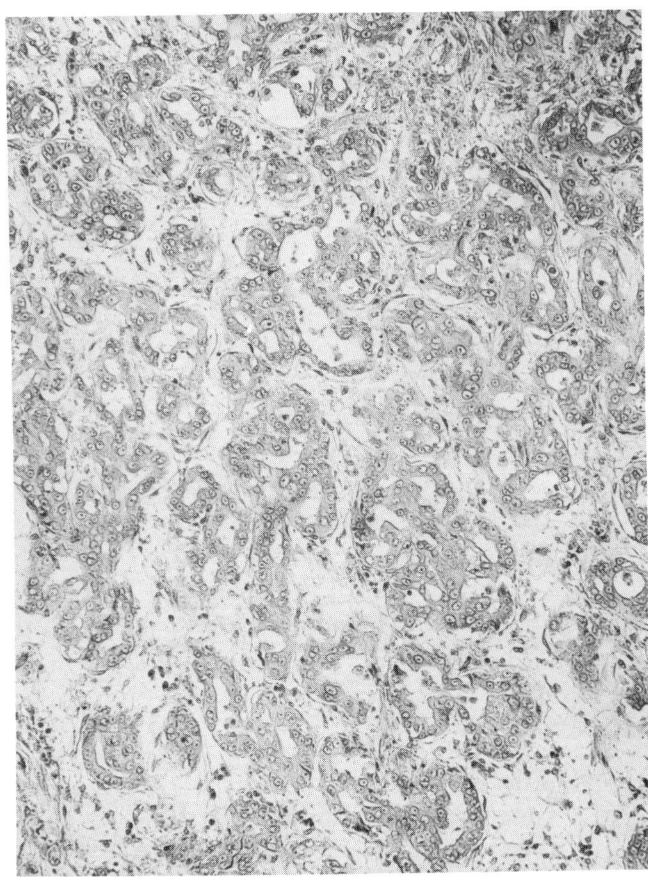

Fig. 3–98. Pine snake *(Pituophis melanoleucus*, male). Pancreas shows atypical regenerative hyperplasia. H and E stain; 130×. (From Cowan, D.F.: Diseases of captive reptiles. J. Am. Vet. Med. Assoc., *153*:848–859, 1968. Photograph courtesy of Dr. D.F. Cowan.)

glycogen content. Pancreatic islet cells were pale and vacuolated, and there was chronic glomerulonephritis. Significant chemical abnormalities in the blood included hyperglycemia (611 mg glucose/dl), hypoproteinemia, hypocalcemia, and elevated levels of cholesterol, blood urea nitrogen (BUN), creatinine, serum glutamic-pyruvic transaminase (SGPT), and alkaline phosphatase.

Renal Diseases. Zwart and Cowan have reviewed renal diseases of reptiles.[68,309] The kidney is frequently damaged in gout (discussed previously). Yellowish-white flecks of urate deposits are seen dispersed in the renal parenchyma (see Fig. 3–90), and there may be blockage of tubules, tophus formation (see Fig. 3–93), and interstitial fibrosis.[68] It is possible that renal damage occurs secondary to the heavy urate deposits in gout rather than as a cause of gout. However, it is likely that renal damage interferes with urate excretion, increasing blood uric acid levels and thus exacerbating the condition in a vicious metabolic circle.

Zwart[309] and Cowan[68] have described a variety of pathologic changes in the reptilian kidney, including acute and chronic glomerulonephritis, glomerulosclerosis, membranous glomerulonephrosis, interstitial nephritis, renal abscesses, acute pyelonephritis, basement membrane disease, renal mycobacterial infection, and renal amebic infection. The studies cited previously dealt mainly with morphologic studies rather than clinical-pathologic correlation. However, by analogy with the comparable diseases in mammals, it is likely that these conditions caused illness and contributed to the demise of these reptiles.

Calculi. Calculi have been found in the urinary bladder of *Hyla aurea*, a New Zealand frog.[242] Some of these calculi filled the entire bladder. They had a soft, friable core surrounded by concentric lamellae of a calcium phosphate salt.

Urinary cystic calculi are also found in turtles and lizards. These calculi have a varied composition; some of them are 98% calcium phosphate. The calculi are easily seen radiographically. Wallach indicates that these calculi are prone to occur in turtles and lizards on diets low in calcium but adequate in vitamin D, and he suggests putting calcium carbonate in the form of limestone, oyster shell, or plaster of paris in their water.[285] Wallach also states that, "Larger carnivorous species require a dietary supplement of 900 mg calcium carbonate for each 100 gm lean red meat fed or 1.5 gm calcium carbonate for each 100 gm fish fed."[285]

Cystic calculi can be removed surgically. Frye has published an excellent description of such a procedure in a desert tortoise *(Gopherus agassizi)*.[95]

Goiter with Hypothyroidism. Amphibians and reptiles are susceptible to goiter with hypothyroidism. Most of these cases have been ascribed to nutritional deficiency of iodine or to goitrogens in the diet, e.g., in lettuce, kale, and spinach fed to tortoises.[285] Giant land tortoises from the Aldabra and Galapagos Islands are particularly susceptible to hypothyroid goiter (Fig. 3–99). It is likely that their natural diet is rich in iodine and, thus, their requirement for iodine may be relatively

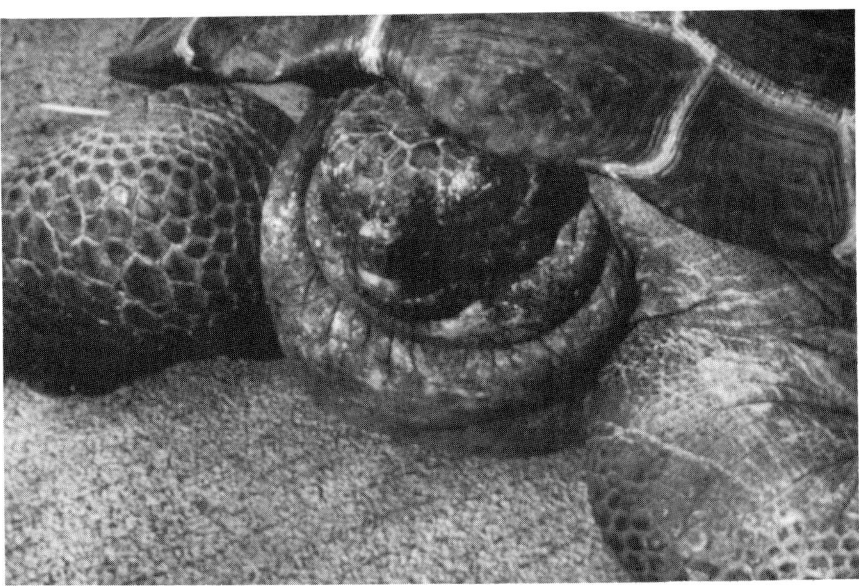

Fig. 3–99. Galapagos tortoise *(Geochelone elephantopus)* with massive hypothyroid goiter. (From Frye, F.L. and Dutra, F.R.: Hypothyroidism in turtles and tortoises. Vet. Med. Small Anim. Clin., *69*:990–993, 1974. Photograph courtesy of Dr. Fredric L. Frye.)

high.[102] Turtles suffering from hypothyroidism may have severe generalized edema.[102]

Amphibians with depressed thyroid function fail to complete metamorphosis. This failure can occur in areas deficient in iodine or from exposure to goitrogens. Dodd and Callan reported that newts *(Triturus helveticus)* in a pond in Scotland failed to mature and had markedly enlarged and hyperplastic thyroids, a condition ascribed to contamination of their pond by feces of rabbits that had been feasting on goitrogenic cabbage.[78] In some areas amphibians normally reach sexual maturity while otherwise maintaining larval characteristics, a physiologic accommodation to their hypothyroid state called neoteny (see p. 8). Hypothyroid tadpoles may reach giant size while failing to mature.[233]

Microscopically, the goiter associated with iodine deficiency has hyperplastic, columnar epithelium and minimum colloid.

Treatment of hypothyroid goiter involves removing goitrogens and supplementing the diet with iodine, e.g., with iodized salt, the recommended level being 0.5% of the total diet. Surgical removal of any of the goiter is contraindicated unless it is secondarily infected or is causing obstruction of a vital organ.

Flaccid Paralysis. Lizards occasionally have flaccid paralysis of the hind limbs and tail. I have seen this condition in skinks and iguanids. The cause is not known, but trauma to the spinal cord should be ruled out by radiographs and examination of the spinal column. There is usually a rapid onset. Reflex withdrawal from a pinch or a needle is reduced or absent. Tremors (probably fasciculations) of the affected limbs are seen. If injury to the cord cannot be demonstrated, then empirical treatment with B complex vitamins, particularly thiamine (B_1), may be useful.[96] Therapeutic trials with calcium gluconate might also be worth trying. The prognosis is poor, and most affected lizards die.

Skin Diseases. Herpetofauna are commonly affected by skin diseases. In addition to specific microbial, parasitic, nutritional, toxic, and neoplastic conditions, there are several idiopathic disorders such as **blister disease, necrotic dermatitis (scale rot),** and **molchpest.**

Blister disease (vesicular pyoderma, pocks, antikeratinic dermatosis) is a vesicular skin disease of snakes that starts with focal accumulation of a clear, viscous fluid between the stratum corneum and stratum germinativum (Fig. 3–100). According to Kiel, pure cultures of a nonhemolytic strain of *Staphylococcus aureus* can routinely be cultured from this fluid.[172] A primary etiologic role for this organism has not been proven, however, and Zwart has not found bacteriologic studies to be definitive.[311] The lesions may become secondarily infected with gram-negative organisms or fungi. Untreated, most snakes die of inanition or septicemia. It is possible that blister disease can result in subcutaneous abscesses (see p. 96), although the relationship of these two conditions is not clear.

A damp environment predisposes to blister disease. In general, terrestrial and arboreal snakes are more susceptible than water snakes.

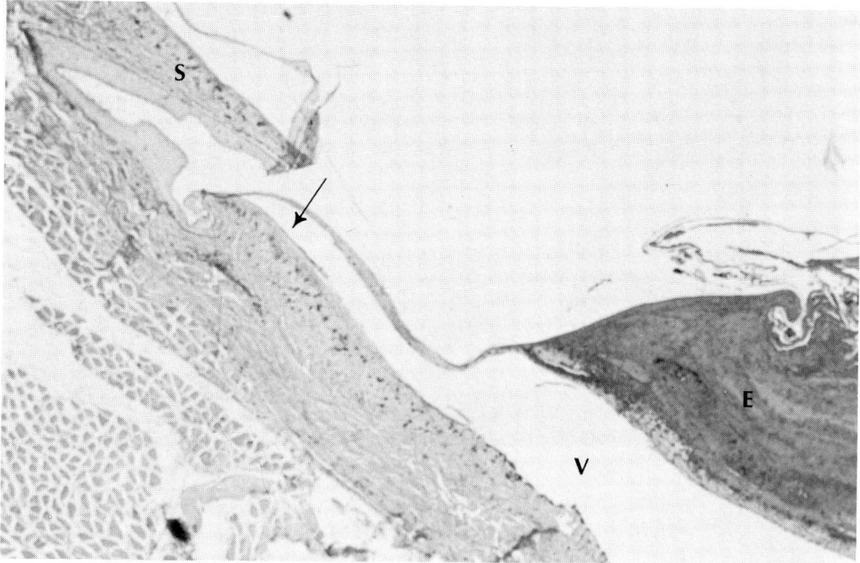

Fig. 3–100. Lesion of blister disease in a Grand Cayman Island water snake *(Tretanorhinus variabilis lewisi)*. A relatively normal scale **(S)** is in the upper left. Schism of the epithelium begins (arrow) between the stratum corneum and stratum germinativum. The layer superficial to the center of the vesicle **(V)** is thickened and contains epithelial nuclear debris, some serum, and some inflammatory cells: i.e., there is an eschar **(E)**. (Armed Forces Institute of Pathology Accession No. 1176342.)

Providing an area in the cage where snakes can dry off is an important preventive measure.

Individual vesicles can be drained. Kiel recommends replacing aspirated fluid with a 2% iodine solution.[172] Bathing in antiseptic solutions or applying mafenamide acetate may be useful. Antibiotics should be used if there is bacterial infection. Supportive therapy, including parenteral fluids or forced feeding, may also be necessary. Zwart recommends vitamin A supplementation which may stimulate shedding and hasten a cure.[311]

Scale rot or **skin rot** is a form of necrotizing dermatitis in snakes which starts as one or more focal lesions that may coalesce to involve large areas of the body. Focal lesions may be associated with incomplete shedding, and healing may be achieved when the retained skin is removed with the aid of a warm water soak.[64] It is possible that some cases are a complication of blister disease, perhaps because of secondary infection. Culture for bacteria and fungi should be taken of lesions not responding to symptomatic therapy such as daily bathing in a quaternary ammonium disinfectant.[64] Cowan considers that skin rot may result from tissue breakdown owing to prolonged starvation.[68] Supportive therapy should include adequate nutrition, provided by forced feeding, and injection of vitamins if the snake is not eating.

Molchpest is an idiopathic fatal disorder of newts and salamanders which can occur as a devastating epizootic in a collection or lab animal colony. Signs include sluggishness, anorexia, disequilibrium, reddening of the skin, and dermal pustules. There is generalized edema, and the skin may be shed in shreds. All affected animals die. A peculiar smell, similar to that of parsley, is said to be diagnostic.[233] The cause of molchpest is not known and there is no cure. Complete disinfection and cleaning of infected quarters is recommended before new animals are introduced.

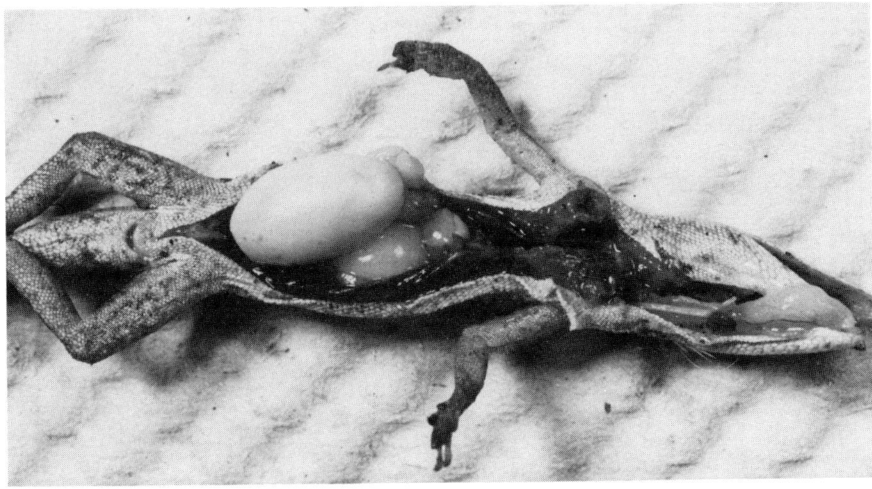

Fig. 3–101. Eggbound anole lizard *(Anolis carolinensis)*.

Egg-laying reptiles can become **eggbound** (Fig. 3–101). This condition, most frequently seen in turtles, should be considered if a female reptile is presented with tenesmus, cloacal prolapse, or a mass in the cloacal region or lower abdomen. The eggs can be shown radiographically. Using nonscreen techniques for turtles, one can also demonstrate decreased lung fields, especially in the craniocaudal position.[110a]

If the egg is accessible from the cloaca, it may be possible to instill an antibiotic ointment as a lubricant to help passage. Usually, however, this will not work because the dystocia is due to inadequate contraction in the oviduct. Since most reptilian eggs have a leathery shell (more mineralized and brittle in turtles), it may be possible to aspirate the egg with a needle and syringe and then pull the collapsed shell out with forceps. If this fails, surgical removal of the egg may be necessary. Excellent description and illustration of the procedure in a turtle is given by Frye and Schuckman.[104] One unit of oxytocin, IM, apparently stimulated egg laying in an eggbound 16-year-old Florida box turtle *(Terrapene carolina bauri)*.[110a]

Occasionally, eggs may be released or may rupture into the body cavity of a reptile instead of following the normal path down the reproductive tract.[147] This might initiate peritonitis, or such eggs may undergo resorption, calcification, or ectopic development. In either of the latter two events the presenting sign of the animal may be a palpable abdominal mass, and the diagnosis might be established radiographically. If indicated clinically, the ectopic egg could be removed surgically. If ovariohysterectomy is done on a reptile or amphibian, the entire ovarian mass must be excised to avoid subsequent release of eggs in the peritoneal cavity.[97]

Toxicology

Disinfectants. Phenol- and cresol-type disinfectants such as Lysol are generally thought to be highly toxic to herpetofauna and should not be used in their vicinity. If animals are exposed, they should be washed copiously with water. If toxic signs such as convulsions develop, symptomatic, supportive treatment can be given. There are no specific antidotes. Appropriate disinfectants are discussed in Chapter 2.

Insecticides. Most insecticides are toxic to herpetofauna if present in sufficient concentration. Chlorinated hydrocarbons such as DDT are especially toxic, and their use on or near reptiles and amphibians is contraindicated. Exposed animals often suffer convulsions and die. Treatment consists of washing off the toxic agent with water and giving supportive therapy.

Even the chemicals most widely recommended and used to control mites can prove toxic (see p. 169). Deaths have been reported in small lizards and snakes exposed to the silica gel, Dri-Die 67. Diazinon 25E has proved toxic for some snakes at recommended dilutions as discussed earlier in this chapter. DDVP has been recommended for mite control, but when I placed a three-inch piece of a cat flea collar in a cage containing anole lizards *(Anolis carolinensis)*, the lizards rapidly developed progressive, generalized, flaccid paralysis which could be reversed by removing the insecticide strips.

Various insecticides and herbicides are toxic for tadpoles.[241] DDT in high doses causes tremors, spasmodic movements, abnormal posturing, and death in adult frogs. Lower doses may cause neurologic and behavioral changes in frogs and tadpoles which make them more subject to predation.[62] There are few, if any, indications for using insecticides therapeutically in captive amphibians, but accidental poisoning with such agents should be considered when there is sudden high mortality in a collection.

In nature, amphibian larvae are exposed to pollutants in water. Insectivorous herpetofauna ingest insecticide-poisoned insects and, in turn, are eaten by larger predators. Because of their likely exposure to toxic agents and their important intermediate position in the food chain, effects on herpetofauna should be incorporated in environmental impact studies of insecticides and herbicides. The article by Cooke is a useful reference source for ecology and toxicology of insecticide poisoning in frogs.[62] The effects of pesticides on reptiles were reviewed by Hall.[120b]

Paint on Turtle Shells. Formerly, it was common for baby aquatic turtles sold in pet stores in the United States to have designs painted on their carapace. This resulted in deformities of the shell and contributed to the high mortality in these animals. The practice of painting turtle shells was banned in most areas. In addition, now that baby turtles cannot be sold in the United States because of the Salmonella hazard (discussed previously), the condition is rarely seen today. The paint should be chipped off without injuring the shell. Paint solvents should not be used because they are toxic for turtles.

Inorganic Ions. Various inorganic ions can prove toxic for amphibians. Kaplan states that leopard frogs *(Rana pipiens)* suffer petechiation and ulceration of the skin when kept in water containing four parts per million (p.p.m.) of chlorine in the form of calcium hypochlorite and that the disease is irreversible and fatal when the concentration is raised to five p.p.m.[158] Frogs kept in distilled or tap water containing 1.10 to 2.75 p.p.m. of chlorine did not get ill. Mud puppies *(Necturus maculosus)* reportedly suffered toxic effects from the chlorine in tap water, manifested by excitement, exhaustion, convulsions, paralysis, and death.[161] I have kept newts *(Notophthalmus viridescens)* in tap water for months without obvious ill effects. Reichenbach-Klinke and Elkan recommend keeping South African clawed toads *(Xenopus laevis)* in 0.4% NaCl (equal to 4000 p.p.m. of NaCl) as a means of reducing mortality in a laboratory colony.[233] The effect of chloride on amphibia or as a disinfectant varies greatly according to its ionic form. If the water appears to be toxic it should be charcoal filtered before use.

Tank water containing more than five p.p.m. of fluoride caused anemia, leukopenia, and gastrointestinal hyperemia and hemorrhage in leopard frogs.[163] Fatalities occurred with concentrations greater than 50 p.p.m., and mortality increased with the level of fluoride concentration.

Lead nitrate solutions were found to be toxic for frogs *(R. pipiens)*, causing sloughing of skin, loss of postural tone, sluggishness, and leukopenia. Deaths occurred with high concentration.[160] Apparently, plumbism could result from keeping amphibians in lead-lined tanks.

Copper sulphate is toxic to leopard frogs *(Rana pipiens);* contact causes excess mucous secretion from the skin and ocular irritation manifested by blinking and rubbing of the eyes. Toxic reactions proportional to ionic concentration are evident when *R. pipiens* is immersed in water containing more than 0.0015% copper sulphate. Bradycardia, cardiac arrhythmias, flaccid paralysis, and death occur at progressively higher concentrations.[164]

Secretions from skin glands of certain frogs and toads may be poisonous to other herpetofauna. The pickerel frog *(Rana palustris)* should not be caged with other amphibians since it may kill them on contact.

Secretions from skin glands of many toads are cardiotoxic. Karstad reported that a fox snake *(Elaphe vulpina)* died within six hours after begin force-fed a live toad *(Bufo americanus),* even though the toad was vomited within two minutes.[165] Symptoms included writhing about and gaping of the mouth. The snake's lungs were collapsed, congested, and edematous, the kidneys were congested, and petechiae were on the gastric serosa. It is interesting that hognose snakes *(Heterodon platyrhinos)* regularly eat toads, apparently with bon appetit and no ill effects.

Many venomous snakes are relatively resistant to poisoning by their own and some other species' venoms, the degree of resistance depending on dose and type of venom. The level of protection is quite high in some snakes, e.g., in kingsnakes that eat pit vipers. The resistance is not owing to humoral immunity. The protective factor can be separated from the globulin and albumin fractions of snake plasma.[265]

Neoplastic Diseases

Benign and malignant tumors of the circulatory system, and of the epithelial and connective tissues have been reported in herpetofauna. Most of their tumors are morphologically similar to neoplasms arising in corresponding tissues in homeotherms. There are major differences in the relative frequency of tumors in different species, however. With some exceptions, neoplasms seem to occur less frequently in reptiles and amphibians than in mammals. This is especially noteworthy since herpetofauna often have a longer life expectancy than mammals of similar size.

Neoplasms of cold-blooded vertebrates were reviewed by Schlumberger and Lucké[244] and by Lucké and Schlumberger.[189] The tumors of amphibians were the subject of two review papers by Balls,[21] and Balls and Clothier,[23] a section of a book chapter by Harshbarger,[121] and a symposium, with the papers later published as a text.[212] The tumors of reptiles were also the subject of recent reviews by Harshbarger,[122] Billups and Harshbarger,[28] and Jacobson.[149c] An extensive bibliography of published case reports and a list of all reptilian tumors accessioned at the Armed Forces Institute of Pathology and at the Registry of Tumors in Lower Animals (RTLA) (discussed at the end of this chapter) may be found in the work of Billups and Harshbarger.[28]

Only the most frequently occurring tumors of herpetofauna are discussed here. Reference should be made to the reviews cited above and to the Registry of Tumors in Lower Animals for case reports of other tumors. These reviews are cited as references in the following discussion. The citation for the original reports can be obtained from the bibliographies in the reviews.

Solid tumors usually are presented as mass lesions. If amenable to surgery, suspected tumors should be excised as soon after discovery as possible. Chemotherapy, radiation therapy, and immunotherapy of neoplasms in herpetofauna have not been investigated.

Renal Adenocarcinoma. Also called the Lucké tumor, renal adenocarcinoma of leopard frogs *(Rana pipiens)* is the most frequently occurring and most intensely studied tumor of herpetofauna. This tumor was first accurately described in 1934 by Baldwin Lucké who spent the next two decades studying it. The tumor has been the subject of many papers, mostly because it is thought to be a model of viral-induced neoplasia.

The prevalence of the Lucké tumor varies geographically. It is relatively common in Vermont, where Lucké obtained most of his frogs. Among the 10,000 frogs he examined, he found 2.7% with tumors. It is also common in Wisconsin, but is rarely seen in southern states. The prevalence in the north-central United States is approximately 8.5%.[204] However, field studies in Minnesota revealed the tumor was much more likely to be seen in certain counties.[205]

The tumor is twice as frequent in males as in females and is bilateral in more than 60% of affected frogs.[227] Tumor-bearing frogs are found in spring and autumn more often than in the summer, perhaps because of higher mortality among tumorous frogs in the summer, e.g., due to predation, or because there might be seasonal regression of the tumor.[205]

Grossly, the Lucké tumor appears as a solid, nodular, fungating growth arising from the kidney (Fig. 3–102). Metastases are infrequently seen in frogs in the wild, presumably because of high mortality. In captivity, however, if the frog is maintained with frequent feedings and is kept relatively warm, metastases are common, most often to the lungs, next most often to the liver, and less often to the bladder, mesentery, peritoneum, pancreas, intestine, ovary, and orbit.[227]

Microscopically, the Lucké tumor is an invasive, nonencapsulated, but usually well-demarcated adenocarcinoma arising from the proximal tubules (Fig. 3–103). All grades of malignancy can be seen in different tumors, from relatively benign to markedly anaplastic. Typically, tubules are formed, lined by few to many cell layers; papillae often project into the lumens.[204]

Cowdry type A intranuclear inclusion bodies are frequently seen in tumors of frogs when they are in a natural or artificial state of hibernation. These so-called "winter tumors" contain large concentrations of a specific herpes virus which is widely accepted as a necessary

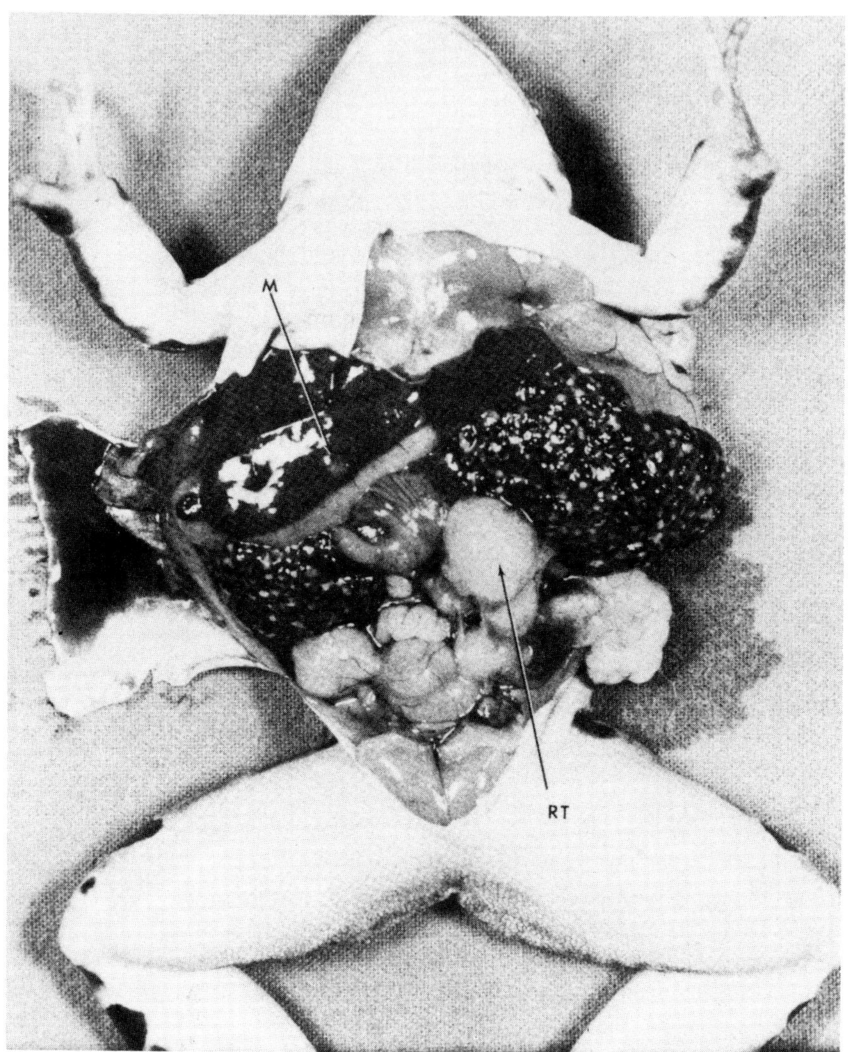

Fig. 3–102. Sexually mature *Rana pipiens* dissected to show large primary renal adenocarcinoma **(RT)** with several metastatic masses in the liver **(M)**. (Tumor-bearing frog courtesy of Professor George M. Nace. From McKinnell, L.M. and Labat, D.D.: Frog renal tumors are composed of stroma, vascular elements and epithelial cells: What type nucleus programs for tadpoles with the cloning procedure? *In* Progress in Differentiation Research. Edited by N. Müller-Bérat. Amsterdam, North-Holland Publishing Co., 1976. Photograph courtesy of Dr. R.G. McKinnell.)

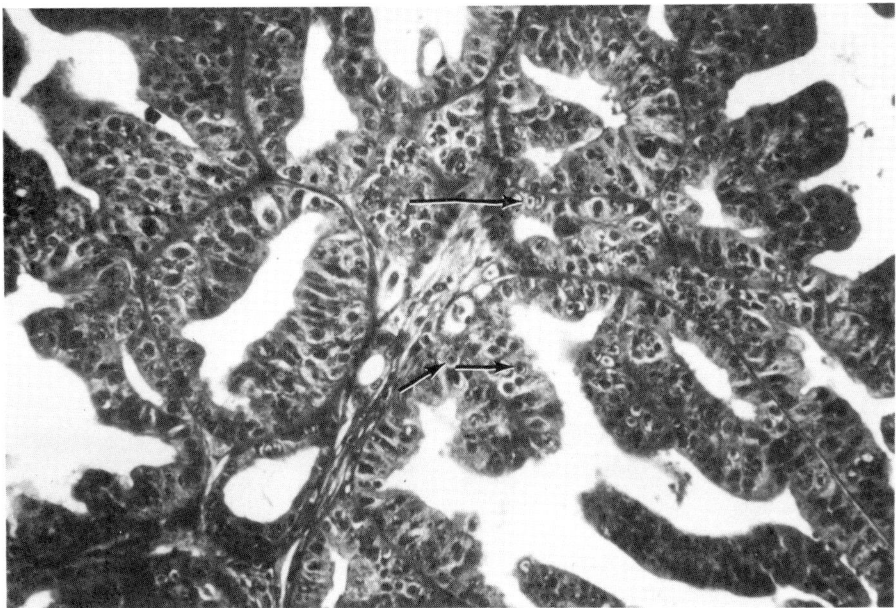

Fig. 3–103. Lucké renal adenocarcinoma ("winter tumor") in a leopard frog *(Rana pipiens)*. Tubules with epithelial lining of varying thickness are formed, and epithelial fronds or papillae project into the tubular lumens. Type A intranuclear inclusions (arrows) are found only in "winter tumors."

causative agent of the Lucké tumor. The virus is shed in the urine of frogs with tumors containing inclusion bodies. Tumors in frogs caught in the summer or maintained at room temperature rarely, if ever, contain such inclusion bodies or virus. The virus is apparently masked or latent in the summer and it is unmasked and replicates with cold weather.[212] "Summer tumors" enlarge rapidly and "winter tumors" grow very slowly.

The Lucké tumor can be transmitted by cell-free filtrates to tadpoles with a developing pronephros[212] and to larger adult frogs if they are kept in a cool environment.[227] It appears that all of the Koch-Henle postulates have been met, proving that the Lucké herpes virus is a necessary etiologic agent of the Lucké tumor.[215] Further work may be necessary to prove it is the only cause.[120] The possible role of a "helper" virus has not been ruled out.[215]

Assuming that the herpes virus is the cause and that the Lucké tumor is transmitted in nature, Rafferty[227] has postulated a life cycle for the disease that seems to be a reasonable theory: The virus replicates in winter tumors in hibernating frogs that are three or more years old. These frogs spawn in the spring as the ice melts at the edge of their lake. Virus is shed in their urine, infecting the eggs or the tadpoles after hatching. The infection is latent until the frog is at least two years old. (Field tumors are almost never seen in younger frogs.) The tumors then become grossly obvious within one or more years, growing rapidly in the summer when the highest mortality directly or indirectly due to the tumor occurs. Frogs with tumors that survived winter hibernation pass virus in their urine to infect the next generation of frogs during the spring spawning season.

The virus requirement for cold temperature to replicate could explain the absence of the Lucké tumor in the southern range of *Rana pipiens*, but this could also be caused by differing susceptibility of different geographic subspecies. It also would not explain why frogs in some northern United States areas rarely get the disease while it is endemic in other areas with a similar temperature range.

Tweedell tried to simulate natural transmission of the Lucké tumor, but was successful only by intraperitoneal injection of cell-free filtrates into female frogs before (induced) ovulation.[280] The progeny in this experiment developed metastasizing tumors when they were five- to 12-month-old adult frogs.

Other than the Lucké tumor, primary renal neoplasms apparently are rare in herpetofauna. Individual cases of malignant renal tumors have been reported in the edible frog *(Rana esculenta)*, the South African clawed toad *(Xenopus laevis)*, the bullfrog *(Rana catesbeiana)*, and the mudpuppy *(Necturus maculosus)*.[23] A boa constrictor with a renal adenocarcinoma is accessioned in the R.T.L.A. (1975 report). A renal adenocarcinoma that metastasized to the liver in a box tortoise *(Terrapene carolina)* and a papillary adenocarcinoma of the kidney in a ring snake *(Tropidonotus natrix)* are cited in the review by Billups and Harshbarger.[28]

A seven-year-old, 14-foot male Indian python *(Python molurus)* that died at the National Zoological Park in Washington, D.C. had an adenocarcinoma of the kidney arising from the renal tubules (Fig. 3–104 A and B). It also had a very anaplastic adenocarcinoma centrally located in the liver, which was either a metastasis from the renal tumor, or a poorly differentiated bile duct carcinoma (Fig. 3–105 A and B). (This python is one of the reptilian tumor cases accessioned at the Armed Forces Institute of Pathology and listed by Billups and Harshbarger.[28])

Hepatomas. There are case reports of hepatomas occurring in an edible frog *(Rana esculenta)*, two leopard frogs *(R. pipiens)*,[23] two iguanas *(Iguana iguana)*, a chameleon *(Chameleo dilepis)*, a tegu *(Tupinambis refescens)*, and a rear-fanged snake, the massuarana *(Pseudoboa cloelia)*.[149c] Other primary hepatic tumors in reptiles include a malignant hepatoma in a skink *(Eumeces fasciatus)*; a bile duct adenoma in a Ricord's iguana *(Cyclura ricordi)*, a boomslang *(Dispholidus typus)*, a garter snake *(Thamnophis sirtalis)*, and a spitting cobra *(Naja nigricollis)*; a biliary adenocarcinoma in a Korean viper *(Agkistrodon halyx)* and a fer-de-lance *(Bothrops atrox)*; and a papillary carcinoma of the bile duct in an East Indian water snake *(Homalopsis bucata)*.[149c]

Hematopoietic Tumors. These tumors in herpetofauna are the subject of reviews by Balls and Ruben,[24] Dawe,[70] and Harshbarger and Dawe.[123] A study set on the comparative pathology of hematopoietic and lymphoreticular tumors is available on loan from The Registry of Experimental Cancers, National Cancer Institute, Bethesda, Maryland,

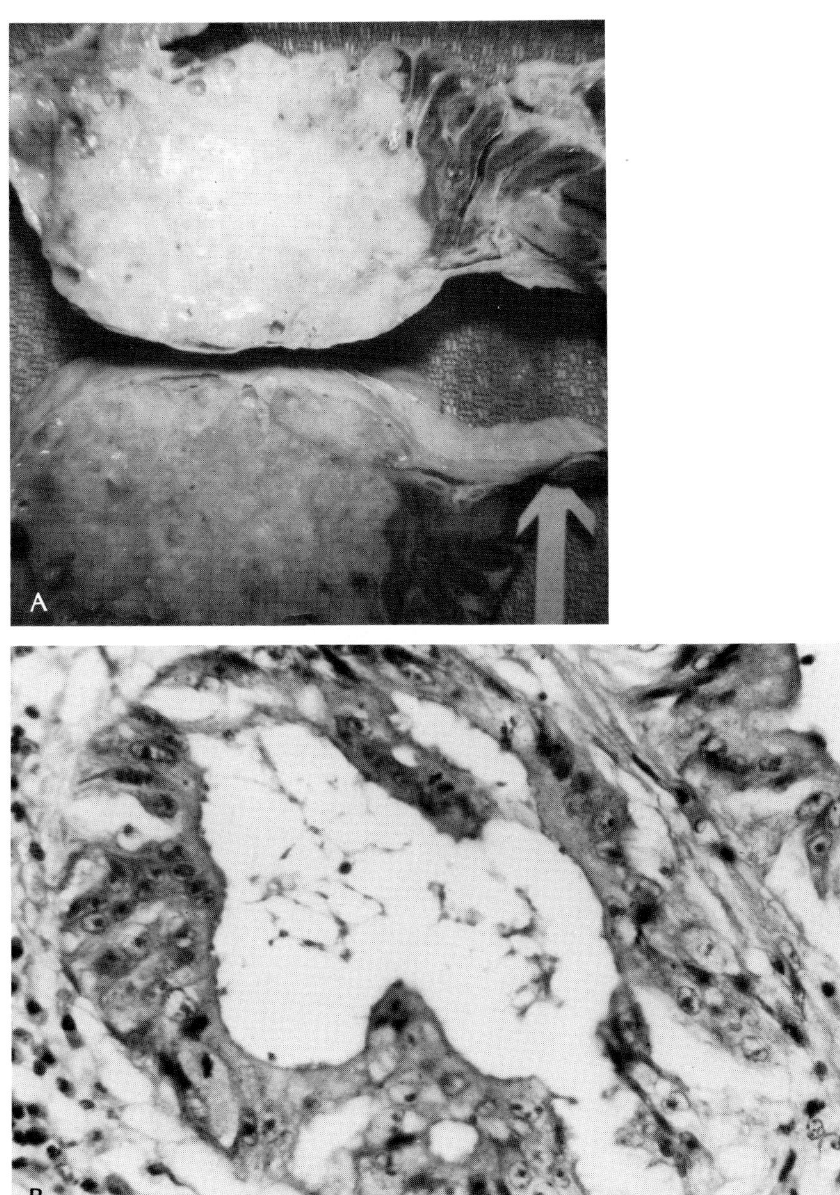

Fig. 3–104. Renal adenocarcinoma in a seven-year-old male Indian python *(Python molurus)*. (Armed Forces Institute of Pathology Accession No. 1172389.) **A.** Remnant of normal kidney is the dark tissue immediately above and to the left of the arrow. The lighter colored tumor has replaced most of the renal parenchyma. **B.** Anaplastic epithelium forming tubules with lining layers of irregular thickness. 130×.

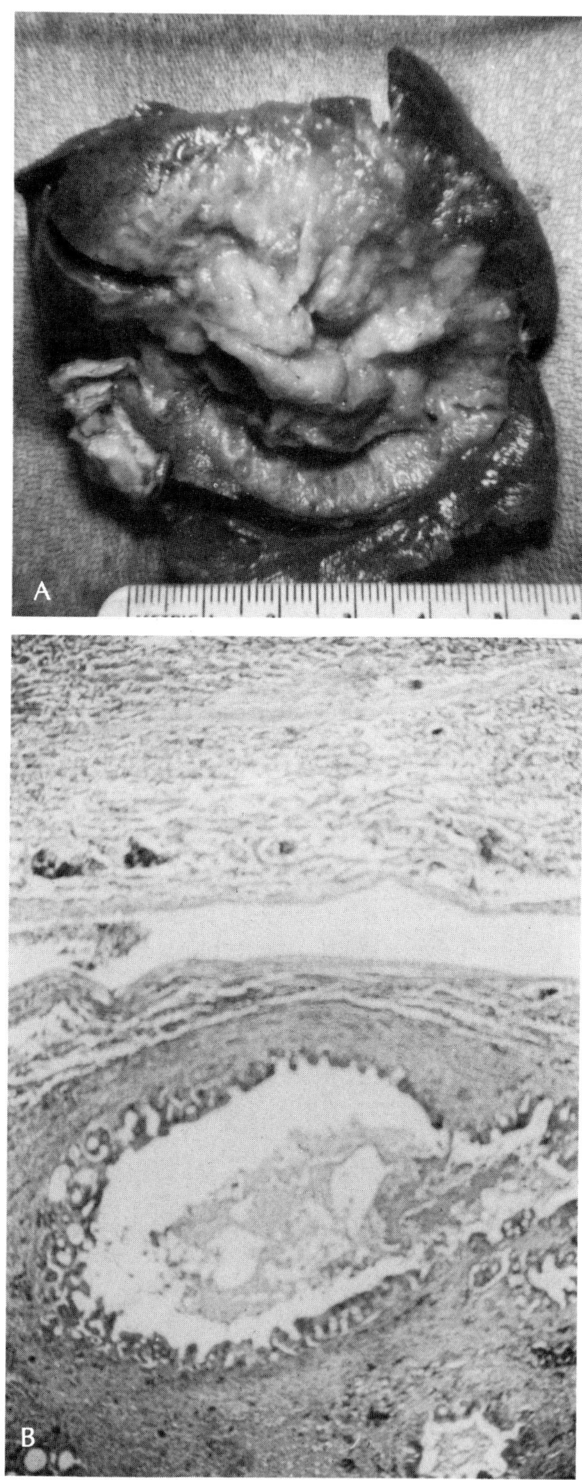

Fig. 3–105. Adenocarcinoma in the liver of the same seven-year-old male Indian python *(Python molurus)* illustrated in Figure 3–104. Several pathologists could not agree whether this was a metastasis from the renal adenocarcinoma or a second primary adenocarcinoma, of bile duct origin. (Armed Forces Institute of Pathology Accession No. 1172389.) **A.** The pale grey tumor tissue occupies the center of the liver. The remaining hepatic parenchyma is the darker tissue seen peripherally. Metric scale. **B.** The tumor formed tubules and induced a desmoplastic reaction. Tumor (bottom) compressed hepatic parenchyma (top). 13×.

20014. This set includes slides of a lymphosarcoma in an axolotl *(Ambystoma mexicanum)*, a reticulum cell sarcoma in an African clawed toad *(Xenopus laevis)*, lymphoid leukemia in a timber rattlesnake *(Crotalus h. horridus)*, and reticulum cell sarcomas in a death adder *(Acanthopis antarticus)* and a hognose snake *(Heterodon platyrhinos)*.[72]

The hematopoietic tumor of herpetofauna that has received the greatest attention is the so-called "lymphosarcoma" of *Xenopus laevis*, which was found as a spontaneous disease in the amphibian colony at Oxford University. Invasive, destructive lesions composed of lymphoid and histiocytic cells, often in nodules, occur in the liver, kidney, spleen, and other organs. The disease is progressive and eventually fatal. It is claimed that the disease is transmissible by contact, that it can be experimentally induced with cell-free filtrates, benzpyrene, methylcholanthrene, or urethan, and can be transmitted to other amphibian species by tissue transplant.[22,24,238]

Some workers think that "lymphosarcoma" in *Xenopus laevis* is a viral-induced tumor, but its viral etiology and neoplastic nature have been challenged. Dawe states that the lesions are histologically compatible with infectious granulomas.[70,71] Acid-fast bacilli (AFB) are often demonstrable in them, and similar lesions can be induced by inoculation of AFB.[70,71] Clothier and Balls have identified the AFB as *Mycobacterium marinum* and present data to show that this organism causes granulomatous disease that is morphologically distinct from lymphosarcoma and that the AFB are only secondary invaders when they are found in the tumor tissue.[59,60]

Even those workers who think the disease in *X. laevis* is a viral tumor acknowledge that what has been described in the fire-bellied newt, *Cynops (Triturus) pyrrhogaster*, as a lymphosarcoma is a mycobacterial disease.[23,24] The cause of lymphosarcoma in *X. laevis* may not be definitively proven until experiments with Mycobacteria-free toads are done.

Dawe found no reports of hematopoietic tumors in reptiles published prior to 1968.[70] (Lawson reported a malignant lymphoma in a Sardinian lizard in 1962.[183]) Billups and Harshbarger cited nine other reported cases plus three registered cases (RTLA) of lymphoid malignancies involving a total of eight snakes (seven species), two lizards, and two turtles (four species).[28] They also cited cases of reticulum cell sarcoma in an anole lizard *(Anolis carolinensis)*, a death adder *(Acanthopis antarticus)*, and a hognose snake *(Heterodon platyrhinos)*. The RTLA had accessioned a case of granulocytic leukemia in a rhinoceros viper *(Bitis nasicornis)* and a possible plasma cell tumor in a Nile monitor *(Varanus niloticus)*.[28] Recorded in the 1975 RTLA report are a plasma cell tumor in a cottonmouth moccasin *(Agkistrodon piscivorus)* and myelogenous leukemia in a helmeted turtle *(Pelomedusa subruta)*.

There are no unequivocal reports of hematopoietic tumors in crocodilians. A possible lymphosarcoma in the liver of a salt water crocodile *(Crocodylus porosus)* is reviewed by Schlumberger and Lucké.[244]

A great variety of solid mesenchymal tumors have been found in herpetofauna. Nine out of 24 such tumors in amphibians reviewed by

Balls and Clothier were fibromas.[23] Fibrocytic tumors are the most common mesenchymal neoplasms found in reptiles and are about evenly divided between benign and malignant forms.

Skin Tumors. These tumors have been reported in herpetofauna, especially amphibians, more frequently than any other neoplasms except for the Lucké renal adenocarcinoma. One reason for this is their obvious external appearance. However, if their real (not just reported) frequency is higher than that of internal tumors, then one possible explanation for their preponderance might be related to the peculiar metabolic role of amphibian skin in respiration and in fluid and electrolyte balance (Chap. 1). Since the amphibian skin is metabolically active in transport mechanisms, it would not be surprising to find it particularly sensitive to certain poisons, including carcinogens.

An epizootic of skin tumors, including epidermal papillomas, benign and malignant melanophoromas, fibromas, and fibrosarcomas, has been found, in that descending order of frequency, among neotenic tiger salamanders *(Ambystoma tigrinum)* in a sewage settling lagoon in Texas.[236,236a] Tiger salamanders from nearby nonsewage pools become sexually mature adults, and tumors have not been found in them. A search is being made for carcinogens in the sewage lagoon.

Papillomas, melanotic tumors, and fibrous tumors have been found in the skin of other urodeles.[23] There is equivocal evidence that a carcinoma of the skin in the newt, *Triton alpestus,* is caused by a transmissible agent.[244]

The most common skin tumors in anurans are adenomas, adenocarcinomas, and squamous cell carcinomas,[244] according to the Activities Report of the Registry of Tumors in Lower Animals from 1965 to 1973. Among "hundreds" of frogs *(Rana pipiens)* examined in two and one-half years at the University of Michigan, 13 had nodular cutaneous growths.[263] Five only had epidermal hyperplasia, seven had squamous cell carcinoma (three of these cancerous frogs also had hyperplastic lesions), and one had a dermal gland adenocarcinoma. The squamous cell carcinomas occurred in frogs that were at least three and one-half to five years old. A squamous cell carcinoma in the digits of a rear leg invaded the underlying bone and muscle. The other squamous cell carcinomas originated in areas where the skin has looser attachment and no invasion of deep structures occurred.

Squamous cell carcinoma has been found in a water moccasin *(Agkistrodon piscivorus)*, two tegu lizards *(Tupinambis nigropunctatus* and *T. teguixin)*, European lizards *(Lacerta* spp.*)*, a Ceylon terrapin *(Geoemyca trijuga),* a European pond turtle *(Emys orbicularis),*[28] and a California kingsnake *(Lampropeltis getulus).*[126] The tumor in *T. nigropunctatus* was of gingival origin. The one in the kingsnake involved the upper jaw and the tumor in the moccasin started near the lips; presumably they also originated in the gingiva. The other reptilian squamous cell carcinomas were of epidermal origin.

The tumor in the European pond turtle was particularly interesting because the primary lesion (Fig. 3–106A) in the intermandibular fossa, was a caseating nodular mass that resembled, and was treated as, an

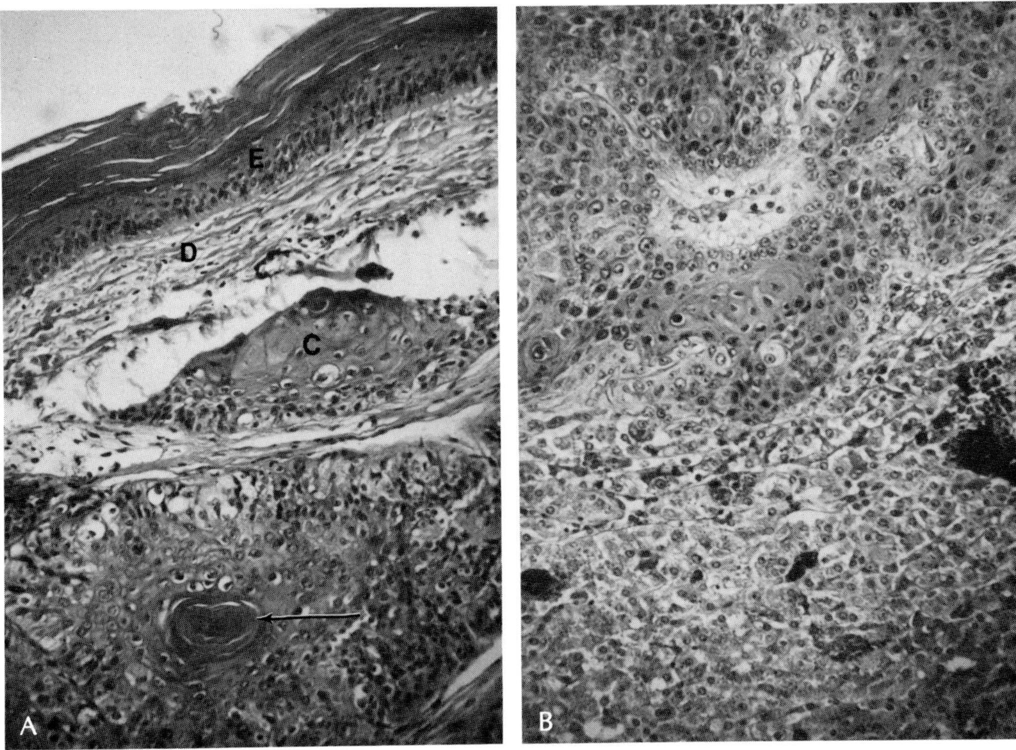

Fig. 3–106. Squamous cell carcinoma from the intermandibular space of a European pond turtle *(Emys orbicularis)* (Armed Forces Institute of Pathology Accession No. 1174550.) **A.** Primary tumor. **E**, Normal epidermis; **D**, dermis; **C**, neoplastic tissue invading the subcutis and forming epithelial pearls (arrow). **B**. Metastasis (top) in the liver. Hepatic parenchyma with normal melanocytes in the bottom half of the picture.

abscess (see p. 96). When the turtle died several months after presentation, multiple metastases were found in the liver (Fig. 3–106B).

Skin tumors are relatively common in *Lacerta* lizards.[28] Hyperkeratotic nodules are formed which can be graded histologically from wart-like papillomas to squamous cell carcinomas. Grossly, these tumors can appear rough and massive, giving rise to the term, "tree bark tumor."[233] Stolk hypothesized these tumors could be caused by a lack of natural sunlight,[264] but more recent evidence indicates they may be viral in origin.[149c] Figure 3–107 illustrates such a growth in a case not previously reported.

Cutaneous fibroepitheliomas up to 25 cm in diameter have been found in green sea turtles *(Chelonia mydas)*. Foreign material such as barnacles, algae, leeches *(Ozobranchus branchiatus)*, and the eggs of flukes *(Distomum [Hapalotrema] constrictum)* have been found in or on these lesions, but no causal associations have been proven.[122,244]

Pigmented Skin Tumors. The pigmented skin tumors that have been reported in anurans include one or more cases each of melanoma, erythrophoroma, guanophoroma, and xanthophoroma (colored black, red, white, or yellow, respectively).[23]

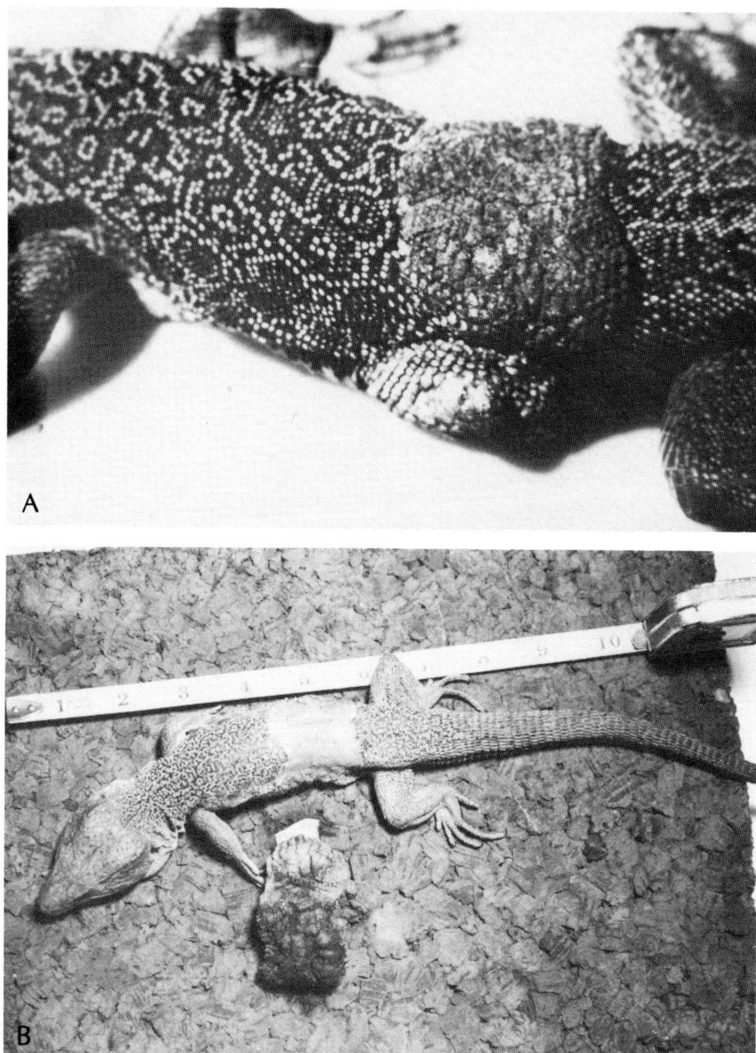

Fig. 3–107. Squamous cell carcinoma ("tree bark tumor") in a jeweled lizard *(Lacerta lepida lepida).* (Specimen provided by Mr. Ernst Hofman.) **A.** The tumor involved the dorsal thoracolumbar area. **B.** Tumor was excised and healing occurred by second intention. There was satisfactory scar formation when the animal was lost to follow-up several months after the surgical procedure. Ruler in inches.

The axolotl, *Ambystoma (Siredon) mexicanum*, often gets melanotic spots on its skin. These can develop into melanophoromas, pigmented tumors that sometimes invade surrounding muscle and connective tissue. The melanophoroma of the axolotl is thought to be hereditary. It is transplantable to other axolotls.[44,244] Further references on melanomas, teratomas, and olfactory neuroepitheliomas in axolotls can be found in the paper by Brunst.[45]

Cutaneous amelanotic melanomas occur spontaneously and can be induced with subcutaneous injection of methylcholanthrene in the newt *Triturus cristatus*. It can be transplanted to other newts with cellular or cell-free extracts. The tumor grows slowly in the winter, rapidly in the summer, and can metastasize widely to internal organs.[185]

Malignant melanomas have been found in several species of snakes, especially pythons, and in a Gila monster *(Heloderma suspectum)*.[28] Three nonmalignant melanomas were found in a 20-foot-long python *(Python reticulatus)* at the Philadelphia Zoo.[244] Multiple subcutaneous malignant melanophoromas containing red and black pigment were found in a western garter snake *(Thamnophis elegans terrestris)*.[100]

Ball reported the occurrence of melanomas in a pair of pine snakes *(Pituophis melanoleucus)* that had been cagemates.[20] The female had a melanoma on the tail which was amputated, but she developed multiple subcutaneous, coelomic, and hepatic metastases and died two and one-half years after the primary lesion was first observed. The male was killed because it was suffering from three large, disfiguring oral tumors: two melanomas and a rhabdomyosarcoma. No internal metastases were found in the male.

Melanomas in reptiles usually appear as pigmented mass lesions in the skin. They usually invade adjacent tissue and can produce widespread metastases. Therefore, early radical excision of the primary tumor is indicated.

Testicular Tumors. Sixteen axolotls over two years old had testicular tumors; there was some evidence that these pedunculated growths secreted androgens.[135] Three other case reports of testicular tumors in amphibians are cited by Balls and Clothier:[23] a teratocarcinoma in a hybrid frog *(Rana pipiens × R. palustris)*, a carcinoma in a giant salamander, *Andrias japonicus (Megalobatrachus maximus)*, and an adenoma in a hellbender *(Cryptobranchus alleganiensis)*. In addition, a Leydig cell tumor in a marbled salamander *(Ambystoma opacum)* is accessioned at the Registry of Tumors in Lower Animals. Only two reptilian testicular tumors are cited by Harshbarger: a Sertoli cell tumor in a garter snake *(Thamnophis sirtalis)* and a seminoma in an American alligator *(Alligator mississippiensis)*.[122]

The Registry of Tumors in Lower Animals serves a useful function by acting as a central facility for accessioning neoplastic material from invertebrates and poikilothermic vertebrates. The Registry also conducts and promotes research on the nature, incidence, and cause of these tumors and disseminates information on these subjects. Examples of neoplastic disease in lower animals can be submitted to the Registry of Tumors in Lower Animals, National Museum of Natural History,

Smithsonian Institution, Washington, D.C., 20560. Specimens are accepted alive, fixed, in blocks, and in slides. Adequate identification and history should accompany the specimen.

REFERENCES

1. Abdulla, P.K., and Karstad, L.: Experimental infections with *Leptospira pomona* in snakes and turtles. Zoonoses Res., *1*:295–306, 1962.
2. Ackerman, L.J., Kishimoto, R.A., and Emerson, J.S.: Nonpigmented *Serratia marcescens* arthritis in a teju *(Tupinambis teguixin)*. Am. J. Vet. Res., *32*:823–826, 1971.
3. Adams, R.M., et al.: Tropical fish aquariums. A source of *Mycobacterium marinum* infections resembling sporotrichosis. JAMA, *211*:457–461, 1970.
4. Addison, J.B., and Jacobson, E.R.: Use of an autogenous bacterin to treat a chronic mouth infection in a reticulated python. J. Zoo Anim. Med., *5*:10–11, 1974.
5. Altman, R., et al.: Turtle-associated salmonellosis: II. The relationship of pet turtles to salmonellosis in children in New Jersey. Am. J. Epidemiol., *95*:518–520, 1972.
6. Andrews, R.D., et al.: Leptospiral agglutinins in sera from southern Illinois herpetofauna. Bull. Wildl. Dis. Assoc., *1*:55–59, 1965.
7. Anonymous: Center for Disease Control National Nosocomial Infections Study. Fourth quarter, 1973 (issued April, 1974): 18–23, 1974.
8. Anonymous: Ban on sale and distribution of small turtles. Fed. Reg., *40*:22543–22546, 1975.

8a. Anonymous: Epidemiologic notes and reports. Q fever–New York. CDC Morbid. Mortal. Weekly Rep., *27*:321–322, 327, 1978.

9. Anver, M.R., Park, J.S., and Rush, H.G.: *Dermatophilus congolensis* in marble lizards *(Calotes mystaceus)*. Am. Assoc. Lab. Anim. Sci. (26th Annual Session), publication 75–2, abstract #87, 1975.
10. Appleby, E.C., and Siller, W.G.: Some cases of gout in reptiles. J. Path. Bact., *80*:427–430, 1960.
11. Ardlie, N.G., and Schwartz, C.J.: Arterial pathology in Australian reptiles: a comparative study. J. Path. Bact., *90*:487–494, 1965.
12. Aronson, J.D.: Spontaneous tuberculosis in snakes. J. Infect. Dis., *44*:215–223, 1929.
13. Ash, L.R., and Beaver, P.C.: A restudy of *Ophidascaris labiatopapillosa* occurring in the stomach of North American snakes. J. Parasitol., *48*(Suppl.):41, 1962.
14. Ayala, S.C.: Lizard malaria in California; description of a strain of *Plasmodium mexicanum* and biogeography of lizard malaria in Western North America. J. Parasitol., *56*:417–425, 1970.
15. Ayala, S.C., and Lee, D.: Saurian malaria: development of sporozoites in two species of Phlebotomine sandflies. Science, *167*:891–892, 1970.
16. Baker, E.F. Jr., Anderson, H.W., and Allard, J.: Epidemiological aspects of turtle-associated salmonellosis. Arch. Environ. Health., *24*:1–9, 1972.
17. Baldauf, R.J.: Another case of parasitic copepods on amphibians. J. Parasitol., *47*:195, 1961.
18. Ball, G.H., Chao, J., and Telford, S.R., Jr.: The life history of *Hepatozoon rarefaciens* (Sambon and Seligmann, 1907) from *Drymarchon corais* (Colubridae), and its experimental transfer to *Constrictor constrictor* (Boidae). J. Parasitol., *53*:897–909, 1967.
19. Ball, G.H., Chao, J., and Telford, S.R., Jr.: *Hepatozoon fusifex* sp. n., a hemogregarine from boa constrictor producing marked morphological changes in infected erythrocytes. J. Parasitol. *55*:800–813, 1969.
20. Ball, H.A.: Melanosarcoma and rhabdomyoma in two pine snakes *(Pituophis melanoleucus)*. Cancer Res., *6*:134–138, 1946.
21. Balls, M.: Spontaneous neoplasms in Amphibia: a review and description of six new cases. Cancer Res., *22*:1142–1154, 1962.
22. Balls, M.: Lymphosarcoma in the South African clawed toad, *Xenopus laevus*: A virus tumor. Ann. N.Y. Acad. Sci., *126*:256–273, 1965.
23. Balls, M., and Clothier, R.H.: Spontaneous tumors in amphibia: a review. Oncology, *29*:501–519, 1974.
24. Balls, M. and Ruben, L.N.: Lymphoid tumors in Amphibia: a review. Prog. Exp. Tumor Res., *10*:238–260, 1968.
25. Barrow, J.H., Jr., and Stockton, J.J.: The influences of temperature on the host-parasite relationships of several species of snakes infected with *Entamoeba invadens*. J. Protozool., *7*:377–383, 1960.

26. Bellairs, A. d'A.: Cleft palate, microphthalmia and other malformations in embryos of lizards and snakes. Proc. Zool. Soc. Lon., *144*:239–251, 1965.
27. Bernstein, J.J.: A clinical view of some reptilian medical problems. J. Zoo Anim. Med., *3*:3–7, 1972.
27a. Bernstein, M.: Personal communication, 1975.
28. Billups, L.H., and Harshbarger, J.C.: Reptiles: Naturally occurring neoplastic diseases of laboratory animals. *In* CRC Handbook of Laboratory Animal Science. Edited by E.C. Melby, Jr., and N.H. Altman. CRC Press, Cleveland, 1976, Vol. III, Section XII.
29. Bisset, K.A.: The effect of temperature upon antibody production in cold-blooded vertebrates. J. Path. Bact., *60*:87–92, 1948.
30. Blok, J.: Eetlusvermindering bij Kameleons. Lacerta, *29*:87–88, 1971.
31. Boam, G.W., et al.: Subcutaneous abscesses in iguanid lizards. J. Am. Vet. Med. Assoc., *157*:617–619, 1970.
31a. Boever, W.L.: *Arizona* septicemia in three boa constrictors. Vet. Med. Small Anim. Clin., *70*:1357–1359, 1975.
32. Boniuk, M., and Luquette, G.F.: Leukokoria and pseudobuphthalmos in snakes. Invest. Ophthalmol., *2*:283, 1963.
32a. Bonney, C.H., Hartfiel, D.A., and Schmidt, R.E.: *Klebsiella pneumoniae* infection with secondary hypopyon in tokay gecko lizards. J. Am. Vet. Med. Assoc., *173*:1115–1116, 1978.
33. Booden, T., Chao, J., and Ball, G.H.: Transfer of *Hepatozoon* sp. from *Boa constrictor* to a lizard, *Anolis carolinensis*, by mosquito vectors. J. Parasitol., *56*:832–833, 1970.
34. Boterenbrood, E.C.: Urodeles. *In* Handbook on the Care and Management of Laboratory Animals. 4th Edition. Edited by UFAW. Williams & Wilkins, Baltimore, 1972, pp. 520–532.
35. Botzler, R.G., Cowan, A.B., and Wetzler, T.F.: Rate of *Listeria monocytogenes* shedding from frogs. J. Wildl. Dis., *11*:277–279, 1975.
36. Botzler, R.G., Wetzler, T.F., and Cowan, A.B.: *Yersinia enterocolitica* and *Yersinia*-like organisms isolated from frogs and snails. Bull. Wildl. Dis. Assoc., *4*:110–115, 1968.
37. Botzler, R.G., Wetzler, T.F., and Cowan, A.B.: *Listeria* in aquatic animals. J. Wildl. Dis., *9*:163–170, 1973.
38. Bovee, E.C., and Telford, S.R., Jr.: *Eimeria sceloporis* and *Eimeria molochis* spp. n. from lizards. J. Parasitol., *51*:85–94, 1965.
39. Boycott, R.S., Taylor, J., and Douglas, S.H.: *Salmonella* in tortoises. J. Path. Bact., *65*:401–411, 1953.
40. Boyer, C.I., Jr., Blackler, K., and Delanney, L.E.: *Aeromonas hydrophila* infection in the Mexican axolotl, *Siredon mexicanum*. Lab. Anim. Sci., *21*:372–375, 1971.
40a. Bowen, G.S.: Prolonged western equine encephalitis viremia in the Texas tortoise *(Gopherus berlandieri)*. Am. J. Trop. Med. Hyg. *26*:171–175, 1977.
41. Bragg, A.N., and Bragg, W.N.: Parasitism of spadefoot tadpoles by *Saprolegnia*. Herpetologica, *14*:34, 1958.
42. Broz, O., and Privora, M.: Two skin parasites of *Rana temporaria: Dermocystidium ranae* Guyenot and Naville and *Dermosporidium granulosum* n. sp. Parasitology, *42*:65–69, 1952.
42a. Brownstein, D.G., et al.: *Cryptosporidium* in snakes with hypertrophic gastritis. Vet. Pathol., *14*:606–617, 1977.
43. Bruce, H.M., and Parkes, A.S.: Rickets and osteoporosis in *Xenopus laevis*. J. Endocrinol., *7*:64–81, 1950.
44. Brunnst, V.V.: The axolotl. II Morphology and pathology. Lab. Invest., *4*:429–449, 1955.
45. Brunnst, V.V.: Structures of spontaneous and transplanted tumors in the axolotl *(Siredon mexicanum)*. *In* Biology of Amphibian Tumors. Edited by M. Mizell. Springer-Verlag, Berlin-Heidelberg-New York, 1969, pp. 215–219.
46. Buchanan, R.E., and Gibbons, N.E.: Bergey's Manual of Determinative Bacteriology. 8th Edition. Williams & Wilkins, Baltimore, 1974.
47. Buhler, G.A.: The post-embryonic development of *Ophiotaenia gracilis* Jones, Cheng and Gillespie, 1958, a cestode parasite of bullfrogs. J. Wildl. Dis., *6*:149–151, 1970.
48. Burrage, B.R.: Observations on the macronyssid mite (order Acarina), *Ophionyssus natricis* (Gervais), on the two iguanid lizards, *Uta stansburiana hesperis* and *Sceloporus occidentalis occidentalis*. Br. J. Herpetol., *3*:275–278, 1966.
49. Bush, M.: Reptilian medicine. Am. Assoc. Zoo Veterinarians, Annual Proc., 68–78, 1974.
50. Caldwell, M.E., and Ryerson, D.L.: A new species of the genus *Pseudomonas* pathogenic for certain reptiles. J. Bacteriol., *39*:323–336, 1940.

51. Camin, J.H.: Mite transmission of a hemorrhagic septicemia in snakes. J. Parasitol., *34*:345–354, 1948.
52. Camin, J.H., et al.: Control of the snake mite, *Ophionyssus natricis* (Gervais), in captive reptile collections. Zoologica, *49*:65–79, 1964.
53. Canning, E.U., Elkan, E., and Trigg, P.I.: *Plistophora myotrophica* spec. nov. causing high mortality in the common toad *Bufo bufo* L. with notes on the maintenance of *Bufo* and *Xenopus* in the laboratory. J. Protozool., *11*:157–166, 1964.
54. Chao, J., and Ball, G.H.: Transfer of *Hepatozoon rarefaciens* (Sanbon and Seligman, 1907) from the indigo snake to a gopher snake by a mosquito vector. J. Parasitol., *55*:681–682, 1969.
55. Cheng, T.C.: The Biology of Animal Parasites. W.B. Saunders Co., Philadelphia, 1964.
56. Clark, H.F., et al.: Comparative studies of amphibian cytoplasmic virus strains isolated from the leopard frog, bullfrog and newt. *In* Biology of Amphibian Tumors. Edited by M. Mizell. Springer-Verlag, Berlin-Heidelberg-New York, 1969, pp. 310–326.

56a. Clark, H.F., and Karzon, D.T.: Iguana virus, a herpes-like virus isolated from cultured cells of a lizard, *Iguana iguana*. Infect. Immun., *5*:559–569, 1972.

57. Clark, W.G.: A veterinarian's challenge. Int. Turtle and Tortoise Soc. J., *1*:12–14, 1967.
58. Clausen, H.J., and Duran-Reynals, F.: Studies on the experimental infection of some reptiles, amphibia and fish with *Serratia anolium*. Am. J. Pathol., *13*:441–451, 1937.
59. Clothier, R.H., and Balls, M.: Mycobacteria and lymphoreticular tumours in *Xenopus laevis*, the South African clawed toad. I. Isolation, characterization and pathogenicity for *Xenopus* of *M. marinum* isolated from lymphoreticular tumor cells. Oncology, *28*:445–457, 1973.
60. Clothier, R.H., and Balls, M.: Mycobacteria and lymphoreticular tumours in *Xenopus laevis*, the South African clawed toad. II. Have Mycobacteria a role in tumour initiation and development? Oncology; *28*:458–480, 1973.

60a. Cohen, M.L., et al.: Turtle-associated salmonellosis in the United States. Effect of public health action, 1970 to 1976. JAMA *243*:1247–1249, 1980.

61. Conti, L.F., and Crowley, J.H.: A new bacterial species, isolated from the chuckwalla *(Sauromalus varius)*. J. Bacteriol., *37*:647–653, 1939.
62. Cooke, A.S.: The effects of pp'DDT on adult frogs *(Rana temporaria)*. Br. J. Herpetol., *5*:390–396, 1974.
63. Cooper, J.E.: Disease in East African snakes associated with *Kalicephalus* worms (Nematoda: Diaphocephalidae). Vet. Rec., *89*:385–388, 1971.
64. Cooper, J.E.: Veterinary aspects of recently captured snakes. Br. J. Herpetol., *5*:368–374, 1973.
65. Cooper, J.E., and Leakey, J.H.: A septicemic disease of East African snakes associated with Enterobacteriaceae. Trans. R. Soc. Trop. Med. Hyg., *70*:80–84, 1976.
66. Cort, W.W., and Brackett, S.: A new strigeid cercaria which produces a bloat disease of tadpoles. J. Parasitol., *24*:263–271, 1938.
67. Coulson, R.A. and Hernandez, T.: Biochemistry of the Alligator. Louisiana State University Press, Baton Rouge, 1964.
68. Cowan, D.F.: Diseases of captive reptiles. J. Am. Vet. Med. Assoc., *153*:848–859, 1968.
69. Crans, W.J.: Preliminary observations of frog filariasis in New Jersey. Bull. Wildl. Dis. Assoc., *5*:342–347, 1969.
70. Dawe, C.J.: Neoplasms of blood cell origin in poikilothermic animals—a review. Natl. Cancer Inst. Monogr., *32*:7–28, 1969.
71. Dawe, C.J.: Some comparative morphological aspects of renal neoplasms in *Rana pipiens* and of lymphosarcomas in Amphibia. *In* Biology of Amphibian Tumors. Edited by M. Mizell. Springer-Verlag, Berlin-Heidelberg-New York, 1969, pp. 429–440.
72. Dawe, C.J., and Berard, W.W.: Workshop on comparative pathology of hematopoietic and lymphoreticular neoplasms. J. Natl. Cancer Inst., *47*:1365–1370, 1971.
73. Deakins, D.E.: Diagnosis and treatment of parasites of amphibia and reptiles. Am. Assoc. Zoo Veterinarians, Ann. Proc.: 37–46, 1972/1973.
74. Deakins, D.E.: Pentastome pathology in captive reptiles. Ph.D. Thesis, University of Oklahoma, 1973.
75. Dhalival, S.S., and Griffiths, D.A.: Fungal disease in Malayan toads: an acute lethal inflammatory reaction. Nature, *197*:467–469, 1963.
76. Diamond, L.S.: The axenic cultivation of two reptilian parasites, *Entamoeba terrapinae* Sanders and Cleveland, 1930 and *Entamoeba invadens* Rodhain, 1934. J. Parasitol., *46*:484, 1960.

77. Diamond, L.S.: A study of the morphology, biology and taxonomy of the trypanosomes of Anura. Wildl. Dis., *44*:85pp (Microfiche), 1965.
77a. Dobbs, J.S., and Vandeford, A.D.: Personal communication.
78. Dodd, J.M., and Callan, H.G.: Neoteny with goiter in *Triturus helveticus*. Q. J. Micr. Sci., *96*:121–128, 1955.
78a. Donaldson, M., et al.: Epizootic of fatal amebiasis among exhibited snakes: epidemiologic, pathologic and chemotherapeutic considerations. Am. J. Vet. Res., *36*:807–817, 1975.
79. Doyle, R.E., and Moreland, A.F.: Diseases of turtles. Lab. Anim. Digest, *4*:3–6, 1968. Reprinted in Int. Turtle and Tortoise Soc. J., *3*:29–31, 1969.
79a. DuPonte, M.W., Nakamura, R.M., and Chang, E.M.L.: Activation of latent *Salmonella* and *Arizona* organisms by dehydration in red-eared turtles, *Pseudemys scripta elegans*. Am. J. Vet. Res., *39*:529–530, 1978.
80. Edgren, R.A., Edgren, M.K., and Tiffany, L.H.: Some North American turtles and their epizoophytic algae. Ecology, *34*:733–740, 1953.
81. Elkan, E.: Some interesting pathological cases in amphibians. Proc. Zool. Soc. Lond., *134*:275–296, 1960.
82. Elkan, E., and Zwart, P.: The ocular disease of young terrapins caused by Vitamin A deficiency. Path. Vet., *4*:201–222, 1967.
83. Ewing, H.E.: A new pit-producing mite from the scales of a South American snake. J. Parasitol., *20*:53–56, 1934.
84. Fantham, H.B., and Porter, A.: The endoparasites of certain South African snakes, together with some remarks on their structure and effects on their hosts. Proc. Zool. Soc. Lond., *120*:599–647, 1950.
85. Fantham, H.B., and Porter, A.: The endoparasites of some North American snakes and their effects on the Ophidia. Proc. Zool. Soc. Lond., *123*:867–898, 1953–1954.
86. Feeley, J.C., and Treger, M.D.: Penetration of turtle eggs by *Salmonella braenderup*. Public Health Rep., *84*:156–158, 1969.
87. Fiennes, R.N. T-W.: Report of the society's pathologist for the year 1957. Proc. Zool. Soc. Lond., *132*:129–146, 1959.
88. Fiennes, R.N. T-W.: Report of the society's pathologist (section on amoebic infection of snakes). Proc. Zool. Soc. Lond., *137*:173–196, 1961.
89. Fiennes, R.N. T-W.: Report of the society's pathologist for the year 1964. J. Zool. (Proc. Zool. Soc. Lond.), *148*:363–380, 1966.
90. Finlayson, R.: Spontaneous arterial disease in exotic animals. J. Zool. (Proc. Zool. Soc. Lond.), *147*:239–343, 1965.
91. Finlayson, R., Symons, C., and Fiennes, R.N. T-W: Atherosclerosis; a comparative study. Br. Med. J., *1*:501–507, 1962.
92. Fischer, L.E.: Absorption of vitamin supplements in lizards. J. Am. Vet. Med. Assoc., *130*:412, 1957.
92a. Fletcher, K.C.: Clinical use of mafenide acetate in reptiles. Am. Assoc. Zoo Veterinarians, Ann. Proc.: 27–32b, 1979.
93. Foekema, G.M.: Ontwikkeling en voortplanting van *Boa constrictor* Linnaeus in een huiskamerterrarium. Lacerta, *31*:131–144, 1973.
93a. Freeman, R.S., et al.: Fatal human infection with mesocercariae of the trematode *Alaria americana*. Am. J. Trop. Med. Hyg., *25*:803–807, 1976.
94. Frenkel, J.K.: Advances in the biology of Sporozoa. Z. Parasitenkd., *45*:125–162, 1974.
95. Frye, F.L.: Surgical removal of a cystic calculus from a desert tortoise. J. Am. Vet. Med. Assoc., *161*:600–602, 1972.
96. Frye, F.L.: Husbandry, Medicine and Surgery in Captive Reptiles. V.M. Publishing, Inc., Bonner Springs, Kansas, 1973.
97. Frye, F.L.: Clinical obstetric and gynecologic disorders in reptiles. Proc. Am. Anim. Hosp. Assoc., 1974, 497–499.
98. Frye, F.L., and Carney, J.: Osteitis deformans (Paget's disease) in a boa constrictor. Vet. Med. Small Anim. Clin., *69*:186–188, 1974.
99. Frye, F.L., and Carney, J.D.: Achondroplastic dwarfism in a turtle. Vet. Med. Small Anim. Clin., *69*:299–301, 1974.
100. Frye, F.L., et al.: Malignant chromatophoroma in a western terrestrial garter snake. J. Am. Vet. Med. Assoc., *167*:557–558, 1975.
101. Frye, F.L., and Dutra, F.: Multiple osteocartilaginous exostoses in a monitor lizard. Vet. Med. Small Anim. Clin., *68*:1414–1416, 1973.
102. Frye, F.L., and Dutra, F.R.: Hypothyroidism in turtles and tortoises. Vet. Med. Small Anim. Clin., *69*:990–993, 1974.
102a. Frye, F.L., and Dutra, F.R.: Articular pseudogout in a turtle *(Chrysemys s. elegans)*. Vet. Med. Small Anim. Clin., *71*:655–659, 1976.

102b. Frye, F.L., et al.: Spontaneous diabetes mellitus in a turtle. Vet. Med. Small Anim. Clin., *71*:935–939, 1976.
102c. Frye, F.L., et al.: Herpesvirus-like infection in two Pacific pond turtles. J. Am. Vet. Med. Assoc., *171*:882–884, 1977.
103. Frye, F.L., and Schelling, S.H.: Steatitis in a caiman. Vet. Med. Small Anim. Clin., *68*:143–145, 1973.
104. Frye, F.L., and Schuchman, S.M.: Salpingotomy and cesarean delivery of impacted ova in a tortoise. Vet. Med. Small Anim. Clin., *69*:454–457, 1974.
105. Garnham, P.C.: Malaria Parasites and Other Haemosporidia. Blackwell, Oxford, 1966.
106. Gebhardt, L.P., et al.: Natural overwintering hosts of the virus of western equine encephalitis. N. Engl. J. Med., *271*:172–177, 1964.
107. Geiman, Q.M., and Ratcliffe, H.L.: Morphology and life cycle of an amoeba producing amoebiasis in reptiles. Parasitology, *28*:208–228, 1936.
108. Georg, L.K., et al.: Mycotic pulmonary disease of captive giant tortoises due to *Beauvaria bassiana* and *Paecilomyces fumosoroseus*. Sabouraudia, *2*:80–86, 1962.
109. Gibbons, L.V., and Kaplan, H.M.: Blood chemistry in frog red leg disease. Anat. Rec., *131*:556, 1958.
110. Gibbs, E.L., Gibb, T.J., and Van Dyck, P.C.: *Rana pipiens:* health and disease. Lab Anim. Care, *16*:142–160, 1966.
110a. Glassford, J.F., and Brown, K.: Treatment of egg retention in a turtle. Vet. Med. Small Anim. Clin., *72*:1641–1645, 1977.
111. Glenn, J.L., Straight, R., and Snyder, C.C.: Vermiplex®, an anthelminthic agent for snakes. J. Zoo Anim. Med., *4*:3–7, 1973. Reprinted, Practicing Veterinarian, *46*:11–13, 1974.
112. Glorioso, J.C., et al.: Laboratory identification of bacterial pathogens of aquatic animals. Am. J. Vet. Res., *35*:447–450, 1974.
113. Glosser, J.W., et al.: Cultural and serologic evidence of *Leptospira interrogans* serotype *Tarassovi* infection in turtles. J. Wildl. Dis., *10*:429–435, 1974.
114. Goin, C.J., and Ogren, L.H.: Parasitic copepods (Argulidae) on amphibians. J. Parasitol., *42*:172, 1956.
115. Goodchild, C.G., and Kirk, D.E.: The life history of *Spirorchis elegans* Stunkard, 1923 (Trematoda: Spirorchiidae) from the painted turtle. J. Parasitol., *46*:219–229, 1960.
116. Goodman, J.D.: Some aspects of the role of parasitology in herpetology. Herpetologica, *7*:65–67, 1951.
117. Graham-Jones, O.: Notes on the common tortoise. IV. Some clinical conditions affecting the North African tortoise ("Greek" tortoise) *Testudo graeca*. Vet. Rec., *73*:317–321, 1961.
118. Gray, C.W., Davis, J., and McCarten, W.G.: Treatment of *Pseudomonas* infections in the snake and lizard collection at Washington Zoo. Int. Zoo Yearbook, *6*:278, 1966.
119. Gray, C.W., et al.: Amoebiasis in the Komodo dragon *Varanus komodoenis*. Int. Zoo Yearbook, *6*:279–283, 1966.
120. Green, M.: Nucleic acid homology as applied to investigations on the relationships of viruses to neoplastic diseases. *In* Biology of Amphibian Tumors. Edited by M. Mizell. Springer-Verlag, Berlin-Heidelberg-New York, 1969, pp. 445–454.
120a. Greer, R.J.: Personal communication, 1975.
120b. Hall, R.J.: Effects of environmental contaminants on reptiles: a review. U.S. Dept. of Interior, Fish and Wildlife Service, Special Scientific Report, Wildlife No. 228, pp. 1–12, 1980.
121. Harshbarger, J.C.: Spontaneous neoplasms in amphibians. *In* Pathology of Laboratory Animals. Edited by K. Benirschke, et al. Springer-Verlag, Berlin-Heidelberg-New York, Vol. II, (in press).
122. Harshbarger, J.C.: Spontaneous neoplasms in reptiles. *In* Pathology of Laboratory Animals. Edited by K. Benirschke, et al. Springer-Verlag, Berlin-Heidelberg-New York, Vol. II, (in press).
123. Harshbarger, J.C., and Dawe, C.J.: Hematopoietic neoplasms in invertebrate and poikilothermic vertebrate animals. *In* Unifying Concepts of Leukemia. (Bibl. Haematol: No. 39) Edited by R.M. Dutcher and L. Chieco-Bianchi. S. Karger, Basel, München, Paris, New York, 1973.
123a. Hazen, T.A., et al.: The parasite fauna of the American alligator *(Alligator mississippiensis)* in South Carolina. J. Wildl. Dis., *14*:435–439, 1978.
124. Heineman, H.S., Spitzer, S., and Pianphongsant, T.: Fish tank granuloma. A hobby hazard. Arch. Intern. Med., *130*:121–123, 1972.
125. Heywood, R.: *Aeromonas* infection in snakes. Cornell Vet., *58*:236–241, 1968.

125a. Hime, J.M.: Eye disease in terrapins. Vet. Rec., *91*:493, 1972.

126. Hill, J.R.: Oral squamous cell carcinoma in a California king snake. J. Am. Vet. Med. Assoc., *171*:981–982, 1977.

127. Hinshaw, W.R., and McNeil, E.: *Salmonella* types isolated from snakes. Am. J. Vet. Res., *6*:264–266, 1945.

128. Hoare, C.A.: Studies on *Trypanosoma grayi* II. Transmission to the crocodile. Trans. R. Soc. Trop. Med. Hyg., *23*:39–56, 1929.

129. Hoare, C.A.: Studies on *Trypanasoma grayi* III. Life cycle in the tsetse fly and in the crocodile. Parasitology, *23*:449–484, 1931.

130. Hoff, G., and Trainer, D.O.: Arboviruses in reptiles: Isolation of a Bunyamwera group virus from a naturally infected turtle. J. Herpetol., *7*:55–62, 1973.

131. Holliman, R.B., and Fisher, J.E.: Life cycle and pathology of *Spirorchis scripta* Stunkard. J. Parasitol. *54*:310–318, 1968.

132. Honigberg, B.M., et al.: A revised classification of the phylum Protozoa. J. Protozool., *11*:7–20, 1964.

133. Huff, C.G.: Exoerythrocytic stages of avian and reptilian malarial parasites. Exp. Parasitol. *24*:383–421, 1969.

134. Hull, R.W., and Camin, J.H.: Haemogregarines in snakes: The incidence and identity of the erythrocytic stages. J. Parasitol., *46*:515–523, 1960.

135. Humphrey, R.R.: Tumors of the testis in the Mexican axolotl *(Ambystoma* or *Siredon mexicanum). In* Biology of Amphibian Tumors. Edited by M. Mizell. Springer-Verlag, Berlin-Heidelberg-New York, 1969, pp. 220–228.

136. Hunt, T.J.: Notes on diseases and mortality in Testudines. Herpetologica, *13*:19–23, 1957.

137. Hunt, T.J.: Influence of environment on necrosis of turtle shells. Herpetologica, *14*:45–46, 1958.

138. Hyland, K.E., Jr.: The life cycle and parasitic habit of the chigger mite *Hannemania dunni* Sambon 1928, a parasite of amphibians. J. Parasitol., *36*:32–33, 1950.

139. Hyland, K.E., Jr.: A new species of chigger mite, *Hannemania hegeneri* (Acarina; Trombiculidae). J. Parasitol., *42*:176–179, 1956.

140. Inman, P.M., Beck, A., Brown, A.E., and Stanford, J.L.: Outbreak of injection abscesses due to *Mycobacterium abscessus*. Arch. Dermatol., *100*:141–147, 1969.

141. Ippen, R.: Vergleichende pathologische Untersuchungen über die spontane und experimentelle Tuberkulose de Kaltblüter. Abh. Deutsch. Akad. Wiss. Berlin Klass Med., *1*:1–90, 1964.

142. Ippen, R.: Vergleichende pathologische Betrachtungen über einige Knochener Krankungen bei Reptilien. Zentralbl. Allg. Path., Bd., *108*:424–434, 1966.

143. Jackson, C.G., Jr., and Fulton, M.: A turtle colony epizootic apparently of microbial origin. J. Wildl. Dis., *6*:466–468, 1970.

144. Jackson, C.G., Fulton, M., and Jackson, M.M.: Cranial asymmetry with massive infection in a box turtle. J. Wildl. Dis., *8*:275–277, 1972.

145. Jackson, C.G., Jr., and Jackson, M.M.: The frequency of *Salmonella* and *Arizona* microorganisms in zoo turtles. J. Wildl. Dis., *7*:130–132, 1971.

146. Jackson, C.G., Jr., Jackson, M.M., and Davis, J.D.: Cutaneous myiasis in the three-toed box turtle, *Terrapene carolina triunguis. Bull. Wildl. Dis. Assoc.*, *5*:114, 1969.

147. Jackson, C.G., Jr., Landry, M.M., and Jackson, M.M.: Reproductive tract anomaly in a box turtle. J. Wildl. Dis., *7*:175–177, 1971.

148. Jackson, M.M., Jackson, C.G., Jr., and Fulton, M.: Investigation of the enteric bacteria of the Testudinata. I: Occurrence of the genera *Arizona, Citrobacter, Edwardsiella* and *Salmonella*. Bull. Wildl. Dis. Assoc., *5*:328–329, 1969.

149. Jackson, O.F.: Reptiles and the general practioner. Vet. Rec., *95*:11–13, 1974.

149a. Jacobson, E.R.: Mycotic diseases of reptiles. *In* Reproductive Biology and Diseases of Captive Reptiles. Edited by J.B. Murphy and J.T. Collins. Symposium, Society for the Study of Amphibians and Reptiles, 1980, pp. 235–241.

149b. Jacobson, E.R.: Viral agents and viral diseases of reptiles. *In* Reproductive Biology and Diseases of Captive Reptiles. Edited by J.B. Murphy and J.T. Collins. Symposium, Society for the Study of Amphibians and Reptiles, 1980, pp. 197–202.

149c. Jacobson, E.R.: Reptile neoplasms. *In* Reproductive Biology and Diseases of Captive Reptiles. Edited by J.B. Murphy and J.T. Collins. Symposium, Society for the Study of Amphibians and Reptiles, 1980, pp. 255–265.

150. Jakowska, S., and Nigrelli, R.F.: *Babesiosoma* gen. nov. and other Babesioids in erythrocytes of coldblooded vertebrates. Ann. N.Y. Acad. Sci., *64*:112–127, 1956.

151. James, H.A., and Ulmer, M.J.: New amphibian host records for *Mesocestoides* sp. (Cestoda: Cyclophyllidea). J. Parasitol., *53*:59, 1967.

152. Jasmin, A.M., and Baucom, J.: *Erysipelothrix insidiosa* infections in the caiman *(Caiman crocodilus)* and the American crocodile *(Crocodilus acutus)*. Am. J. Vet. Clin. Path., *1*:173–177, 1967.
153. Joiner, G.N., and Abrams, G.D.: Experimental tuberculosis in the leopard frog. J. Am. Vet. Med. Assoc., *151*:942–949, 1967.
154. Jubb, K.V., and Kennedy, P.C.: Bones, joints and synovial structures. *In* Pathology of Domestic Animals. 2nd Edition. Academic Press, New York, 1970, Vol. I, p. 9.
155. Kane, K.K., Corwin, R.M., and Boever, W.J.: Impaction due to oxyurid infection in a Fiji Island iguana (a case report). Vet. Med. Small Anim. Clin., *71*:183–184, 1976.
156. Kaplan, H.M.: Septicemic, cutaneous ulcerative disease of turtles. Proc. Anim. Care Panel, *7*:273–277, 1957.
157. Kaplan, H.M.: Treatment of escherichiosis in turtles, frogs and rabbits. Proc. Anim. Care Panel, *8*:101–106, 1958.
158. Kaplan, H.M.: Toxicity of chlorine for frogs. Proc. Anim. Care Panel, *12*:259–262, 1962.
159. Kaplan, H.M.: Parasites of laboratory reptiles and amphibians. *In* Parasites of Laboratory Animals. Edited by R.J. Flynn. Iowa State University Press, Ames, 1973, pp. 507–644.
160. Kaplan, H.M., Arnholt, T.J., and Payne, J.E.: Toxicity of lead nitrate solution for frogs *(Rana pipiens)*. Lab. Anim. Care, *17*:240–246, 1967.
161. Kaplan, H.M., and Glaczenski, S.S.: Salamanders as laboratory animals: *Necturus*. Lab. Anim. Care, *15*:151–155, 1965.
162. Kaplan, H.M., and Light, L.: Evaluation of chemicals used in control and treatment of disease in fish and frogs caused by *Pseudomonas hydrophila*. Am. J. Vet. Res., *16*:342–344, 1955.
163. Kaplan, H.M., Yee, N., and Glaczenski, S.S.: Toxicity of fluoride for frogs. Lab. Anim. Care, *14*:185–188, 1964.
164. Kaplan, H.M., and Yoh, L.: Toxicity of copper for frogs. Herpetologica, *17*:131–135, 1961.
165. Karstad, L.: Fatal poisoning of a fox snake *(Elaphe vulpina)* by feeding a toad *(Bufo americanus)*. Bull. Wildl. Dis. Assoc., *3*:73–74, 1967.
166. Kauffeld, C.F.: Mites and ticks in captive snakes with remarks on cage sanitation. Herpetologica, *10*:103–107, 1954.
167. Kaufmann, A.F., Feeley, J.C., and DeWitt, W.E.: *Salmonella* excretion in turtles. Public Health Rep., *82*:840–842, 1967.
168. Kaufmann, A.F., et al.: Turtle-associated Salmonellosis III. The effects of environmental salmonellae in commercial turtle breeding ponds. Am. J. Epidemiol., *95*:521–528, 1972.
169. Kaufmann, A.F., and Morrison, Z.L.: An epidemiologic study of salmonellosis in turtles. Am. J. Epidemiol., *84*:364–370, 1966.
170. Kaura, Y.K., et al.: Snakes as reservoirs of *Arizona* and *Salmonella*. Zentralbl. Bakteriol. (Orig. A) *219*:506–513, 1972.
170a. Kazacos, K.R., and Fisher, L.F.: Renal styphlodoriasis in a boa constrictor. J. Am. Vet. Med. Assoc., *171*:876–878, 1977.
171. Kennedy, M.E.: *Salmonella* isolations from snakes and other reptiles. Can. J. Comp. Med., *37*:325–326, 1973.
172. Kiel, J.L.: A synopsis of some common bacterial diseases in snakes. Southwestern Veterinarian, *27*:33–36, 1974.
173. Kreier, J.P., and Ristic, M.: Diseases caused by protista. *In* Infectious Blood Diseases of Man and Animals. Edited by D. Weinman and M. Ristic. Academic Press, New York, 1968, Vol. II, pp. 387–472.
174. Kulp, W.L., and Borden, D.G.: Studies on *Proteus hydrophilus*, the etiological agent in 'Red Leg' disease of frogs. J. Bacteriol., *44*:673–685, 1942.
175. Kutzer, E., and Grünberg, W.: Parasitologie und Pathologie der Spulwurmkrankheit der Schlangen. Zbl. Vet., *12*(b):155–175, 1965.
176. Kwapinski, J.B., and Kwapinski, E.H.: Immunological reactions of *Mycobacterium leprae* and *Mycobacterium leprae-murium* grown in cayman. Can. J. Microbiol., *19*:764–766, 1973.
177. Kwapinski, J.B., Kwapinski, E.H., and McClung, N.M.: The growth of *Mycobacterium leprae* in snakes. Can. J. Microbiol., *20*:420–422, 1974.
177a. Lainson, R., Landau, I., and Shaw, J.J.: Observations on non-pigmented haemosporidia of Brazilian lizards, including a new species of *Saurocytozoon* in *Mabuya mabouya* (Scincidae). Parasitology, *69*:215–223, 1974.
177b. Lainson, R., and Shaw, J.J.: A new haemosporidian of lizards, *Saurocytozoon tupinambi* gen. nov., sp. nov., in *Tupinambus nigropunctatus* (Teiidae). Parasitology, *59*:159–162, 1969.

178. Lainson, R., Shaw, J.J., and Landau, I.: Some blood parasites of the Brazilian lizards *Plica umbra* and *Uranoscodon superciliosa* (Iguanidae). Parasitology, *70*:119–141, 1975.
179. Lainson, R., Shaw, J.J., and Ward, R.D.: *Shellackia landauae* sp. nov. (Eimeriorina: Lankasterellidae) in the Brazilian lizard *Polychrus marmoratus* (Iguanidae): experimental transmission by *Culex pipiens fatigans*. Parasitology, *72*:225–243, 1976.
180. Lamm, S.H., et al.: Turtle-associated salmonellosis. I. An estimation of the magnitude of the problem in the United States, 1970–1971. Am. J. Epidemiol., *95*:511–517, 1972.
181. Langham, R.F., Zydeck, F.A., and Bennett, L.R.: Steatitis in a captive Marley garter snake. J. Am. Vet. Med. Assoc., *159*:640–641, 1971.
182. Lautenschlager, E.W.: Meningeal tumors of the newt associated with trematode infection of the brain. Proc. Helminthol. Soc., *26*:11–14, 1959.
183. Lawson, R.: A malignant neoplasm with metastases in the lizard *Lacerta sicula çetti* Cara. Br. J. Herp., *3*:22–24, 1962.
184. Lee, S.H.: The life cycle of *Skrjabinoptera phrynasoma* (Ortlepp) Schulz, 1927 (Nematoda Spiruroidea), a gastric nematode of Texas horned toads, *Phrynosoma cornutum*. J. Parasitol., *43*:66–75, 1957.
185. Leone, V.G., and Zavanella, T.: Some morphological and biological characteristics of a tumor of the newt, *Triturus cristatus* Laur. *In* Biology of Amphibian Tumors. Edited by M. Mizell. Springer-Verlag, Berlin-Heidelberg-New York, 1969, pp. 184–194.
185a. Levine, N.D., and Nye, R.R.: *Toxoplasma ranae* sp. n. from the leopard frog *Rana pipiens* Linnaeus. J. Protozool, *23*:488–490, 1976.
186. Lewis J. F., and Wagner, E.D.: *Hepatozoon sauromali* sp. n., a haemogregarine from the chuckwalla *(Sauromalus* spp.) with notes on the life history. J. Parasitol., *50*:11–14, 1964.
187. Lie Kian Joe, et al.: *Basidiobolus ranarum* as a cause of subcutaneous mycosis in Indonesia. Arch. Dermatol., *74*:378–383, 1956.
188. Lopez, J.F., Quesada, V., and Saied, A.: Bacteremia and osteomyelitis due to *Aeromonas hydrophila*. Am. J. Clin. Pathol., *50*:587–591, 1968.
189. Lucké, B., and Schlumberger, H.G.: Neoplasia in cold blooded vertebrates. Physiologic Rev., *29*:91–126, 1949.
190. MacCallum, G.A.: Epidemic pneumonia in reptiles. Science, *54*:279–281, 1921.
190a. Mace, T.F., and Anderson, R.C.: Development of the giant kidney worm, *Dioctophyma renale* (Goeze, 1782) (Nematoda, Dioctophymatoidea). Can. J. Zool., *53*:1552–1568, 1975.
191. Machicao, N., and LaPlaca, E.: Lepra-like granulomas in frogs. Lab. Invest., *3*:219–227, 1954.
192. MacKerras, M.J.: Hematozoa of Australian reptiles. Aust. J. Zool., *9*:61–122, 1961.
193. Mann, K.H., and Tyler, M.J.: Leeches as endoparasites of frogs. Nature, *197*:1224–1225, 1963.
194. Marcus, L.C.: Diseases of snakes and turtles. *In* Current Veterinary Therapy III. Edited by R.W. Kirk. W.B. Saunders Co., Philadelphia, 1968, pp. 435–442.
195. Marcus, L.C.: Infectious diseases of reptiles. J. Am. Vet. Med. Assoc., *159*:1626–1631, 1971.
196. Marcus, L.C.: Parasitic diseases of captive reptiles. *In* Current Veterinary Therapy VI. Edited by R.W. Kirk. W.B. Saunders Co., Philadelphia, 1977, pp. 801–806.
197. Marcus, L.C., Stottmeier, K.D., and Morrow, R.H.: Experimental infection of anole lizards *(Anolis carolinensis)* with *Mycobacterium ulcerans* by the subcutaneous route. Am. J. Trop. Med. Hyg., *24*:649–655, 1975.
198. Marcus, L.C., Stottmeier, K.D., and Morrow, R.H.: Experimental alimentary infection of anole lizards *(Anolis carolinensis)* with *Mycobacterium ulcerans*. Am. J. Trop. Med. Hyg., *25*:630–632, 1976.
199. McConnachie, E.W.: Studies of *Entamoeba invadens* Rodhain, 1934 *in vitro* and its relationship to some other species of *Entamoeba*. Parasitology, *45*:452–481, 1955.
200. McConnell, E.E., Garner, F.M., and Kirk, J.H.: Hartmanellosis in a bull. Path. Vet., *5*:1–6, 1968.
201. McCoy, R.H., and Seidler, R.J.: Potential pathogens in the environment: isolation, enumeration and identification of seven genera of intestinal bacteria associated with small green pet turtles. Appl. Microbiol., *25*:534–538, 1973.
202. McGhee, R.B.: Diseases caused by protista. *In* Infectious Blood Diseases of Man and Animals. Edited by D. Weinman and M. Ristic. Academic Press, New York, 1968, Vol. I, pp. 307–341.
203. McKenzie, R.A., and Green, P.E.: Mycotic dermatitis in captive carpet snakes *(Morelia spilotes variegata)* J. Wildl. Dis., *12*:405–408, 1976.
204. McKinnell, R.G.: Incidence and histology of renal tumors of leopard frogs from the North Central States. Ann. N.Y. Acad. Sci., *126*:85–98, 1965.

205. McKinnell, R.G.: Lucké renal adenocarcinoma: epidemiological aspects. *In* Biology of Amphibian Tumors. Edited by M. Mizell. Springer-Verlag, Berlin-Heidelberg-New York, 1969, pp. 254–260.
206. Mead, R.W., and Olsen, O.W.: The life cycle and development of *Ophiotaenia filaroides* (LaRue, 1909) (Proteocephala: Proteocephalidae). J. Parasitol., *57*:869–874, 1971.
206a. Medical Letter: *16*:7, 1974.
207. Meerovitch, E.: A new host of *Entamoeba invadens* Rhodain, 1934. Can. J. Zool., *36*:423–427, 1958.
208. Meerovitch, E.: Some biological requirements and host parasite relations of *Entamoeba invadens*. Can. J. Zool., *36*:513–523, 1958.
209. Meerovitch, E.: Infectivity and pathogenicity of polyxenic and monoxenic *Entamoeba invadens* to snakes kept at normal and high temperatures and the natural history of reptile amoebiasis. J. Parasitol., *47*:791–794, 1961.
210. Migaki, G., and Frye, F.L.: Mycotic granuloma in a tiger salamander. J. Wildl. Dis., *2*:525–528, 1975.
211. Mittleman, M.B.: Letter to the editor. Phila. Herp. Soc. Bull. *10*:9, 1962.
212. Mizell, M.: State of the art: Lucké tumor. *In* Biology of Amphibian Tumors. Edited by M. Mizell. Springer-Verlag, Berlin-Heidelberg-New York, 1969, pp. 1–25.
212a. Montali, R.J., Bush, M., and Smeller, J.M.: The pathology of nephrotoxicity of gentamicin in snakes: a model for reptilian gout. Vet. Path.,*16*:108–115, 1978.
213. Montali, R.J., Smith, E.E., Davenport, M., and Bush, M.: Dermatophilosis in Australian bearded lizards. J. Am. Vet. Med. Assoc., *167*:553–555, 1975.
213a. Munday, B.L., et al.: *Sarcocystis* and related organisms in Australian wildlife: II. Survey findings in birds, reptiles, amphibians and fish. J. Wildl. Dis., *15*:57–73, 1979.
213b. Munday, B.L. and Mason, R.W.: *Sarcocystis* and related organisms in Australian wildlife: III. *Sarcocystis murinotechis* sp. n. life cycle in rats (*Rattus, Pseudomys*, and *Mastocomys* spp.) and tiger snakes (*Notechis ater*). J. Wildl. Dis. *16*:83–87, 1980.
214. Murphy, J.B.: The use of macrolide antibiotic tylosin in the treatment of reptilian respiratory infections. Br. J. Herp., *4*:317–321, 1973.
215. Naegele, R.F., Granoff, A., and Darlington, R.W.: The presence of the Lucké herpes virus genome in induced tadpole tumors and its oncogenicity: Koch-Henle postulates fulfilled. Proc. Natl. Acad. Sci. (USA) *71*:830–834, 1974.
216. Nelson, D.J.: A treatment for helminthiasis in Ophidia. Herpetologica, *6*:57–59, 1950.
217. Nickerson, M.A., and Hutchison, J.A.: The distribution of the fungus *Basidiobolus ranarum* Eidam in fish, amphibians and reptiles. Am. Midland Naturalist, *86*:500–502, 1971.
218. Nigrelli, R.F., and Mararentano, L.W.: Pericarditis in *Xenopus laevis* caused by *Diplostomulum xenopi* sp. nov., a larval strigeid. J. Parasitol. *30*:184–190, 1944.
219. Olson, G.A., and Woodard, J.C.: Miliary tuberculosis in a reticulated python. J. Am. Vet. Med. Assoc., *164*:733–735, 1974.
220. Otis, V.S., and Behler, J.L.: The occurrence of Salmonellae and *Edwardsiella* in the turtles of the New York Zoological Park. J. Wildl. Dis., *9*:4–6, 1973.
221. Page, L.A.: Experimental ulcerative stomatitis in king snakes. Cornell Vet., *51*:258–266, 1961.
222. Page, L.A.: Diseases and infections of snakes: a review. Bull. Wildl. Dis. Assoc., *2*:111–126, 1966.
223. Pearson, A.D., and Tamarind, D.L.: Acarine parasites on the lizard, *Lacerta vivipara* Jacquin. Br. J. Herp., *5*:352–353, 1973.
224. Pfuetze, K.H., and Hubble, R.: Non-tuberculous mycobacterial infections. Disease-a-Month, September, 1968, pp. 1–39.
225. Pienaar, U. De V.: Haematology of some South African reptiles. Witwatersrand University Press, Johannesburg, 1962.
226. Pollack, E.D.: A simple method for the removal of protozoan parasites from *Rana pipiens* larvae. Copeia:557, 1971.
227. Rafferty, K.A., Jr.: Kidney tumors of the leopard frog: a review. Cancer Res., *24*:169–185, 1964.
228. Ratcliffe, H.L.: Carcinoma of the pancreas in Says pine snake *Pituophis sayii*. Am. J. Cancer, *24*:78–79, 1935.
229. Ratcliffe, H.L.: Neoplastic disease in the pancreas of snakes (Serpentes). Am. J. Pathol. *19*:359–369, 1943.
230. Ratcliffe, H.L., and Geiman, Q.M.: Spontaneous and experimental amebic infection in reptiles. Arch. Pathol., *25*:160–184, 1938.

231. Rebell, G., et al.: Fusariosis in marine turtles. Bacteriol. Proc. (Abstracts of the 71st. Annual Meeting. Am. Soc. Microbiol.) 1971, p. 121.
232. Refair, M., and Rohde, R.: *Salmonella* in reptiles in zoological gardens. Zbl. Vet-med., *16*B:383–386, 1969.
233. Reichenbach-Klinke, H., and Elkan, E.: The Principal Diseases of Lower Vertebrates. Academic Press, New York, 1965, pp. 209–568.
234. Robbins, S.L.: The musculoskeletal system. *In* Pathology. 3rd. Edition. W.B. Saunders Co., Philadelphia, 1967, pp. 1313–1367.
235. Robert, V.B., and Rorke, L.B.: Primary amebic encephalitis, probably from Acanthamoeba. Ann. Intern. Med., *79*:174–179, 1973.
236. Rose, F.L.: Tumorous growths of the tiger salamander, *Ambystoma tigrinum*, associated with treated sewage effluent. Prog. Exp. Tumor Res., *20*:251, 1976.
236a. Rose, F.L., and Harshbarger, J.C.: Neoplastic and possibly related skin lesions in neotenic tiger salamanders from a sewage lagoon. Science, *196*:315–317, 1977.
237. Rothman, N., and Rothman, B.: Course and cure of respiratory infections in snakes. Phila. Herp. Soc. Bull., *8*:No. 5, 19–23, 1960.
238. Ruben, L.N.: Possible immunological factors in amphibian lymphosarcoma development. *In* Biology of Amphibian Tumors. Edited by M. Mizell. Springer-Verlag, Berlin-Heidelberg-New York, 1969, pp. 368–384.
239. Ryckman, R.E.: Lizards: A laboratory host for Triatominae and *Trypanasoma cruzi*, Chagas. Trans. Am. Microsc. Soc., *73*:215–218, 1954.
240. Sadek, I.M.: Salmonellosis in U.A.R. with special reference to reptiles. J. Egypt. Vet. Med. Assoc., *30*:97–107, 1970.
241. Sanders, H.O.: Pesticide toxicities to tadpoles of the western chorus frog *Pseudacris triseriata* and Fowler's toad *Bufo woodhousii fowleri*. Copeia, No. 2, 246–251, 1970.
242. Scarpelli, D.G.: Survey of some spontaneous and experimental disease processes of lower vertebrates and invertebrates. Fed. Proc., *28*:1825–1833, 1969.
243. Schad, G.A.: Studies on the genus *Kalicephalus* Nematoda: Diaphanocephalidae I. On the life histories of the North American species *K. parvus, K. agkistrodontis* and *K. rectiphilus*. Can. J. Zool., *34*:425–452, 1956.
244. Schlumberger, H.G., and Lucké, B.: Tumors of fish, amphibians and reptiles. Cancer Res., *8*:657–754, 1948.
245. Schmidt, F.L.: *Entonyssus vitzthumi* (Acarina), a new ophidian lung mite. J. Parasitol., *26*:309–313, 1928.
246. Schmittner, S.M., and McGhee, R.B.: The intra-erythrocytic development of *Babesiosoma stableri* n. sp. in *Rana pipiens pipiens*. J. Protozool., *8*:381–386, 1961.
247. Schuchman, S.M., and Taylor, D.O.: Arteriosclerosis in an iguana *(Iguana iguana)*. J. Am. Vet. Med. Assoc., *157*:614–616, 1970.
248. Schultz, H.: Human infestation by *Ophionyssus natricis* snake mite. Br. J. Dermatol., *93*:695–697, 1975.
249. Schwabacher, H.: A strain of *Mycobacterium* isolated from skin lesions of a cold-blooded animal, *Xenopus laevis*, and its relation to atypical acid-fast bacilli occurring in man. J. Hyg., *57*:57–67, 1959.
250. Schweinfurth, W.: Perorale Behandlung der Amöbiasis bei Schlanger. Salamandra, *6*:44–45, 1970.
251. Self, J.T.: Biological relationships of the Pentastomida; a bibliography of the Pentastomida. Exp. Parasitol. *24*:63–119, 1969.
252. Self, J.T., and Kuntz, R.E.: Host-parasite relations in some pentastomida. J. Parasitol., *53*:202–206, 1967.
252a. Shakespeare, W.: Hamlet, Act IV, Scene iii, line 20, 1604.
253. Shalev, M., Murphy, J.C., and Fox, J.G.: Mycotic enteritis in a chameleon and a brief review of phycomycosis of animals. J. Am. Vet. Med. Assoc., *171*:872–875, 1977.
254. Sharma, V.K., Kaura, Y.K., and Singh, I.P.: Frogs as carriers of *Salmonella* and *Edwardsiella*. Antonie van Leeuwenhoek, *40*:171–175, 1974.
255. Shilkin, K.B., et al.: Infection due to *Aeromonas hydrophila*. Med. J. Aust., *1*:351–353, 1968.
256. Shortridge, K.F., et al.: Arbovirus infections in reptiles: immunological evidence for a high incidence of Japanese encephalitis virus in the cobra *Naja naja*. Trans. R. Soc. Trop. Med. Hyg., *68*:454–460, 1974.
257. Shotts, E.B., et al.: *Aeromonas*-induced deaths among fish and reptiles in an eutrophic inland lake. J. Am. Vet. Med. Assoc., *161*:603–607, 1972.
258. Simmons, G.C., Sullivan, N.D., and Green, P.E.: Dermatophilosis in a lizard *(Amphibolurus barbatus)*. Aust. Vet. J., *48*:465–466, 1972.
259. Smith, S.W.: Chloromycetin in the treatment of "red leg." Science, *112*:274–275, 1950.

260. Sprent, J.F.: Studies on ascaridoid nematodes in pythons: The life history and development of *Ophidascaris moreliae* in Australian pythons. Parasitology, *60*:97–122, 1970.
261. Sprent, J.F.: Studies on ascaridoid nematodes in pythons: The life history and development of *Polydelphis anoura* in Australian pythons. Parasitology, *60*:375–397, 1970.
262. Sprouls, R.W., Farris, H.E., and Frith, C.H.: Salmonellosis in laboratory frogs. Am. Assoc. Lab. Anim. Sci. (26th Annual Session), Publication 75–2, Abstract #84, 1975.
263. Steen, van der, A.B., et al.: Cutaneous neoplasms in the leopard frog *(Rana pipiens)*. Lab. Anim. Sci., *22*:216–222, 1972.
264. Stolk, A.: Hyperkeratosis and carcinoma planocellulare in the lizard *Lacerta agilis* L. (Preliminary note). Proc. Koninkl. Med. Akad. Wetensch. Ser. C., *56*:157–163, 1953.
265. Straight, R., Glenn, J.L., and Snyder, C.C.: Antivenom activity of rattlesnake blood plasma. Nature, *261*:259–260, 1976.
266. Suenaga, O., and Miyagi, I.: Low susceptibility of common snakes in Japan to Japanese encephalitis virus. Trop. Med., *11*:27–32, 1969.
267. Telford, S.R., Jr.: A comparative study of endoparasitism among some southern California lizard populations. Ph.D. Thesis, U.C.L.A., 1964. (Reprinted in Am. Midland Naturalist, *83*:516–554, 1970.)
268. Telford, S.R., Jr.: Some observations on the effects of varying ambient temperatures in vivo on filarial worms of snakes. Jpn. J. Exp. Med., *35*:291–300, 1965.
269. Telford, S.R., Jr.: A study of filariasis in Mexican snakes. Jpn. J. Exp. Med., *35*:565–586, 1965.
270. Telford, S.R., Jr.: Morphological observations on Haemosporidian parasites of some Southern California and Mexican lizards. Jpn. J. Exp. Med., *36*:237–250, 1966.
271. Telford, S.R., Jr.: Exoerythrocytic gametocytes of saurian malaria. Q. J. Fla. Acad. Sci., *33*:77–79, 1970.
272. Telford, S.R., Jr.: Saurian malarial parasites in eastern Panama. J. Protozool., *17*:566–574, 1970.
273. Telford, S.R., Jr.: Parasitic diseases of reptiles. J. Am. Vet. Med. Assoc., *159*:1644–1652, 1971.
274. Thompson, P.E.: Effects of quinine on saurian malarial parasites. J. Infect. Dis., *78*:160–166, 1946.
275. Thompson, P.E., and Huff, C.G.: A saurian malarial parasite, *Plasmodium mexicanum*, n. sp., with both elongatum- and gallinaceum-types of exoerythrocytic stages. J. Infect. Dis., *74*:48–79, 1944.
276. Thorson, T.E.: Salmonellosis in pet turtles. Mod. Vet. Pract., *55*:31–32, 1974.
277. Tiffney, W.N.: The identity of certain species of the Saprolegnaceae parasitic to fish. J. Elisha Mitchell Scientific Soc., *55*:134–151, 1939.
278. Toft, J.D. II, and Schmidt, R.E.: Pseudophyllidean tapeworms in green tree pythons *(Chondropython viridis)*. J. Zoo Anim. Med., *6*:25–26, 1975.
279. Trevino, G.S.: Cephalosporiosis in three caimans. J. Wildl. Dis., *8*:384–388, 1972.
280. Tweedell, K.S.: Simulated transmission of renal tumors in oocytes and embryos of *Rana pipiens*. *In* Biology of Amphibian Tumors. Edited by M. Mizell. Springer-Verlag, Berlin-Heidelberg-New York, 1969, pp. 229–239.
281. Ungureanu, C., et al.: Hemorrhagic septicemia in tortoises and snakes in captivity at the Zoological Garden of Bucharest. Arch. Vet., *8*:Fasc. 2, 85–96, 1972.
282. Vastesaeger, M.M., Delcourt, R., and Gillot, P.H.: Spontaneous atherosclerosis in fishes and reptiles. *In* Comparative Atherosclerosis. Edited by J.C. Roberts, Jr., and R. Straus. Harper and Row Publishers, New York, 1965, pp. 129–149.
283. Vogel, H.: Mycobacteria from cold-blooded animals. Am. Rev. Tuberc., *77*:823–838, 1958.
284. Wallach, J.D.: Hypervitaminosis D in green iguanas. J. Am. Vet. Med. Assoc., *149*:912–914, 1966.
285. Wallach, J.D.: Medical care of reptiles. J. Am. Vet. Med. Assoc., *155*:1017–1034, 1969.
286. Wallach, J.D.: Diseases of reptiles and their clinical management. *In* Current Veterinary Therapy IV. Edited by R.W. Kirk. W.B. Saunders Co., Philadelphia, 1971, pp. 433–439.
287. Wallach, J.D.: Environmental and nutritional diseases of captive reptiles. J. Am. Vet. Med. Assoc., *159*:1632–1643, 1971.
287a. Wallach, J.D.: The pathogenesis and etiology of ulcerative shell disease in turtles. Aquatic Mammals, *4*:1–4, 1976.
287b. Wallach, J.D.: Ulcerative shell disease in turtles: identification, prophylaxis and treatment. Int. Zoo Yearbook, *17*:170–171, 1977.
288. Wallach, J.D., and Hoessle, C.: Visceral gout in captive reptiles. J. Am. Vet. Med. Assoc., *151*:897–899, 1967.

289. Wallach, J.D., and Hoessle, C.: Steatitis in captive crocodilians. J. Am. Vet. Med. Assoc., *153*:845–847, 1968.
290. Wallach, J.D., and Hoessle, C.: Fibrous osteodystrophy in green iguanas. J. Am. Vet. Med. Assoc., *153*:863–865, 1968.
291. Wallach, J.D., Hoessle, C., and Bennett, J.: Hypoglycemic shock in captive alligators. J. Am. Vet. Med. Assoc., *151*:893–896, 1967.
292. Walton, A.C.: The parasites of amphibia. J. Wildl. Dis., #39 and #40 (Micro cards), 1964.
293. Walton, A.C.: Supplemental catalogue of the parasites of Amphibia. J. Wildl. Dis., #48 (Micro card, 58 pp.), 1966.
294. Walton, A.C.: Supplemental catalogue of the parasites of Amphibia. J. Wildl. Dis., #49 (Micro card, 10 pp.), 1967.
295. Ward, H.B.: A new blood fluke from turtles. J. Parasitol., *7*:114–128, 1921.
296. Wardle, R.A., and McLeod, J.A.: The Zoology of Tapeworms. University of Minnesota Press, Minneapolis, 1952.
297. Weber, A.: Über einen Behandlungsversuch bei latent mit Salmonellen infizierten SchildKröten. Kleintier-Praxis, *18*:48–50, 1973.
298. Weinstein, P.P., Krawczyk, H.J., and Peers, J.H.: Sparganosis in Korea. Am. J. Trop. Med. Hyg., *3*:112–130, 1954.
299. White, F.H.: Leptospiral agglutinins in snake serums. Am. J. Vet. Res., *24*:179–182, 1963.
300. White, F.H., Simpson, C.F., and Williams, L.E., Jr.: Isolation of *Edwardsiella tarda* from aquatic animal species and surface waters in Florida. J. Wildl. Dis., *9*:204–208, 1973.
301. Widmer, E.A.: Development of third-stage *Physaloptera* larvae from *Crotalus viridis* Rafinesque, 1818 in cats with notes on pathology of the larvae in the reptile. (Nematoda, Spiruroidea) J. Wildl. Dis., *6*:89–93, 1970.
302. Wieczorowski, E.: Parasitic lesions in turtles. J. Parasitol., *25*:395–399, 1939.
303. Williams, A.O.: Pathology of phycomycosis due to *Entomophthora* and *Basidiobolus* species. Arch. Pathol., *87*:13–20, 1969.
304. Williams, R.W.: Observations on the life history of *Rhabdias sphaerocephala* Goodey, 1924 from *Bufo marinus* L. in the Bermuda Islands. J. Helminthol., *34*:93–98, 1960.
304a. Wilson, D.E., et al.: Induction of amoebiasis in tissues of white mice and rats by subcutaneous inoculation of small free-living, inquilinic and parasitic amebas with associated coliform bacteria. Exp. Parasitol., *21*:277–286, 1967.
305. Wittenberg, G., and Gerichter, C.: The morphology and life history of *Foleyella duboisi* with remarks on allied filariids of Amphibia. J. Parasitol., *30*:245–256, 1944.
306. Wittner, M., and Rosenbaum, R.M.: Role of bacteria in modifying virulence of *Entamoeba histolytica*. Studies of amebae from axenic cultures. Am. J. Trop. Med. Hyg., *19*:755–761, 1970.
307. Wolf, K., et al.: Tadpole edema virus: pathogenesis and growth studies and additional sites of virus infected bullfrog tadpoles. *In* Biology of Amphibian Tumors. Edited by M. Mizell. Springer-Verlag, Berlin-Heidelberg-New York, 1969, pp. 327–336.
308. Woo, P., and Soltys, M.A.: The experimental infection of reptiles with *Tryponasoma brucei*. Ann. Trop. Med. Parasitol., *63*:35–38, 1969.
308a. Yadav, M.P., and Sethi, M.S.: Poikilotherms as reservoirs of Q-fever *(Coxiella burnetii)* in Uttar Pradesh. J. Wildl. Dis., *15*:15–17, 1979.
309. Zwart, P.: Studies on renal pathology in reptiles. Pathol. Vet., *1*:542–566, 1964.
310. Zwart, P.: Intraepithelial protozoon, *Klossiella boae* n. sp. in the kidneys of a boa constrictor. J. Protozool., *11*:261–263, 1964.
311. Zwart, P.: Ziekten van reptielen I: ectoparasieten, huidaandoeningen. Lacerta, *30*:41–48, 1972.
312. Zwart, P.: Ziekten van reptielen II: aandoeningen van de ogen, de oren, de mondholte en de longen. Lacerta, *30*:72–79, 1972.
313. Zwart, P.: Ziekten van reptielen III: aandoeningen van de maag, de darmen, de lever, de geslachtsorganen en de nieren. Lacerta, *30*:121–127, 1972.
314. Zwart, P.: Ziekten van reptielen V: infectieziekten. Lacerta, *31*:116–120, 1973.
315. Zwart, P.: Ziekten van reptielen VI: deficiëntieziekten. Lacerta, *31*:117–182, 1973.
316. Zwart, P., and Jansen, J.: Treatment of lungworm in snakes with tetramisole. Vet. Rec., *84*:374, 1969.
317. Zwart, P., and van de Watering, C.C.: Disturbance of bone formation in the common iguana *(Iguana iguana* L.*)*. Pathology and etiology. Acta Zool. Pathol. Antverp., *48*:333–356, 1969.

Index

Numerals in *italics* indicate a figure; "t" following a page number indicates a table.